S. HRG. 105–449

THE MANY FACES OF LONG-TERM CARE: TODAY'S BITTER PILL OR TOMORROW'S CURE

AF709351

HEARING

BEFORE THE

SPECIAL COMMITTEE ON AGING UNITED STATES SENATE

ONE HUNDRED FIFTH CONGRESS

FIRST SESSION

LAS VEGAS, NV
JANUARY 12, 1998

RENO, NV
JANUARY 13, 1998

Serial No. 105–14

Printed for the use of the Special Committee on Aging

362.16 Un3m
United States. Congress.
Senate. Special Committee
The many faces of long-term
care

U.S. GOVERNMENT PRINTING OFFICE
47–539 WASHINGTON : 1998

For sale by the U.S. Government Printing Office
Superintendent of Documents, Congressional Sales Office, Washington, DC 20402
ISBN 0-16-056532-4

SPECIAL COMMITTEE ON AGING

CHARLES E. GRASSLEY, Iowa, *Chairman*

JAMES M. JEFFORDS, Vermont
LARRY CRAIG, Idaho
CONRAD BURNS, Montana
RICHARD SHELBY, Alabama
RICK SANTORUM, Pennsylvania
JOHN WARNER, Virginia
CHUCK HAGEL, Nebraska
SUSAN COLLINS, Maine
MIKE ENZI, Wyoming

JOHN B. BREAUX, Louisiana
JOHN GLENN, Ohio
HARRY REID, Nevada
HERB KOHL, Wisconsin
RUSSELL D. FEINGOLD, Wisconsin
CAROL MOSELEY-BRAUN, Illinois
RON WYDEN, Oregon
JACK REED, Rhode Island

THEODORE L. TOTMAN, *Staff Director*
KENNETH R. COHEN, *Minority Staff Director*

CONTENTS

LAS VEGAS, NV, JANUARY 12, 1998

CHRONOLOGICAL LIST OF WITNESSES

RENO, NV, JANUARY 13, 1998

CHRONOLOGICAL LIST OF WITNESSES

APPENDIX

9/25/00

THE MANY FACES OF LONG-TERM CARE: TODAY'S BITTER PILL OR TOMORROW'S CURE?

MONDAY, JANUARY 12, 1998

U.S. SENATE,
SPECIAL COMMITTEE ON AGING,
Las Vegas, NV.

The committee met, pursuant to notice, at 9 a.m., in the West Charleston Library, 6301 West Charleston, Las Vegas, NV, Hon. Harry Reid presiding.

Present: Senator Reid.

OPENING STATEMENT OF SENATOR HARRY REID

Senator Reid. Good morning, ladies and gentlemen. Can you hear to the back of the room? Is this any better? Good.

Again, ladies and gentlemen, good morning. I call this Senate Aging Committee to order and welcome everyone here to this hearing titled, "The Many Faces of Long-Term Care: Today's Bitter Pill or Tomorrow's Cure." Everyone is welcome. Appreciate those in the audience. We hope that you are able to hear the witnesses.

I want to first of all take this time to thank Aging Committee Chairman Charles Grassley of Iowa who has graciously allowed this hearing to take place. Also, we have the staff director, Ted Totman, who is responsible for all Aging Committee activities, present with us. He is to my far left.

He has helped arrange this hearing. He will also travel with us to Reno and, of course, package this material and distribute it to the other members of the Aging Committee. We also have with us the staff director of the ranking member of the Aging Committee, John Breaux from Louisiana. Ken Cohen, two seats over from me, is here with us and has been heavily involved in this as has been, as I have indicated, Ted Totman.

Next to me is my staff assistant, Jerry Reed, who specializes in matters relating to aging and veteran's affairs. He has been working on this hearing for several months and I appreciate his good work.

I recently became aware of a couple of studies in the long-term care area that when viewed together really concern me. One study pointed out that 43 percent or two out of five of us will, upon reaching the age of 65, require the assistance of long-term care facilities such as nursing homes and assisted living facilities.

But a second survey published in the Journal of American Geriatrics, suggested that almost a third of those polled said they would rather die than live in a nursing home. It does not take a real bright person to see that a significant portion of the public has lost faith in the potential of our long-term care facilities. I believe it is important to examine these concerns and to do what it takes to restore confidence in such a large segment of our overall health care delivery system for older Americans.

For the past 15 years, four years in the House and 11 years in the Senate, a total of 15 years, I have been on aging committees in both the House and the Senate. I served in the House under the able leadership of my friend and mentor, Claude Pepper. I have learned much while living and serving on these committees about the many dimensions of long-term care.

One thing I have learned is the importance of Federal standards in nursing homes. I was a strong supporter of the Federal nursing home standards enacted in 1987 and remain a supporter of those Federal standards today. While most facilities deliver compassionate and professional health care to its residents, a system of well-defined standards with annual review is vital if we are to ensure the maintenance of quality in these institutions.

Today there are 33.9 million or, let's say, 34 million older Americans that represent almost 13 percent of our population. But by the year 2030, there will be 70 million older persons, more than twice our population today. This group will make up about 20 percent of the population, or said another way, one in five Americans will be over the age of 65 by the year 2030.

The need for long-term care will grow along with our population and it is not an option for us to hide our head in the sand on this topic. Along with these changing demographics, the face of long-term care is also changing. Today long-term care is no longer just care provided in nursing homes. Home health care, assisted living, hospice care in addition to institutional care have become popular alternatives to nursing homes.

Although these industries are booming, our public policy has not kept pace with these changes. We must begin to answer critical questions. What should be the Federal role, the State role, and the role of families which is so important? How do we ensure quality in programs and safety of residents? Should a patient's eligibility for assistance dictate the care to be received, or should the patient's condition be the determining factor?

In short, should money be the determining factor or how the institutions are going to be paid, or should the condition of the patient be the concern? Of course, we all agree it should be the condition of the patient, but frankly, that is not the way it is much of the time in America today.

At this point, let me briefly address the safety of residents issue. Senators Grassley, Kohl, and I have introduced legislation, S. 1122, The Patient Abuse and Prevention Act, to require the establishment of a national registry for confirmed abusers of seniors in long-term care facilities and require that staff undergo full background checks before working in these facilities.

In effect, what we are trying to stop is people who are laid off, fired in rest homes and other institutions who simply go on to work someplace else after having abused people in various places in a community, the State or around the country. It happens and that is too bad.

With this national registry, this would stop. I believe patients and families deserve this protection. I am hopeful that Aging Committee Chairman Grassley will convene a hearing on this topic in Washington very early this next session.

Now back to today's hearing. I want to talk a little bit about why I wanted to have this hearing in Nevada. Nevada is in a unique position to show the rest of the nation how to build a future for those who require long-term care. I say this because our senior population is the fastest growing in the nation and our long-term care infrastructure will, by sheer demand, be forced to grow with it.

In 1996, there were about 210,000 senior citizens over the age of 65 in Nevada. This number is projected to grow to almost 350,000 by the year 2020. The over-85 group in the Silver State numbered just 10,000 in 1993. This will reach about 35,000 a short 20 years from now. It is this group for whom long-term care options become crucial.

In spite of this growth, as recently as a month ago, it was reported that the state's growing senior population is putting a strain on the long-term care system. While the occupancy of available nursing home beds is over 90 percent, it is expected the demand will far exceed availability as the baby boomers retire.

Vice President Humphrey said, "The true moral test of government is how it treats those in the dawn of life, the children; those in the twilight of life, the aged; and those who are in the shadow of life, the sick, the needy, and the disabled." That is what this hearing is all about.

We must do all we can to assure quality, safety, affordability, and accessibility in our nation's long-term care facilities. This must be done in partnership between Federal and State Government and the long-term care industry and must include the voice of the consumers of long-term care.

Our first panel today will address the Federal and State perspective as it relates to long-term care. We will also hear about the prevalence of Alzheimer's and other dementia among older Americans and the impact these diseases will have on our future long-term care needs.

Our second panel will tell the story from the patient's perspective, as well as the perspective of those who are charged with overseeing the quality and safety of care provided.

On our third and final panel, we will hear from various witnesses, some of whom will speak from the perspective of those who provide long-term care in nursing homes, assisted living facilities, and home and community care settings. We will also hear about the type of long-term care delivery systems that should be in place to prepare for the future.

I would now like to begin the testimony from our witnesses. I would like to remind all witnesses that their testimony will be limited to five minutes. You will see these lights here that we brought especially from Washington. Green, everything is okay; the yellow, you have a minute to go; the red, you are all through. Your written testimony will be made part of the official record. There are a number of witnesses who have elaborated upon their oral statements. This will be made a part of the official record.

For those in the audience, we have passed out question cards. If you would like to submit questions for a response from one of the witnesses, please complete the card and hand it to one of the staff members standing throughout the room. We will collect them and answer as many as we can within our time constraints.

Also, the reason we found that question cards work better, some people ask the same question over and over again and it is best just to pick out the best question phrased dealing with that topic. Those that we do not answer here will receive written responses.

Our first witness today is Jeanette Takamura, Assistant Secretary of Aging, Department of Health and Human Services. We appreciate very much Dr. Takamura being here. She served as the First Deputy Director of Hawaii Department of Health. Prior to that, she served as the Director of the Hawaii Executive Office of Aging from 1987 to 1994 where she developed numerous programs to prepare Hawaii's diverse population for an aging society.

She is a graduate of the University of Hawaii where she earned a Bachelor's degree and a Master's degree in social work. She has a Ph.D. in social policy from Brandeis University. It might be interesting, Dr. Takamura, when I leave here today, I am going to go to speak to Brandeis University alumni here in Las Vegas.

Secretary TAKAMURA. Oh, wonderful.

Senator REID. They are having a meeting and I learned a lot about Brandeis last night preparing for that. It is a brand new university. It is 50 years old, but rated as one of the finest research facilities in America. In fact, out of all the schools in America, it is ranked number nine in research. So you have great credentials there.

We also have with us on our first panel Dr. Charles Bernick. He is a professor of neurology and Chief of the Division of Neurology, University of Nevada School of Medicine. He is the founder and director of the University of Nevada's Alzheimer's Disease Diagnostic and Treatment Centers.

Dr. Bernick is a member of the Alzheimer's Disease National Education Initiative. He serves on the advisory board of the National Geriatric Council. He is not only well-qualified academically, but has a great background for having worked personally with patients with diseases such as Alzheimer's. Dr. Takamura.

[The prepared statement of Senator Reid follows:]

UNITED STATES SENATOR FOR NEVADA

HARRY REID

OPENING STATEMENT FOR SENATOR HARRY REID
"THE MANY FACES OF LONG TERM CARE:
TODAY'S BITTER PILL OR TOMORROW'S CURE?"

Good Morning and welcome to this morning's Special Committee on Aging Field Hearing entitled "The Many Faces of Long-Term Care: Today's Bitter Pill or Tomorrow's Cure?" I welcome all of you and our distinguished panel of witnesses.

Recently, I became aware of two studies in the long-term care area that when viewed together really concerned me. One study commented that projections suggest that 43%, or 2 out of 5 of us will - upon reaching the age of 65 - require the assistance of long-term care facilities such as nursing homes or assisted living facilities in our lifetime. A second survey published in *the Journal of the American Geriatrics Society* suggested that 30% of those polled said they would rather die than live in a nursing home. Knowing of the tremendous need for long-term care in the future, I decided it was time to see where we are and what needs to be done. It does not take a rocket scientist to see that a significant portion of the public has lost faith in the potential of our long-term care facilities even though 43% of us knowingly will come to rely on such care. Some of this public concern may be due to misinformation, anecdotal news reports, or personal experience. Regardless of the source, I believe it is important to examine these concerns and do what it takes to restore confidence in such a large segment of our overall health care delivery system for older Americans. A system that will become even more crucial in the years to come.

I have visited many long-term care facilities and attended many hearings on this subject over my years in Congress and my overall opinion is that like anything else, there are some excellent, some good, some average and some questionable programs. However, when it comes to our nation's seniors, questionable or average is just not good enough. I always ask myself, and would ask you to do the same, if it were your parent or your spouse, would questionable or average be acceptable?

For the past 12 years I have served on the Senate Special Committee on Aging and before that during my four years in the House of Representatives I served on the House Aging Committee under the leadership of my friend and mentor the late Claude Pepper. I have learned much while serving on these Committees about the many dimensions of long-term care. One thing I have learned is the importance of federal standards for our nursing homes. I was a strong supporter of the federal nursing home standards enacted back in 1987 and remain a supporter of these federal standards today. While most facilities deliver compassionate and professional health care to residents, a system of well-defined standards with annual review is vital if we are to ensure the maintenance of quality. The enforcement of these standards, with penalties as necessary, is key if these standards are to be taken seriously. Seniors deserve nothing less.

LONG-TERM CARE A GROWING PROBLEM

Today, there are 33.9 million older Americans representing 12.8% of the U.S. population. By 2030, there will be approximately 70 million older persons, more than twice our population today. This group will make up 20% of the population, or said another way, 1 in 5 Americans will be over the age of 65 by 2030. The need for long-term care will grow right along with the population and it is not an option for us to hide our head in the sand on this topic. It is time we discuss our current long-term care system, both its strengths and its weaknesses, and hear from users, providers, advocates and state and federal officials about what needs to be considered for the future.

The face of long-term care is changing. Today, long-term care is no longer just care provided in nursing homes. Home health care, assisted living, and hospice care, in addition to institutional care have become popular alternatives to nursing homes. Although these industries are booming, our public policy has not kept pace with these changes. We must begin to answer critical questions. What role will long-term care insurance play in the future? What should be the federal role, state role, or the role of families? Should spending down to qualify for Medicaid be the national expectation? How do we ensure quality in programs and safety of residents? Should a patient's eligibility for assistance dictate the care to be received or should the patient's condition be the determining factor?

Today, we will cover many aspects of long-term care--including accessability, affordability, quality, and safety. We will hear from several witnesses who will discuss what we should consider as we craft long-term care policy for the future. It is not my intention to focus on abuse and neglect issues, affordability issues, the role of private or public funding sources, or to engage in an attack on any industry or provider, but instead to discuss where we are today and where we need to be in the future regarding long-term care.

PATIENT ABUSE

I would like to briefly mention that Senators Grassley, Kohl and I have introduced legislation, S. 1122 "The Patient Abuse Prevention Act," to require the establishment of a national registry for confirmed abusers of seniors in long-term care facilities and require that staff undergo thorough background checks before working in these facilities. I believe patients and families deserve this protection. I am hopeful that Aging Committee Chairman Grassley will convene a hearing on this topic in Washington in the next session and look forward to working with he and Senator Kohl, the sponsor of this important legislation, in planning the hearing.

NEVADA - A MODEL FOR THE NATION

Now back to today's hearing. I want to talk a little about why I wanted to have this hearing in Nevada. Nevada is in a unique position to show the rest of the nation how to build a future for those who will require long-term care. I say this as our senior population is the fastest growing in the nation and our long-term care infrastructure will by sheer demand be forced to grow with it. We have the opportunity to engage in efforts to shape our future rather than maintaining the status quo. As we already know, for Nevadans with long-term care needs, status quo is not an option as demand will far exceed availability in the years to come.

When looking to the future and the growth in the senior population that can already be seen, I am reminded of the old saying, "we ain't seen nothing yet." If our current system cannot accommodate the nation's growing long-termcare needs, how will we be able to do so when the senior population doubles.

Here in Nevada, in 1996, we had 209,000 senior citizens over the age of 65, and this number is projected to grow to 333,000 by the year 2020. The over 85 group in the Silver State numbered 10,000 in 1993, and will reach 34,000 in 2020. It is this group for whom long-term care options become so crucial.

In spite of this growth, as recently as one month ago, it was reported that the state's growing senior population is putting a strain on the long-term care system. While occupancy of available nursing home beds is over 90%, it is expected that demand will far exceed availability as the baby boomers retire. It is therefore worth our time to examine Nevada's experience as we determine what our future national policy should consider to accommodate the rapidly growing senior population. I am grateful that Senator Grassley, Chairman of the Senate Aging Committee, and Senator Breaux, the ranking minority member, approved bringing the Committee's work to Nevada.

THE PANELS

Our first panel will address the federal and state perspective as it relates to long-term care. We will also hear about the prevalence of Alzheimer's and Parkinson's among older Americans and the impact these diseases will have on our future long-term care needs. Our second panel will tell the story from the patient's perspective as well as from the perspective of those who are charged with overseeing the quality and safety of the care provided. In our third and final panel we will hear from various witnesses, some of who will speak from the perspective of those who provide long-term care in nursing homes, assisted living facilities and home and community care settings. We will also hear about the type of long-term care delivery systems that should be in place to prepare for the future.

I am aware that Nevada's Interim Finance Committee recently held a hearing on "Long-Term Health Care Needs of Persons Living in Nevada." I compliment them on their initiative. It is not my intention today to duplicate that effort. My objective is to hear from Nevadans who interact with long-term care on a daily basis and learn from their experience as we address national policy concerns and theappropriate role of the federal government in this policy formulation.

I do not expect today's hearing to provide all the answers. It is more my hope that we will gain an understanding of the right questions to be asking. With my seat on the Aging Committee, and representing the state with the fastest growing senior population in the nation, I am in a unique position to look to the future on this issue.

Hubert Humphrey once said that "the true moral test of government is how it treats those in the dawn of life-the children; those in the twilight of life-the aged; and those who are in the shadow of life-the sick, the needy and the disabled." We must do all we can to ensure quality, safety, affordability and accessibility in our nation's long-term care facilities. This must done in partnership between federal and state government and the long-term care industry. For this reason I am pleased that today's witnesses have agreed to join me as we seek to identify the right questions to be asking.

I would now like to begin hearing testimony from our witnesses. I would like to remind all witnesses to keep their comments to 5 minutes. Written testimony will be made a part of the official record. For those in the audience, we have passed out question cards. If you would like to submit a question for response from one of the witnesses, please complete the card and hand it to one of the staff members standing throughout the room. We will collect them and ask as many as we can within our time constraints. I will provide those we do not get a chance to ask today to the witnesses and ask that written responses be provided to the Committee by February 2nd for inclusion in the official record.

At this point I would like to introduce our first witness.

STATEMENT OF JEANETTE C. TAKAMURA, ASSISTANT SECRETARY FOR AGING

Ms. TAKAMURA. Thank you, Chairman Reid, and members of the subcommittee. It is a really great privilege for me to be here today on behalf of Secretary Donna Shalala. I am indeed honored, as the Assistant Secretary for Aging, to be participating in this very important forum with someone who is regarded to be a long-standing true friend and a dedicated and effective advocate and leader within the U.S. Senate for older Americans, and that is, of course, no other person than the Honorable Harry Reid.

I have been asked today to provide insights into the current and future state of the extraordinarily complex and challenging domain of long-term care. I will attempt to provide a framework of Federal long-term care programs, indicate some of the key long-term care issues facing policy-makers at all levels, note Health and Human Services' initiatives, and suggest possible future directions.

I will also include a brief description of the long-term care needs of older persons and of families, stressing the importance of advocacy to ensure the emergence of a consumer-oriented, cost-effective long-term care system. As I do this, may I ask you to keep in mind several trends.

First of all, as the Senator mentioned earlier, by the year 2020, there will be more than 70 million older persons in this country, or more than twice the number today. Thus, despite all the recent evidence that there is improved health status among our older Americans, we know that the need for long-term care services will continue to expand.

Second, let me mention that women dedicate a significant amount of time as primary care givers providing elder care to their spouses, fathers, and brothers. Indeed, some experts have indicated that women spend more years providing elder care than child care. Concomitantly, women tend to be the primary consumers of long-term care services because they generally out-survive their male relatives.

Third, let me mention that the elderly population is rapidly becoming more diverse as minorities live longer and will account for 25 percent of all older Americans by 2030. Let me go on to mention also that baby boomers are now grappling with long-term care concerns related to their parents and will join the ranks of older Americans starting in 2011. As a baby boomer, I can tell you I am very concerned about that.

Let me very briefly highlight some of the important federally-funded programs which serve our older Americans who require long-term care. As you know, the Administration on Aging, the agency which I head, grants and authorizes the expenditure of funds under the Older Americans Act to states and local communities for infrastructure development and the building of comprehensive and coordinated service delivery systems.

What I do know is that the Older Americans Act provides for the provision of gap-filling services such as transportation and nutrition services as well as advocacy, coordination, and other activities which help meet the needs and protect the rights of older adults. Here in Nevada alone, the Division of Aging Services under the very able leadership of my colleague, Carla Sloan, fulfills these responsibilities.

Currently, Nevada receives 1.6 million in Federal dollars for supportive services, including about $50,000 for protective elder rights services, such as the long-term care ombudsman and elder abuse activities; 2 million for congregate meals; $600,000 for home-delivered meals; $87,000 for disease prevention, health promotion activities; and $52,000 for the provision of in-home services for the frail elderly.

With respect to Federal funding for long-term care, the Health Care Financing Administration administers the Medicaid program, and I think all of you are familiar with this particular program. About 28 million for nursing home care comes to the elderly in Nevada and more money also comes here for home health, personal care, and home and community-based care services.

HCFA also administers the Medicare program, a program which primarily covers acute care benefits, but also some chronic and post-acute care under its home health care benefits package. There are other agencies for sure that provide very essential funding for services that support us in long-term care, and I would mention two of them very briefly.

One of them is HUD, the Department for Housing and Urban Development, and the other is Social Security Administration, which administers a variety of income security programs including the Supplemental Security Income program, which provides essential cash assistance to the aged, blind, and disabled individuals and their dependent family members.

Many older persons use their Social Security Administration benefits, including SSI, to pay out-of-pocket long-term care expenses including board and care. There is so much that I could say about long-term care and I think, Chairman, that you have pointed out that this is a critical area for our examination and certainly action.

Let me note that Carla Sloan, again my colleague, will be testifying about the long-term care ombudsman program. We know that there are several long-term care policy issues which really deserve our attention at this time. Certainly we are seeing assisted living facilities sprout out and bloom all across the country and this is an area of great interest to all of us in aging.

In addition to that, I think you know, and you have certainly been a leader in this regard, that the administration has been very concerned about fraud and abuse, and really with the Operation Restore Trust, we are now beginning to address many of the concerns which have long been of interest to us across the country.

I would like to mention that another area of great concern to people all across the country, and you have once again been a leader in this regard, is the need for a seamless, cost-effective system of care. Not just Federal officials, but also State officials have been working for a very long time to make this a reality.

Within the aging network, managed care is an area of great interest. Consumers must be given every opportunity to understand how to utilize managed care systems.

Under the new 1997 Health Insurance Portability and Accountability Act, we are seeking to clarify the tax treatment of private long-term care insurance. Accordingly, the Department of Treasury is now preparing regulations for such purposes in partnership with, of course, the Department of Health and Human Services.

For 30 years now, the Older Americans Act has authorized the Administration on Aging to serve as a partner with our state and local communities in the provision of an array of long term care services deemed necessary to meet the needs of our older Americans. Many of these services are very heavily relied upon and it is truly with leadership from people such as you—and yours have been outstanding, that we are able to fund services that make such a difference in communities across the country.

An ideal home and community-based care system, of course, would include services such as personal care, homemaker and chore services, congregated home-delivered meals, adult day care, transportation, and others, and certainly we could spend a lot of time on these but I know——

Senator REID. Dr. Takamura, your time is up.

Ms. TAKAMURA. Yes, our time is up.

Senator REID. Because you are a guest here, I have been very lenient.

Ms. TAKAMURA. I am sorry. [Laughter.]

Senator REID. But we have already received questions from the audience and——

Ms. TAKAMURA. OK, great. I would be more than willing to take those questions.

Senator REID. I appreciate very much your statement.

[The prepared statement of Ms. Takamura follows:]

DEPARTMENT OF HEALTH & HUMAN SERVICES

Washington, D.C. 20201

STATEMENT OF

JEANETTE C. TAKAMURA

ASSISTANT SECRETARY FOR AGING

DEPARTMENT OF HEALTH AND HUMAN SERVICES

BEFORE THE

SENATE SPECIAL COMMITTEE ON AGING

FIELD HEARING

JANUARY 12, 1998 - LAS VEGAS, NEVADA

JANUARY 13, 1998 - RENO, NEVADA

Mr. Chairman and Members of the Subcommittee:

It is a great privilege to be here with you today on behalf of Secretary Donna Shalala. I am indeed honored as the Assistant Secretary for Aging to be participating in this important forum with a true friend and advocate within the U.S. Senate for older Americans — the Honorable Harry Reid.

I have been asked today to provide insights into the current and future state of long-term care (LTC) at the national level. This is indeed an ambitious task, because LTC as a policy and program area is extraordinarily complex. I will attempt to provide a framework of federal LTC programs; indicate some of the key LTC issues facing policy makers at all levels; note HHS initiatives; and suggest possible future directions for LTC. I will also include a brief description of the LTC needs of older persons and their families and the importance of advocacy to ensure the emergence of a consumer-oriented, cost-effective LTC system. As I do this, I would ask you to keep in mind a number of trends. That is: 1) The older population will continue to grow. By the year 2020, there will be more than 70 million older persons in this country or more than twice the number today. The older population also is getting frailer. Despite recent evidence of declines in disability rates related to longevity, the need for LTC services will continue to expand. 2) Women, the family members who most often serve as the primary caregivers, are spending a significant amount of time providing eldercare. Indeed, some experts have indicated that women spend more years providing eldercare than child care. Concomitantly, women tend to be the primary consumers of LTC services because they generally survive their spouses, fathers, and brothers. 3) The older population is rapidly becoming more diverse as minorities live longer. For example, in 1990, 13 percent of persons 65 years and older were minorities. This percentage is projected to rise to 25 percent by 2030, almost doubling in 35 years. 4) Baby boomers, many of whom are now beginning to grapple in growing numbers with LTC concerns related to their parents, will join the ranks of our older Americans starting in 2011. By that time their own potential LTC needs will have taken on a measure of reality.

Let me briefly highlight some of the important federally funded programs which serve older Americans who require LTC beginning with those in the Department of Health and Human Services (DHHS). The Administration on Aging (AoA), the agency which I head, grants and authorizes the expenditure of funds under the Older Americans Act (OAA) to states and local communities for infrastructure development and the building of comprehensive and coordinated service delivery systems. These systems directly lend support to LTC needs through efforts to improve the coordination of other programs and funding streams. For example,

OAA funds provide gap-filling services such as transportation and nutrition services and are used for advocacy, coordination and other activities which help meet the needs and protect the rights of older adults. Here in Nevada, the Division on Aging Services under the leadership of my colleague, Carla Sloan, fulfills these responsibilities. Currently, Nevada receives $1.6 million for supportive services, including $50,000 for protective elder rights services such as the LTC Ombudsman and elder abuse activities; $2 million for congregate meals; $600,000 for home delivered meals; $87,000 for disease prevention, health promotion activities; and $52,000 for the provision of in-home services for the frail elderly. I have attached for the record a summary of some other programs administered by DHHS that address LTC.

With regard to federal funding of LTC, the Health Care Financing Administration (HCFA) administers the Medicaid program -- the largest source of public financing for LTC services for older adults. In FY 1996, approximately $16.7 billion in federal funds were expended for care in nursing facilities for the elderly. This included approximately $28.2 million for nursing home care for the elderly in Nevada. Approximately an additional $2 billion in federal funds was spent nationally for home and community-based alternative care for the elderly, including home health, personal care, and home and community-based waivers. Nevada received approximately $2.2 million of these funds. HCFA also administers Medicare, a program which mainly covers acute care benefits. However, the Medicare home health benefits cover some chronic care as well as post-acute care. In FY 1996, more than $16.7 billion was spent for home health benefits to meet chronic and post-acute care needs. A share of these funds has gone to serve the needs of older persons in this state.

Among the important agencies involved in LTC services outside DHHS are the Department of Housing and Urban Development (HUD) and the Social Security Administration (SSA). HUD, for example, administers the Supportive Housing Program for the Elderly (Section 202). In FY 1997, $645 million was appropriated to support this program nationally. SSA administers a variety of income security programs including the Supplemental Security Income (SSI) program to provide cash assistance to aged, blind, and disabled individuals and their dependent family members. Many older persons use their SSA benefits, including SSI, to pay out-of-pocket LTC expenses, including board and care.

At the federal level we are also emphasizing quality through a number of means. Last Spring, the President appointed a Commission on Consumer Protection and Quality in the Health Care Industry for which Secretary Shalala serves as a co-chair. This Fall, the Commission approved a Consumer Bill of Rights which was endorsed by the President. Additional Commission recommendations are expected later this Winter addressing requirements for protecting consumers in managed care and fee-for-service plans.

These recommendations and their implementation will have important implications for consumers of LTC.

The OAA authorizes state LTC ombudsman programs. In all 57 states and territories and 550 localities, LTC ombudsmen investigate and resolve complaints related to the care of nursing home and board and care residents. In a number of states, ombudsmen also monitor the quality of home care. This program provides a community presence in long-term care facilities by monitoring private and publicly-subsidized care.

The LTC issues which face national, state and local officials are complex. To offer a sense of this, let me just list a few major LTC policy issues.

Assisted living facilities are one of the fastest growing residential care options for older persons. Many states are wrestling with how much regulation is necessary to protect residents and ensure quality of care while assuring sufficient flexibility to sustain a home-like environment, accommodate individual residents' preferences, and avoid discouraging developers.

Industry-driven Medicare home health benefits are being utilized increasingly to meet the LTC needs of older adults. However, the Office of the Inspector General (OIG) and the General Accounting

Office have found this benefit to be very susceptible to abuse. The OIG evaluated a sample of 3,745 services in 250 home health claims in four states and estimated that 40 percent of the services did not meet Medicare reimbursement requirements.

Over at least the last two decades, Medicaid spending on nursing homes has risen. States are making efforts to control costs and increase the provision of home and community-based services. The rates of increase for nursing home expenditures have been declining and nursing home utilization rates are beginning to come down. However, estimates of nursing home expenditures continue to increase at rates beyond the overall inflation rate, e.g., 7.8 percent in FY 1995. Nursing home spending continues to be a significant part of total Medicaid expenditures for older persons, e.g., almost 64 percent in FY 1995, with an additional 8 percent spent on home care.

Out of an interest in creating a more seamless, cost-effective system of care, federal and state officials alike are giving increased attention to strategies for integrating acute and LTC through mechanisms such as managed care, especially for those older persons who are dually eligible for Medicare and Medicaid. Managed care organizations, primarily concerned with primary and acute care in the past, generally do not have an established track record in LTC and many advocates are concerned about this lack of experience. For these reasons, we need to monitor closely provider performance.

From the beginning of his administration, the President has maintained a strong and continuing commitment to health care reform. This commitment has been reflected in LTC efforts by DHHS and other federal agencies. At the 1995 White House Conference on Aging, President Clinton unveiled Operation Restore Trust (ORT) to combat fraud and abuse in the Medicare and Medicaid programs, targeting in particular nursing homes and home health agencies with questionable fiscal and care practices. Within DHHS, the Office of the Inspector General, HCFA, and AoA, partnered, along with the Department of Justice, to carry out ORT demonstrations in five states. The ORT demonstration has proved so successful that a full-scale national effort is now underway.

The Administration supported the 1996 Health Insurance Portability and Accountability Act (HIPAA) authored by Senators Kassebaum and Kennedy. The HIPAA clarifies tax treatment of private LTC insurance and directs the Department of Treasury to prepare regulations for the implementation of these provisions in consultation with DHHS.

Through the 1997 Balanced Budget Act (BBA), the President took important steps toward improving and expanding health care access and quality. The BBA includes provisions for developing a prospective payment system for home care and skilled nursing home facilities under Medicare and the repeal of the Boren Amendment under Medicaid, all of which are expected to reduce nursing home and home health costs. The BBA also provides for an expansion of the PACE program, which represents one model for integrating LTC and acute care using Medicare, Medicaid, and other dollars.

The AoA has been engaged for the last three decades in partnership with State and Area Agencies on Aging in the development of a LTC infrastructure. More than half of all State Units on Aging nationwide are administering Medicaid waiver programs, two-thirds are administering the widely-appreciated Health Insurance Counseling and Assistance Program, and one half are administering programs for adults with disabilities. Many area agencies have taken on similar responsibilities at the local level.

While the scope and operation of LTC systems are complex and the issues pertaining to the system of services, costs and quality of care are challenging, the needs of most frail older Americans and their families are relatively simple. The majority of older Americans live at home or in small community residential settings. As survey after survey has shown, older adults and their families — the payers of the major portion of LTC costs, prefer to have services provided in their homes and communities rather than in institutions. Long-term care, particularly when it is delivered in the community, does not generally involve expensive medical care. For the most part, it entails basic assistance with dressing, eating, using the bathroom, and other activities of daily living. Personal care, meal preparation, or chore services – whether provided by one of the millions of volunteer caregivers, family members, neighbors, friends, or by a paid service provider – can help older persons remain in their homes as long as possible. As simple as the needs of a frail older person may be, some basic infrastructure must be in place and accessible to them. For instance, an ideal home and community-based care system would include the following services, as appropriate: personal care, homemaker, and chore services; congregate and home-delivered meals; adult day care; rehabilitative care; assisted transportation; home health care; supportive services for caregivers; and assisted living. Because older Americans often have multiple and changing health and social service needs, effective HCB service programs also require administrative arrangements that facilitate the coordination of and access to HCB and institutional services, including discharge planning, case management, pre-admission screening, and linkages to medical providers.

In light of the gift of longevity with which a growing majority of Americans are now blessed, we must engage as a nation in ensuring that we have an architecture for longevity in place; i.e., a design for the future which acknowledges long life as a reality, is sensitive to the needs of current elders, and is informed by the likely requirements and contributions of the largest cohort of older adults this world has yet to see – the baby boomers. Let me thus suggest four areas where more attention must be focused at the federal level if we are to empower all Americans as well as develop a LTC system which resonates with the broadest spectrum of our population.

- **We must ready America for longevity.** That is, those of us in federal positions of responsibility must be sure that all Americans are aware of and prepared for the challenges and opportunities which lie ahead for our communities, families, and ourselves as the gift of longevity begins to manifest itself in even more pronounced ways. To the extent that life expectancy is increasing and disability rates among the elderly are declining, we need to foster a climate of "active aging", where society can continue to draw on the talents of its older citizens. At the same time, frail elders with disabilities need access to appropriate long-term care services in their communities.

- **We must give greater emphasis to consumer education and protection.** Although increased choices are leading to healthy market competition and in most cases improved potential consumer options, the number and magnitude of these choices is bewildering to many older persons. As you know, HCFA is launching a number of consumer education efforts around the new preventive benefits and managed care options under the BBA. We support these and are working closely with them. In addition, last year we transmitted to the aging network our managed care principles which suggested broad roles in advocacy, information and assistance, benefits counseling, quality assurance, care management, and consumer protection, including adopting the ombudsman function in managed care. Because the aging network is so concerned about the relationship of managed care to LTC, it is important that we encourage them to establish a clear understanding of what approaches they will adopt in relation to managed care organizations, particularly in regard to advocacy and consumer protection.

● **We must encourage public-private partnerships as well as partnerships among federal agencies which can generate more resources, new creative approaches, and which recognize and address the diverse needs of a longevous population.** There is hardly enough that we can do in this regard, particularly if we are committed to fostering the development of more coordinated and effective services. The AoA and I take the coordination and advocacy responsibilities seriously. We are already beginning to plan how these might be carried out through partnerships with others.

● **We need vigorous experimentation and testing to determine what is working and at what cost.** The HCB waiver program has expanded dramatically and supports reforms that can make HCB services a more attractive alternative to institutional care. I submit that the Title IV research and demonstration program under the OAA is another important vehicle for doing the type of demonstrations that are needed in LTC, particularly for non-nursing home eligible older persons. As most people in the field recognize, Title IV has been the testing ground for many important developments in LTC, e.g., On Lok (the predecessor of PACE), case management (particularly under the channeling projects), the LTC Ombudsman Program, and national LTC resource centers and state planning grants.

This concludes my assessment of the current state of LTC at the national level and some of the future possibilities for improving services for older persons. Obviously there is much we all must do at every level of government to institute needed changes in the way LTC is organized, financed and delivered. The AoA is just one of many agencies that has an important role to play in this endeavor. Nonetheless, it is an important role. The OAA authorizes the AoA to be an "effective and visible advocate for older persons" within DHHS and other departments and agencies, and to coordinate federal, state local and private programs to "establish a nationwide network of comprehensive and coordinated services" for older persons. As the new Assistant Secretary for Aging, I am anxious to begin initiating discussions with others with the goal of promoting the development of more effective LTC systems for older persons and all those needing LTC.

Finally, I would like to thank you, Senator Reid, for providing me with this opportunity to be here with you in Nevada and to present testimony before the Senate Special Committee on Aging on this important topic. I look forward to the rest of this morning's hearing, and working with you as we move forward toward improving LTC services. I will be happy to answer any questions you might have.

ATTACHMENT 1

SUMMARY OF OTHER DHHS PROGRAMS RELATED TO LTC

The Administration for Children and Families (ACF) administers the Social Services Block Grants which are awarded to states and may be used to provide a broad array of supportive, social, and personal care and assistance services to persons in need of home and community-based assistance, including the elderly. In FY 1997, $13.9 million was allocated to Nevada.

The Substance Abuse and Mental Health Services Administration (SAMSHA) administers, among other programs, the Community Mental Health Block Grants which are formula grants to each state to carry out comprehensive community mental health services for all populations regardless of age. In FY 1997, Nevada received $1.4 million under this program.

The Health Resources and Services Administration (HRSA) has administered since 1992 a State Alzheimer's Disease Demonstration Program which is designed to demonstrate new approaches to providing home and community-based services to Alzheimer's victims and their families. Currently, $6 million is allocated to 15 states. While Nevada is not one of these states, the new approaches under development will be of use in planning community-based approaches to addressing the issues of Alzheimer's disease.

The Office of the Assistant Secretary for Planning and Evaluation (ASPE) funds a large number of national policy research studies relative to disability, aging and LTC. Currently, two of their most significant ones are the evaluation of the Cash and Counseling demonstrations funded by the Robert Wood Johnson Foundation and a national study of assisted living. The cash and counseling demonstrations are designed to test new methods of providing consumer-directed services for the elderly and the disabled. The assisted living study is examining the state-of-the-art of the emerging area of assisted living and how it fits into the development of LTC systems around the country. Both of these studies have important policy implications for Nevada and other states.

Senator REID. Dr. Bernick.

STATEMENT OF CHARLES BERNICK, M.D., DEPARTMENT OF INTERNAL MEDICINE DIVISION OF NEUROLOGY, UNIVERSITY OF NEVADA SCHOOL OF MEDICINE

Dr. BERNICK. Senator Reid and members of the field hearing committee, I, too, very much appreciate this opportunity to address the committee regarding actually the unique demands of patients that are afflicted with Alzheimer's disease and other dementias on long-term care systems.

I think it is well-recognized that Alzheimer's disease is a major public health problem. The numbers speak for themselves. Ten percent of those over the age of 65 have Alzheimer's disease or some other form of dementia, and as you mentioned, in the group over 85, which is the fastest growing segment of the population here in Nevada and in the nation, it is estimated that close to 40 percent of people will have Alzheimer's disease.

Using those figures, it is projected that by the year 2050, the number of elderly that will be affected will grow from 4 million, which it is now, to close to 14 million people. I think beyond the numbers, the impact of Alzheimer's disease really involves the nature of the disease, which is a progressive impairment and loss of memory and other cognitive abilities and everyone, everyone with that disease will at some point during the disease require 24-hour care and supervision and many will require institutionalization.

Now, the type of care that Alzheimer's disease patients will require really depends on the point in the course of the disease itself. I think many recognize that close to 50 percent of people in nursing homes have Alzheimer's disease, but what is not as well-recognized is that most of the care that's provided to Alzheimer's patients is at home. Seventy percent of people who have Alzheimer's disease are cared for at home.

That amount of care really also changes. Initially people may just need supervision with finances and medications, but as the disease progresses, other troublesome behaviors occur, aggressiveness, agitation, wanderings, sleeplessness.

It is not really surprising when you look at the figures that a third of the people that are caregivers have to either give up work or reduce their employed work to become caregivers, and 50 percent of caregivers themselves are depressed by having the burden of this type of care.

The unfortunate part is that the services that are available to these home caregivers is rather sparse. Most people either have to depend on other family members, on adult day care activities, on home health aides and paid companions. These services are not always available. I think the geographic separation of families these days make family members not always available.

If you live in rural areas, these services are not available especially here in Nevada, which has a lot of rural areas. We do not have adult day care in a lot of these places. Even if they are available, most people cannot afford them, or many cannot. These are not benefits of Medicare, adult day care and services such as home health aides. To pay out of pocket for these things is again a real burden to caregivers.

Eventually most patients with Alzheimer's disease will need to go into some type of residential care. I think that is a difficult decision for caregivers for several reasons. One is the cost and another the quality and appropriateness of care that these people are going to be given in group care homes, assisted living, and in skilled nursing facilities.

I think that is for good reason because there is often a gap between what these patients need and the services that are provided in these type of residential care facilities. There are concerns about the training of staff, about the programs that are available. Nursing homes in particular have traditionally been aimed at treating physical illness and not the type of things that you see in Alzheimer's disease.

Of course, there is the burden of payment which these people have to pay either out of pocket or spend down to Medicaid levels and lose pretty much all that they have had and earned throughout their life to be cared for. So in summary, I think Alzheimer's disease is going to really provide a significant burden to the long-term care and I think we are going to need ways to support families and caregivers at home, because this could be a damn against the flood of Alzheimer's patients and the care they are going to need.

I think we are going to need to look at strategies to improve the residential-type care that is available because people are certainly going to need that, and, of course, alternative ways to finance these systems to make it affordable to individuals with Alzheimer's disease in the community. Thank you.

[The prepared statement of Dr. Bernick follows:]

UNIVERSITY OF NEVADA
SCHOOL OF MEDICINE

Dept. of Internal Medicine
Division of Neurology
901 S. Rancho Lane
Suite 105
Las Vegas, Nevada 89106
(702) 474-0532
Fax # (702) 477-0033

THE MANY FACES OF LONG TERM CARE: TODAYS BITTER PILL OR TOMMORROWS CURE?

Testimony before the

Senate Special Committee on Aging Field Hearing

January 12, 1998
West Charleston Library
Las Vegas, Nevada

January 13, 1998
Washoe Medical Center Auditorium
Reno, Nevada

Presented by
Charles Bernick, M.D.

Senator Reid and members of the field hearing committee. My name is Charles Bernick and I am the director of the University of Nevada Alzheimer's Disease Diagnostic and Treatment Centers for the state of Nevada. I very much appreciate this opportunity to address the committee regarding the unique demands placed by patients afflicted with Alzheimer's Disease and related dementias on long term care systems.

That Alzheimer's Disease is a major public health problem is widely acknowledged. Close to 10% of individuals over the age of 65, and 40% of those over 85 years of age, suffer from Alzheimer's Disease and other forms of dementia (which I will subsequently lump together with Alzheimer's Disease in this testimony).With the 85 and older age group being the fastest growing segment of the population in Nevada and the nation, it is estimated that the number of patients with Alzheimer's Disease (AD) will rise from the 4 million currently affected to 14 million by the year 2050.

More than just the numbers, AD has a significant impact on long term care due to the nature of the condition. Alzheimer's Disease relentlessly and progressively impairs memory and other cognitive function; every individual with AD will at some point in their disease require 24 hour care and supervision, with many eventually needing institutionalization.

47-539 98 - 2

The type of care needed by AD patients changes with disease progression. Though it is often recognized that 50% of nursing home patients have AD, what is less known is that unpaid family caregivers represent a critical and hidden part of long term care in the United States. Approximately 80% of AD patients are cared for at home by family. Initially, caregivers may only have to supply moderate supervision such as managing finances and medication, in addition to dealing with the repetitiveness and frustration that may come with memory decline. As the disease advances, caregivers may need to cope with more troublesome behaviors such as wandering, paranoia, agitation, physical abusiveness, sleep impairment and need for assistance with self care tasks (eg bathing, dressing and feeding). Some family member leave or reduce paid employment to assume the caregiving role. It is not surprising that studies show 50% of caregivers are themselves depressed and suffer from impaired health.

Services to shore up this fragile part of the long term care spectrum are sparse. Most caregivers must either depend on other family members, adult day care services or paid home health aides or companions for badly needed respite time. Unfortunately, these resources may not be available or financially feasible for all caregivers. For example, adult day care or sitter services are not covered by Medicare and only on a limited basis by Medicaid programs. Furthermore, in rural areas that are far from a major city, as we have in Nevada, there may not be any respite services short of family and friends.

When family caregivers are no longer able to provide care at home, the AD patient is placed into some type of residential care, either a group home or nursing home. Placement decisions are extremely difficult for caregivers due to both emotional and economic concerns.

One recurring worry of caregivers is the quality and appropriateness of care provided by these facilities, and for good reason. These is frequently a gap between the services available and the care an AD patient needs. In the case of group homes, there is a concern regarding the type of training staff members receive in handling dementia patients, along with the social activities provided. Some of the same issues apply to nursing homes, which traditionally have emphasized care of residents with physical illness in need of skilled nursing facilities. Nursing homes have in the past been accused of "warehousing" AD patients, using strategies such as isolation and employment of physical and pharmacological restraint in response to disruptive behaviors.

The past ten years has seen a proliferation of Special Care Units (SCU) in nursing homes. These units purport to offer programs more tailored to dementia patients. The efficacy of SCUs has not yet been systematically demonstrated. More disturbing, studies indicate that not all SCUs offer the same degree of specialized care, with some units only differing from the rest of the facility by being locked.

The cost of residential care becomes another tremendous burden for families. Group home care must be payed out of pocket. Because Medicaid will fund nursing home care, families are often forced to spend down their assets to qualify for welfare. This is indeed a "bitter pill to swallow" for many who have worked their entire life, yet accumulated limited savings. The potential exists for private insurance policies to cover long term care. However, many policies offer only restricted coverages or are too expensive for most elderly persons.

In summary, in the coming years, AD will place an increasing burden on long term care. Several issues deserve further consideration:

1) Because institutionalization of AD patients is often determined by the interplay between disease progression and caregiver vulnerability, programs and services aimed at assisting families with caregiving are needed. More recognition should be directed at family caregivers, as this unpaid force is a dam against the flood of AD cases that are anticipated.

2) Strategies to reduce the gap between the care required by a dementia patient and services provided by residential facilities need further development. These strategies might include alternative forms of residential care, programs to increase social activities and new design principles in refurbishing or building new facilities.

3) Alternative ways to finance the care of AD patients should be evaluated. Some of the reforms that have been proposed include increasing the availability of long term care insurance, extending the health maintenance organization model of prepaid financing to cover long term care services, allowing AD patients to cash in life insurançe policies early, allowing more flexibility in funds from Medicaid to cover group home and home health services, and providing tax credits or other forms of relief for family caregivers.

4) Research into treatments for AD needs to be continually supported. A treatment that would simply delay the onset of the disease for 5 years would reduce in half the number of individuals afflicted with AD.

Thank you for your consideration.

Senator REID. Let me explain to the audience. This is a typical congressional hearing. The first panel has completed their testimony. We will now ask questions.

Dr. Bernick, it was really impressive when I heard that almost half the patients of the 1.6 million people in rest homes around the country are there because of Alzheimer's and Parkinson's disease. I guess from an academic standpoint—Dr. Takamura, if you want to add something, you certainly can—what is being done that you know of in the way of scientific research to delay the onset of either one or both of these diseases?

It is obvious from your testimony and that of Dr. Takamura that not only would huge amounts of money be saved if we could delay the onset of these diseases, but the human pain and suffering not only of the person that has the disease, but of the caregiver would be relieved. So what is being done academically to delay the onset of these diseases or hopefully cure them someday?

Dr. BERNICK. Actually, Senator Reid, quite a bit. Probably as you know, it has been estimated that if we did not cure the disease but just had a treatment to delay the onset for five years, we would reduce in half the number of people with this disease simply because it is a disease of aging. I think there is a lot of work going into looking at strategies to delay the onset of the disease, and even now there are treatments available to improve symptoms and hopefully keep people functioning better longer.

So there is a lot of research in the biomedical part, and I think what really we need, too, is more research into strategies to assist people to stay at home longer and be able to improve their function by perhaps even non-pharmaceutical measures. But I think this really is a big area for research and hopefully will continue to be funded.

Senator REID. Are there programs underway sponsored by the National Institutes of Health or Centers for Disease Control or some Federal agency that is focusing on these diseases that you know of?

Dr. BERNICK. Oh, absolutely. I think there is a number of long-term programs that are being looked at. The Federal budget does support a number of Alzheimer's centers that are looking at longitudinal changes in the disease and doing pharmaceutical interventions and other types of research. I think this truly is one of the hottest areas of research now that is going on.

Senator REID. Dr. Takamura, would you add anything to that?

Ms. TAKAMURA. Yes. I think what Dr. Bernick said was absolutely correct. The other thing, though, that we need to be aware of is that people are so often terrified of Alzheimer's that oftentimes they are reluctant even to attempt to ascertain whether they have the disease. Treatment interventions cannot be offered until diagnoses are made. Fortunately, we have monies under the Older Americans Act to assist families with community-based care for Alzheimer's patients. We are indeed very grateful for this funding.

Senator REID. One of the things you both mentioned is something that I have seen very recently. Friends of mine are caring for their mother and mother-in-law. She is in her 80s. One of the things they need—they are very caring, good people. They are willing to take care of their loved one. But they need a little bit of time off once in a while where they could go someplace, take a drive for a weekend, maybe go to a movie.

I think one of the things we need to look into, and I would like comments from both of you, is some help for respite care. Once a month there would be a place that they could call and say, "I have been here 28 days. I would like a couple days off. Could you send somebody over to watch mom for the weekend?" Wouldn't a program like that be helpful?

Dr. BERNICK. Absolutely. There actually have been studies that show that the use of respite care will delay placement. So there is no question that is an effective management tool. Again, I think a lot of this has to do with funding, because that is not a benefit of Medicare, for people to utilize it in a useful manner. We are going to have to develop some programs and ways to fund it to allow these services to be used by the community that needs them.

Senator REID. Excuse me, Dr. Takamura. We know that some of the programs that would seem to be very simplistic in nature, to be a senior companion and some of those programs, have really been effective in delaying people going into an extended care facility. I think this would also be something we should jump on. Dr. Takamura.

Ms. TAKAMURA. I think your point is very well taken. The Interfaith Council is another group that has done a lot of work in bringing forward volunteers to help caregivers. I think there are many opportunities there. It is an excellent point.

Senator REID. I was in Carson City last week and went to a senior lunch program and participated in the lunch and walked around tables and said hello to people. One couple said to me, "Senator, you know, we have been paying for many years on an insurance policy that would provide protection for us if one of us had to go into a rest home." They said, "We checked and it pays $280 a month." They, in effect, have wasted their money. They might just as well have put that money someplace else.

Dr. Takamura, do we have programs underway to work with the insurance industry for private insurance to protect people in their golden years, if, in fact, one of them has to go into a rest home?

Ms. TAKAMURA. We have a health insurance counseling program which is funded by Federal monies, this is, of course, one resource. The entire aging network is very cognizant of the extent to which private long-term care insurance can and cannot be used. I think our network certainly is ready to work with our consumers on that particular issue.

Senator REID. Everyone, if you have a chance, if you cannot see it from here where you are, we have a chart up here that indicates who pays for nursing home care at the present time. Medicaid pays for more than half of it, and in that, people are indigent to qualify for Medicaid. Some people pay out of their own pocket, about a third. The Veteran's Administration pays for 4 percent. Private insurance pays for 2 percent. And, of course, Medicare 9 percent.

So we really have to—I think Congress really has to take a look at this to find out if it is going to be a burden of the Federal Government, State government, private sector, or combination of all because I do not think we have the luxury of just letting this ramble on as we have in recent years.

One thing I would like you to elaborate on, Dr. Takamura, is this Operation Restore Trust. Tell us what this is all about.

Ms. TAKAMURA. This is actually a wonderful program that was in demonstration for a while and will now be launched on a nationwide basis. It gives us the opportunity to combat fraud and abuse, particularly with respect to nursing home care, but also with respect to home health care. I think we have been able to identify quite a bit of money that we can save as a result.

So it is a very good consumer protection effort. It also makes us very aware of the extent to which we can do good work to assure quality of care.

Senator REID. One of the things we held a hearing on in Washington during the month of November was on fraud, waste, and abuse in the Medicare system. One of the things we learned there is that when home health care started, approximately ten years ago in America, 60 percent of every claim that was filed was reviewed. Today at most 2 percent.

So 98 percent or more of claims that are submitted for home health care are not reviewed by anybody. I think we have to take a close look at that, also. We want to make sure that Medicare and Medicaid does not become any more burdensome through paperwork than it is now, but I certainly think that we have to start reviewing more of these claims than just 2 percent of them.

Dr. Bernick, let me ask you another question or so. We are going to hold a hearing comparable to this in Reno tomorrow and we are going to have it simulcast into seven rural areas. You have talked briefly about the difficulty that people have in urban areas, and surprisingly, for people here in Nevada, we are the most urban State in America, Nevada is. Ninety percent of the people, Dr. Takamura, live in the metropolitan Reno and Las Vegas areas. Only about 10 percent live in rural Nevada, but rural Nevada covers vast areas.

Tell me, Dr. Bernick, if services are not perfect in urban Nevada, what must they be like in rural Nevada?

Dr. BERNICK. Senator, I would hate to even look. I think this is not true only for Nevada. I think this is probably true for a lot of the western states where things are spread out. I think it is a two-edged sword.

One of the advantages of rural areas is there usually is family around to help take care of people that may—family members that may have a chronic disease like Alzheimer's disease. On the other hand, they do not have programs such as adult day care and some of these other things that are available in urban areas.

Now, fortunately, here in our State, we have a very strong Division for Aging Services that has provided services to these rural areas, but still, there is a gap. There has to be a gap and I think that is one of the areas, for example, it is one of our interests to look at means or ways to deliver services, either through using televised means to provide information to providers there in these communities and workshops and other things. I think it is a real gap, again, in the services that we provide to the elderly.

Senator REID. Dr. Bernick, Dr. Takamura, thank you very much for your testimony here today. As they are leaving and the next panel of witnesses are coming forward, I would announce that the second panel will consist of Josephine George, who is a Las Vegas resident, and her daughter, Rose Marie George, whose mother is in need of nursing home placement, but is unable to find placement due to long waiting lists for Medicaid patients.

We will also hear from the Attorney General of the State of Nevada, Frankie Sue Del Papa; Carla Sloan, who has already been mentioned in the testimony, who is the Administrator for the Division of Aging Services, Department of Resources for the State of Nevada; and Rick Panelli, who is the Chief of the Bureau of Licensure and Certification in the Nevada State Health Division.

If I could have these four witnesses come forward, it would be appreciated. They are going to talk about patient safety and law enforcement in long-term care facilities; and they are going to talk about ombudsmen programs, patient advocates, the 1987 OBRA Act, licensing requirements, and other facets of facility regulation and oversight.

The perspectives offered here will be diverse, discussing patient rights from both personal and professional experiences. We will first hear from Josephine George, actually, and her daughter, Rose Marie. Rose Marie, would you please proceed?

STATEMENT OF JOSEPHINE GEORGE, LAS VEGAS RESIDENT, AND HER DAUGHTER, ROSE MARIE GEORGE

Ms. GEORGE. My name is Rose George and this is my mother, Josephine. We would like to thank the United States Senate Special Committee on Aging for the opportunity to testify at today's hearing.

My mother is 79 years old and has been living with rheumatoid arthritis for 20 years. I am the Development Coordinator for the Las Vegas branch of the Arthritis Foundation. Arthritis is the nation's most common chronic health problem and the number one cause of disability. My mother has one of the most severe forms of rheumatoid arthritis and although we are very appreciative of the support we have received, due to the length of mom's illness, we find that some of the benefits are just not enough and some of them are being taken away.

Additionally, we have found that when you are considered "middle class," you do not qualify for some of the needed benefits. Over the years, mom's arthritis and general health has deteriorated. She is in constant pain and has experienced loss of movement. To attempt to alleviate some of her pain, she has had joint replacements in her hands, both shoulders, both hips, and both knees. This has only been moderately successful and she is unable to have any more surgeries due to her current state of health.

For the past ten years, my mother has been unable to care for herself. She cannot cook, get out of bed, bathe or dress herself, or go to the bathroom. For a while, our family took on all these duties, but ten years ago when my mother reached the point of needing 24-hour care, we found it necessary to obtain live-in aides to care for her.

The cost for such care for ten years has been financially devastating to our family. My mother, brother, sister, and I have gone through our savings to cover these costs. Unfortunately, we are unable to obtain any assistance from Medicare, Medicaid, or my mom's insurance for the cost of these live-ins. We have had to sell our house, cars, cash in life insurance policies, sell furniture, et cetera, to come up with the money.

The cost for the live-in has been anywhere from $300 a week to $275 a day depending on how ill my mother is. Let me just address some of the experiences with the live-ins. A home health care agency is very expensive, about $175 a day or $50 for an hour for a live-in. Therefore, we have had to advertise in the newspaper or depend on referrals.

We have had some very bad experiences with some of the aides. Some have been abusive, both verbally and physically, and some have left mom to sit on the toilet for hours. Some have been alcoholics, stole money and jewelry, ran up phone bills, and one had a nervous breakdown and had to be committed to a mental institution while caring for my mother. One simply just left out the window one night. They do not stay very long and we have to scramble to find replacements.

Due to the level of care mom now needs, the problems with the live-ins and due to lack of funds, our family began pursuing long-term care options. First we looked into subsidized senior housing, but when you add the cost of the live-in to the rent, it was not feasible. Next we looked into assisted living centers. Some were $3,000 per month and the resident had to be able to take care of themselves.

Next we looked into group homes. The fee is usually about $1,800 a month and my mother's income just does not cover it. Then we learned that if she went in a group home, she would lose her Medicaid benefits and my mother's medical bills are so astronomical we could not afford to do that.

Also, group home facilities like to accept individuals who do not require as much care as my mother needs. But if we did find a nursing home, she would have to requalify for Medicaid, which is a lengthy process and the beds are only available a day or so, and then she cannot afford to lose her Medicaid benefits.

In the pursuit of other assistance, I've been informed that my mother makes too much money, $11 too much to qualify for certain programs. Next we checked into nursing homes. This is a very hard step to take as nobody wants to put their parent in a nursing home. Some were very undesirable, but some were nice, but when we stated that mom was on Medicaid, we were informed that there were only so many Medicaid beds available and that there was a two-year waiting list.

We recommend that when a nursing home puts you on a waiting list, they follow the order of the list. I contact these facilities every week to see if there are any beds and I am continually told no. I have been advised that due to the increase in the senior population, the beds are simply not there.

Also, I would just like to make the following recommendations due to our experiences. More Medicaid beds need to be available in long-term care facilities. Long-term care facilities need to abide by the order of the waiting list. We feel that you can balance the budget without cutting necessary Medicaid programs.

Provide funding for group homes and assisted living centers that are less costly than nursing homes. More beds, make beds available even if an individual is not in the hospital for three days. Live-in home care should be available to the disabled in their homes. The cost would be far less than a nursing home and their quality of life would improve.

Also, I would like to take this opportunity to say how thankful we are to the CHIPS program for all the assistance that they have given us. We would like to thank you for this opportunity and mom would like to just say a few words.

Mrs. GEORGE. Thank you and I hope everything turns out all right for my sake and everybody like me. Thank you. [Applause.]

[The prepared statement of Ms. George follows:]

December 23, 1997

Senator Harry Reid
Senator John Breaux
Senator Charles E. Grassley
United States Senate
Special Committee on Aging
Washington, DC 20510-5400

Dear Senators and Committee:

In March of 1996, I helped to coordinate "At the Table", a nationwide women's outreach effort by the White House Office for Women's Initiatives and Outreach with the Treasurer of the United States, the Honorable Mary Ellen Withrow. Our roundtable discussion group was held in Las Vegas and consisted of women from Las Vegas, wherein we discussed issues of importance, and our report was submitted to Betsy Myers, Deputy Assistant to the President & Director of the White House Office for Women's Initiatives and Outreach and President Clinton. It is now an honor to be able to participate in "The Many Faces of Long-Term Care: Today's Bitter Pill or Tomorrow's Cure?"

I have been advised that the purpose of this hearing is to examine long-term care and that it is your hope to identify the strengths and weaknesses of our current national policy on long-term care during this discussion and solicit possible solutions and recommendations for future improvements. My mother, Josephine George and I will be participants in Panel 2 - "Today's Perspective" of the hearing.

My mother is 79 years old and a person living with rheumatoid arthritis for 20 years. I am the Development Coordinator for the Las Vegas Branch of the Arthritis Foundation and I can state with certainty that arthritis is the nation's most common chronic health problem and the number one cause of disability. Nearly 40 million Americans have some form of arthritis. Close to seven million Americans are disabled by arthritis in its most severe form. My mother has one of the most severe forms of arthritis I have ever seen. Although we are very appreciate of the support we have received from the government, due to the length of Mom's illness, we have found that the benefits are just not enough and some of them are being rescinded. Additionally, we have found that when you are considered "middle class" you do not qualify for some of the needed benefits.

Before I address our concerns regarding long-term care, I feel it is important to give you some background on my mother's health history. She was diagnosed with rheumatoid arthritis 20 years ago. Over the years, her arthritis and general health has deteriorated. I have witnessed her regress from a cane to a walker to a wheelchair and bedridden at times. She is in constant pain and has experienced loss of movement due to the arthritis. To attempt to alleviate some of the pain she has had joint replacements in her hands, both shoulders, both hips and both knees. These surgeries were only moderately successful and some of the replacements need to be replaced and the arthritis continues to ravage her entire body. However, she is unable to have any more surgeries as the doctors inform us she may not survive due to her current state of health.

For the past ten years, my mother has been unable to take care of herself. She cannot cook, get out of bed, bath or dress herself, to go the bathroom, etc. For a while, our family took on all those duties. But when my mother reached the point of needing 24-hour care, we found it necessary to obtain live-in aides to care for her. The cost of such care for ten years has been financially devastating to our family. My mother, brother, sister and I have gone through our savings to cover these costs. Unfortunately, we are unable to obtain any assistance from Medicare, Medicaid or my mother's insurance to help with these costs.

We have had to sell our house, cars, cash in life insurance policies, sell furniture, etc. to come up with the money to pay for the live-in aides and other expenses. The cost just for the live-ins has been anywhere from $300 a week to $175 a day plus room and board depending on how ill my mother is, as some days she has required nursing care.

Let me just address some of our experiences with the live-ins. Going through a home health care agency is very expensive - about $175 a day or $50 a hour just for a live-in. Therefore, we have had to advertise in the newspaper or depend on referrals. We have had some bad experiences with some of the aides - some have turned out to be very mean to my mother, leaving her to sit on the toilet for hours, verbally and physically abusive. Some have been alcoholics, stole money and jewelry, ran up phone bills, one had a nervous breakdown and had to be committed to a mental health facility while caring for my mother, one simply left out the window one night and left my mother alone. I don't know if it's the nature of the job, but most do not stay very long and we have to scramble to find replacements.

Due to the fact that Mom is now needing more care than she can receive at home, the problems with the live-ins and due to lack of funds, our family began pursuing long-term care options. First we looked into subsidized senior housing but when you add the cost of live-ins to the rent, it was not feasible. Next we looked into assisted living facilities. Some were $3,000 per month and the resident had to be able to take care of themselves. This was not an option. Next we looked into group homes. The fee is usually $1,800 per month. My mother's income is $611 in Social Security benefits and $288 in P.E.R.S. (Public Employees Retirement System - my father's pension), for a total of $899 per month. Therefore, we would need to come up with $1,000 per month in addition to her income. Then we learned that if she went into a group home she would loose her Medicaid benefits. Her medical bills can be astronomical at times. Also, the group home facilities like to accept individuals who do not require as much care as my mother needs. Then, if we did find a nursing home, she would have to requalify for Medicaid which is a lengthy process and the beds are only available for a day or so. She cannot afford to loose her Medicaid benefits. In the pursuit of other assistance I have been informed that my mother makes too much money ($11 too much) to qualify for certain programs.

Our next step was to check into nursing homes or convalescent facilities. This is a very hard step to take as no one wants to put their parents in a nursing home. We looked at many. Some were very undesirable. Some were very nice but when we stated that Mom was on Medicaid we were informed that there were only so many Medicaid beds available and that there was a 2-year waiting list to get in. In one instance, we visited a particular facility and when we asked the admissions representative how the long the wait was she stated 2 months. The next day another admissions representative at the same facility stated it was 2 years.

It is my recommendation that when a nursing home puts you on a waiting list that they follow the order of the list. I have heard through the grapevine that these facilities accept admissions more on the dollar amount they will receive as opposed to what number you are on the list. Simply put, they pick and choose their admissions based on how much money they will make. In another instance, one home was ready to admit my mother in 3 days time. We made arrangements, and the day before she was to be admitted, they contacted us and said they had given her bed away. My feeling is they had someone who had needed a higher level of care than my mother and could make more money so they gave her bed away.

I contact these facilities every week to check to see if there are any beds and am continually told, **NO**. I have also been advised that due to the increase in the senior population in Nevada, the beds are simply not there. Additionally, I have been advised that if my Mom were a patient in the hospital for three (3) days we would have an easier time getting her into a nursing home. This is also very perplexing to me. I don't understand why that is the case. If there are no beds now, what will happen when I am a senior and may be in need of such care? Also, I understand that Congress and the Senate want to balance the deficit, but cutting $163 million from the Medicaid budget does not seem like the answer, especially to those who are dependent on the assistance.

Another concern to our family is that my mother has a Hickman tube in her chest. Several years ago, mother fell and broke both her legs and ribs. She went into the hospital and came home with leg casts up to her pelvis. She developed a bacterial infection while in the hospital and developed pneumonia, blood poising, dehydration and went into septic shock. It required her being hospitalized 8 times and she almost died those eight times. Due to the fact that she had no veins left for intravenous drugs it was necessary to insert a Hickman tube in her chest for the antibiotics and medications. The tube has to be flushed daily by a nurse. The doctor decided to leave the tube in as occasionally she needs to have blood tests and he was concerned that if the tube was removed she would not survive the operation, or she may get ill again and require the tube as she still has no available veins to access. Medicaid will no longer pay for the nurse. Therefore, she is having the tube removed at the end of this month with a local anesthetic even though they recommend general anesthesia.

My mother no longer receives "Ensure", a nutritional supplement, she may also loose her diapers and chux and now they want to take away her hospital bed which is about the only form of independence she has. If you would look at my mother, you would see that she really is in need and is not trying to cheat anyone. I have heard stories from some of the home health care agencies of some of their clients who are bedridden and the nurse only visits them once a day and the people must lay in their bed all day with only one meal and can't move or get their diaper changed until the nurse visits them the following day.

Our family has been very supportive, but we are burnt out and tapped out financially due to the length and seriousness of Mom's health problems. We are also very grateful to the State of Nevada Division for Aging Services for all their assistance but their hands are tied in a lot of these matters. The paperwork in obtaining some of these programs is unbelievable. My heart goes out to those seniors who have no family and are alone and attempt to complete the magnitude of paperwork.

Based on the above information, our recommendations would be as follows:

- More Medicaid beds need to be available at long-term care facilities;
- Long-term facilities need to abide by the order of the waiting list and be more concerned about the patient and not the money or who pays the money;
- Live-in home health care should be available to the disabled in their homes, the cost would be far less than a nursing and their quality of life would improve (the cost could be $1,000-$1,550 a month as opposed to $3,000-$4,000 in a nursing home);
- Balance the budget without cutting necessary Medicaid programs for those in need;
- Provide funding for group home facilities and assisted living centers that are less costly than nursing homes;
- Address fraud as opposed to cutting benefits to the disabled;
- More funding should be available on a state level to address these needs; and
- Make beds available even if a individual is not in the hospital for 3 days.
- The current system forces individuals and their families to deplete their assets and forces the disabled into nursing homes, this robs the disabled and their families of their self-esteem, but the nursing homes cannot accommodate them. Custodial care in the home would save money and the disabled would have a better quality of life.

In closing, we thank you for this opportunity. We hope this will help not only those with arthritis, but the six million Medicaid program recipients who are disabled and in need of long-term health care. Should you have any questions, I may be reached at 702-367-1626 at the Arthritis Foundation. I hope we can make a difference!

Very truly yours,

Rose M. George

Rose Marie George
6335 Annie Oakley Dr., #226
Las Vegas, NV 89120
702-456-5664 (Home)
702-367-1626 (Work)

Biography of
Rose Marie George

A native of Warren, Ohio, Rose Marie George is the Development Coordinator for the Las Vegas Branch of the Arthritis Foundation. Her duties include coordination of special events, fund-raisers and public relations. Arthritis Foundation events for 1998 include: Oscar Night America™, Professional Secretaries Day, 11th Annual Golf Classic, 12th Annual Bachelor Auction and the 18th Annual Turkey Trot™. She is the former Development Coordinator for AFAN (Aid for AIDS of Nevada) and prior to that was a model, talent and entertainment agent in Las Vegas for many years.

She is member and former board member of Women in Communications and active in the National Society of Fundraising Executives and the Las Vegas Chamber of Commerce.

Senator REID. We know how hard it was for you to come and talk about your mom and how hard for you Mrs. George to be here. We appreciate it very much. One of the things I would comment on, we are going to have some questions for you if you will just be patient. One of the things that we have to take a close look at is, the rules now are if you are in the hospital for three days, you can go to an extended care facility.

There are a lot of unusual things being done to make sure that people spend three days in the hospital before going into one of these rest homes. It is just a ping-ponging effect, and you can only stay in a rest home so long after being in a hospital three days. So a lot of times, they put you back in the hospital unnecessarily, run up costs, very inconvenient for everyone. This is something we really need to take a close look at. Attorney General Del Papa.

STATEMENT OF FRANKIE SUE DEL PAPA, ATTORNEY GENERAL, STATE OF NEVADA

Ms. DEL PAPA. Senator Reid and members of the committee, we all know here that Nevada has the fastest growing population of persons 65 years of age and older, and I would say in response to that that Nevada is still the Silver State because of the valuable silver-haired citizens who live here and who, in significant numbers, are continuing to choose to make Nevada their home.

Our office has the Medicaid Fraud Control Unit responsibility. We were the 40th state in the country. That was one of the big priorities when I was first elected seven years ago. In addition to going after medical providers, which obviously is a very important responsibility, particularly when you look at the economic pie of the money that is spent in the State of Nevada because we spend about 55 cents of every dollar on education.

We spend about 28 percent, approximately, on human resources and the big ticket item within that 28 percent category is, of course, Medicaid for providing medical services to those that are indigent. So our responsibility I take very seriously and it has been a really good unit for us.

In addition to the provider fraud that we attack, we also have primary jurisdiction to investigate and prosecute patient abuse, and that is both fiscal and physical patient abuse, primarily in long-term care facilities. Our Medicaid Fraud Control Unit has received almost a 50 percent increase in the number of complaints and referrals of patient abuse and neglect, for instance, in the last year.

Over the last two years, the Medicaid Fraud Unit has reviewed over 130 complaints and referrals and opened over 20 criminal investigations. These numbers may reflect the need to address the serious problem of patient abuse and neglect in our state, but I think also that these numbers reflect the increased reporting of abuse cases thanks to an ongoing public education effort and awareness efforts that we have participated in, along with others who sit at this table with me and many who are in the audience today.

In the fall of 1995, the Attorney General's Office, in conjunction with the Department of Human Resources and county social service agencies formed a long-term care task force to help meet the needs of a rapidly growing senior population.

That task force produced this particular document called "Long-Term Care, Choices for Seniors." This document addressed the following: the need to develop choices among a range of service options many of which she has just referred to here which are more responsive to our seniors' needs.

Responsibility to assure the availability of these choices and settings for quality of care can be assured, and the commitment to educate all factions of the community regarding elder abuse, neglect, and exploitation. To help in this commitment, what we have done is a simple little guide to long-term care. It is a pamphlet that includes tips on how to choose long-term care facilities, information on the rights of residents, and information on alternatives to nursing home care.

In order to better meet the growing need, long-term need of senior Nevadans who require varying degrees of assistance and medical attention, the State and Federal Government, I think, need to explore the possibility of extending the Medicaid/Medicare funds to assist seniors who could live in less restrictive settings than skilled nursing facilities.

Additionally, I think it is really critical—and this is something, Senator, that I would really urge and I know you are interested in it because your staff has contacted me in the past in this regard. The jurisdiction of the Medicaid Fraud Control Units in this country needs to be expanded.

The National Association of Attorneys General has asked for flexibility, in some cases relaxation of the rules in order to better coordinate with other law enforcement agencies. As more and more seniors come to Nevada to make their home, I think it is important to provide strong systems for their safety.

In the fall of 1996, we joined forces with Betsy Kolkoski, the elder rights attorney from the Division for Aging Services, to come up with a more comprehensive plan to address the issue of elder abuse. That task force is viable. Elder abuse is a crime. It is something that we take very seriously in our state.

We had some good luck at this last legislative session as far as making intentional and unjustified isolation of the elderly a crime. We have created double damages and authorized recovery of attorney's fees in civil litigation involving elder abuse, neglect, and exploitation.

There are other bills obviously that passed. We have had good luck with a guide for mandated reporters. This is something that literally we are making thousands of copies of and every document that we have we tell everyone to please plagiarize it and put it as far and wide a distribution as possible.

This is obviously a very serious subject. We have developed protocols to better coordinate law enforcement's response in this regard. We have also done the "RX for Abuse", which is a patient abuse video. There are many other things that we have tried to do. I know that you will hear from others and I see that my time is up and so I will yield the floor there and be happy to answer any questions.

Senator REID. I do have some questions for you at the right time, General Del Papa.

[The prepared statement of Ms. Del Papa follows:]

STATE OF NEVADA
OFFICE OF THE ATTORNEY GENERAL
100 N. Carson Street
Carson City, Nevada 89701-4717
Telephone (702) 687-4170
Fax (702) 687-5798

FRANKIE SUE DEL PAPA
Attorney General

BROOKE A. NIELSEN
Assistant Attorney General

TESTIMONY OF ATTORNEY GENERAL FRANKIE SUE DEL PAPA BEFORE THE SENATE SPECIAL COMMITTEE ON AGING FIELD HEARINGS HELD JANUARY 12 AND 13, 1998.

Thank you for the opportunity to address this important issue, one that is critical to Nevada. Our state was originally nicknamed "The Silver State" because of the valuable silver ore buried deep beneath the Nevada soil. Today, with the fastest growing population of persons 65 years of age and over, Nevada is still the "The Silver State" because of the valuable silver haired citizens who live here and who, in significant numbers, are continuing to choose to move here and make Nevada their home their home and to live through their twilight years by enjoying the multiple forms of recreation and relaxation our state offers.

In Nevada, the Medicaid Fraud Control Unit of the Attorney General's Office has primary jurisdiction to investigate and prosecute patient abuse cases in long term care facilities. Our MFCU has received almost a 50% increase in the number of complaints/referrals of patient abuse and neglect in the last year. Over the last two years, the MFCU has reviewed over 130 complaints/referrals and opened over twenty criminal investigations. On the one hand, these numbers may reflect the need to address the serious problem of patient abuse and neglect in our state. But on the other hand, these numbers may also reflect increased reporting of abuse cases thanks to ongoing public education and awareness efforts.

In the fall of 1995, the Attorney General's Office in conjunction with the Department of Human Resources and County Social Services Agencies formed a Long Term Care Task Force to help meet the needs of a rapidly growing senior population. That task force produced the report "Choices for Seniors," a copy of which has been provided to you. This report addressed the following:

- The need to develop choices among a range of service options which are responsive to senior's needs.
- The responsibility to assure the availability of these choices in settings where quality of care can be assured.
- The commitment to educate all factions of the community regarding elder abuse, neglect and exploitation.

To help in this commitment, the Attorney General's Office published "A Practical Guide to Long Term Care," a pamphlet containing tips on how to choose a Long Term Care Facility, information on the rights of residents and information on Alternatives to Nursing Home care.

In order to better meet the growing long term care needs of senior Nevadans who require varying degrees of assistance and medical attention, the state and federal governments need to explore the possibility of extending Medicaid/Medicare funds to assist seniors who could live in less restrictive settings than skilled nursing facilities. Additionally, it is critical that the jurisdiction of the Medicaid Fraud Control Units be similarly expanded. In fact, the National Association of Attorneys General has asked for flexibility, or some relaxation of the rules, in order to better coordinate with other law enforcement agencies.

As more and more seniors make Nevada their home, it is important to provide strong systems for their safety and well being whether or not they reside in a long term care facility. In the fall of 1996, my office joined forces with Betsy Kolkoski, the Elder Rights Attorney from the Division for Aging Services to come up with a more comprehensive plan to address the growing problem of elder abuse, neglect and exploitation. We met with, among others, senior advocates from both private and public sectors, and used their input to publish "An Action Plan to Better Protect Nevada's Elderly." A copy of that plan has also been provided to you. Committees were formed to implement the goals of the Action Plan which was made public in March of 1997. Since then, much has been accomplished on behalf of our state's elderly population:

- Passage of legislation proposed in the Action Plan including:

AB 242 which made Nevada one of the first states to recognize the intentional and unjustified isolation of the elderly as a serious crime;

SB 80 which created double damages and authorized recovery of attorneys fees in civil litigation involving elder abuse, neglect, exploitation and isolation.

AB 9, Assemblyman Mark Manendo's bill to increase the minimum penalty for criminal elder abuse was amended to add funeral home employees as mandatory elder abuse reporters and to authorize an elder abuse reporting hotline.

AB 155, which was proposed by Assemblywoman Vivian Freeman and Assemblyman Jack Close was strongly supported by participants in the Action Plan. This bill requires the fingerprinting and mandatory criminal background checks for long term care employees.

In addition to the legislation I have just mention, implementation of the goals of the Action Plan has led to:

- The publication of the "Guide for Mandated Reporters of Elder Abuse." This guide is a resource for all persons concerned about the elderly and explains the role and responsibility of state and local agencies who respond to reports of elder abuse, neglect and intimidation. You have all been provided with a copy of the guide which should also help you better understand the roles of various state and local agencies involving cases of Elder Abuse.

- Development of Protocols to help law enforcement and protective services agencies better coordinate and communicate their response to, and investigation of, reports of Elder Abuse. Last week, these Protocols were signed by representatives from eleven different state and local agencies with varying responsibilities to respond to reports of Elder Abuse. A copy of those Protocols has been provided to you.

- Statewide distribution of the video "Rx for Abuse," which was produced by the Division For Aging Services to provide health care professionals with information on how to detect and report cases of elder abuse. The video stars Shirley Jones and Marty Ingles.

- Public Service Announcements to encourage better reporting of Elder Abuse which aired both in the north and the south.

- Guardianship survey, in which providers and advocates statewide were surveyed regarding the need for guardianship.

- Obtained funding for additional Elder Abuse videos and materials to provide education to law enforcement officers throughout the state.

- Creation of an Elder Abuse reporting Hotline in Northern Nevada.

In conclusion, I would like to applaud Senators Reid, Kohl and Grassley who are co-sponsoring the Patient Abuse Prevention Act and encourage Congress to pursue the establishment of a national registry identifying persons who have been convicted of patient abuse, neglect and other related crimes.

Finally, we must support every local, state and national effort to educate the public about long term care alternatives, how and where to report abuse and neglect and what resources already exist for relatives and friends of family and other loved ones who will be or who are already receiving long term care. Thank you.

Senator REID. We will now hear from Carla Sloan.

STATEMENT OF CARLA SLOAN, ADMINISTRATOR, DIVISION FOR AGING SERVICES, DEPARTMENT OF HUMAN RESOURCES

Ms. SLOAN. Thank you, Senator Reid. I am honored to participate on this panel to present Nevada's long-term care ombudsman program for patient advocacy. The position of ombudsman was originally created by the Swedish government in 1809. This government official was given independence, power, and prestige for the impartial hearing and resolution of citizen complaints.

It was not until after World War II that the idea of an ombudsman position grew throughout the rest of the world. This was tied to a growing popular feeling that there was an increasing distance between government and citizens.

Media attention in the 1960s about accounts of abuse in nursing homes brought attention to the need for advocates for institutionalized seniors in the United States. In 1978, amendments to the Older Americans Act required each state to establish an ombudsman program. Long-term care ombudsmen take on a variety of roles at different levels.

Under the direction of the resident, ombudsmen act on their concerns and violation of their rights. In addition to resolving individual problems, the work of the ombudsmen lay the foundation for systemic change within the long-term care system. Aggressive enforcement of government regulation of the industry is essential for the protection of residents.

We applaud the commitment and commend the work that the Nevada Health Division does on a daily basis to ensure regulatory compliance of the long-term care industry. Aging Services collaborates with the Health Division and provides feedback on a regular basis to the survey process. The divisions frequently conduct joint investigations.

During the last three years, we have seen a 3 percent increase in the number of complaints in nursing homes. Seventy-three percent of the complaints received come from facility staff. As the number of nursing facilities has not increased, this high level of self-reporting shows a cooperative effort by the industry to coordinate complaint investigation and resolution.

Residential facilities for groups are rapidly growing in Nevada to meet the ever-increasing demand for long-term care alternatives. Inappropriate level of care complaints have increased by 22 percent during the last three years. Since this segment of the industry is relatively new, self-reporting of incidents and complaints has not reached the same level as in nursing homes. There is much education to be done with this part of the continuum of care.

Fifty-five percent of the complaints investigated by Nevada ombudsmen were substantiated during the past year. The major complaint categories were care plan and assessment; staff supervision; accidents and improper handling; abuse, neglect, and exploitation; dignity, respect, and staff attitudes.

Our program is one of the few nationally that investigates complaints of abuse, neglect, and exploitation, and in a 1995 survey of ombudsmen programs by the Administration on Aging, Nevada was responsible for investigating 13 percent of abuse and neglect complaints reported nationally.

The ombudsman program's focus on expanding community presence into nursing homes and other residential care settings has become the most effective vehicle for combating the abuse and neglect of residents, and promoting quality of care and quality of life. The program is unlike any other. Its sole purpose is supporting and protecting the resident.

The State of Nevada, through Governor Bob Miller and the legislature, have been very supportive of this critical program. A Federal Older Americans Act grant funds 38 percent of our program. State funding of 62 percent of the program expense allows the division to provide professional service to the most vulnerable of our elderly population.

Nevada's sincere commitment to elders and long-term care is evident by its continual support of the ombudsman program. Nevada is also committed to volunteerism. Governor Miller and the 1997 legislature approved a new state annual appropriation of nearly $250,000 for senior volunteer programs.

The retired senior volunteer programs in southern and northern Nevada have agreed to provide the volunteer management for a pilot program called the Silver Stripers. The Silver Striper program seeks to enhance the quality of life of residents in long-term care facilities by providing them with an opportunity to experience friendship and support from trained older volunteers.

While volunteer initiatives such as the Silver Striper program are essential to enriching the lives of elders, as the patient advocacy demands of the senior population increase, we will see continued and increased support from the Administration on Aging, the Congress, the state legislature, and from local community partners to preserve and expand ombudsmen services.

Thank you for this opportunity to speak on behalf of the elders served by the Nevada Department of Human Resources, Division for Aging Services. As the state with the fastest growing 65 and older population, we are pleased to offer our experience to the Senate Special Committee on Aging's effort to identify the strengths and weaknesses of national policy on long-term care. We pledge our continued partnership in seeking solutions and recommendations for future improvements.

[The prepared statement of Ms. Sloan follows:]

UNITED STATES SENATE
SPECIAL COMMITTEE ON AGING
FIELD HEARINGS
JANUARY 12 AND 13, 1998

"THE MANY FACES OF LONG-TERM CARE: TODAY'S BITTER PILL OR TOMORROW'S CURE?"

PANEL 2
TODAY'S PERSPECTIVE
NEVADA'S LONG TERM CARE OMBUDSMAN PROGRAM
FOR PATIENT ADVOCACY

PRESENTED BY:
CARLA SLOAN, ADMINISTRATOR
NEVADA DIVISION FOR AGING SERVICES
340 N. 11TH STREET, SUITE 203
LAS VEGAS, NEVADA 89101
PHONE (702) 486-3545
FAX (702) 486-3572

The Many Faces of Long Term Care: Today's Bitter Pill or Tomorrow's Cure?

Panel 2 - Today's Perspective
Nevada's Long Term Care Ombudsman Program for Patient Advocacy

Carla Sloan, Administrator
Nevada Division for Aging Services
Department of Human Resources

Introduction

The position of ombudsman was originally created by the Swedish government in 1809. This government official was given independence, power, and prestige for the impartial hearing and resolution of complaints by citizens. The classical definition of an ombudsman is described as a neutral third party who investigates and makes reports regarding grievances.

A broad conceptualization of an ombudsman is a "citizen defender" who advocates between citizens and the authority, with the power to personalize bureaucratic red tape, to increase government responsiveness, to implement a complaint resolution system, and to recognize appropriate services for citizens.

It was not until after World War II that the idea of an ombudsman position spread throughout the rest of the world. This has been tied to the growing popular feeling that there was an increasing distance between government administration and citizens and their needs.

Media attention in the 1960s about accounts of abuse in nursing homes brought attention to the need for advocates for institutionalized seniors in the United States.

The Office of the Long-Term Care Ombudsman was federally mandated in 1971. President Nixon proposed initiatives in 1975 creating ombudsman units whose focus would be on individual residents, thus compensating for the limitations of quality assurance and regulation. In 1978, amendments to the Older Americans Act required each state to establish an ombudsman program. In 1981, decisions by Congress added board and care facilities to the ombudsman federal mandate. Although this legislation did not change the qualities of the ombudsman program, it greatly increased the population that required ombudsman services.

The scope of the ombudsman program's responsibilities and authority are described in Title VII, Chapter 2 of the Older Americans Act. The programs are directed at responding to needs of institutionalized seniors by:

1) Investigating and resolving complaints made by or on behalf of residents of long term care facilities;

2) Establishing procedures for ombudsman access to facilities and patients' records;

3) Creating a statewide reporting system to collect and analyze data relating to complaints;

4) Mandating procedures to assure client confidentiality;

5) Providing information to public agencies regarding the problems of long term care facilities' residents; and

6) Other responsibilities include educating the public, training staff and volunteers, and helping to develop resident and family councils in facilities.

Ombudsmen take on a variety of roles at different levels. Two levels of advocacy include resident-level and systems-level. On a systems-level, ombudsmen attempt to solve broader or underlying causes of problems by advocating for policy change. This is done by evaluating laws and regulations, educating public and facility staff, analyzing program data, and promoting resident and family councils. On a resident-level, the ombudsmen's responsibilities include working cooperatively with outside agencies and providing assistance and training to facility staff. It is important that ombudsmen ensure residents have timely access to the ombudsman program and resolution to complaints.

In pursuit of these activities, the ombudsman must maintain relationships involving tension between the individual and the system. On the one hand, the ombudsman must be critical of the facilities and other agencies they review, and then be able to work cooperatively with the same agencies to ensure that residents receive proper services and protection of rights. This can be difficult considering that ombudsmen have the ability to affect administrators and staff and to induce change within the long term care system.

Whatever power the ombudsman has, whether real or perceived, adds to the tension of the ombudsman relationship. The long term care ombudsman's powers range from conciliatory to coercive action, including education, coordination with other agencies, win/win negotiations, pursuing the involvement of regulatory agencies, administrative and civil, or criminal, legal actions, or public disclosure activities such as using the media.

Impact of 1987 OBRA

The Division for Aging Services supports a strong survey and enforcement process that assures that each resident receives the care and services that he or she needs to achieve the highest attainable level of well-being. Because of the Nevada Division of Health's survey process, we feel the long term care industry in Nevada has improved and continues to provide a commitment to quality of care and quality of life.

We applaud the commitment and commend the work that the Health Division does on a daily basis to ensure that residents of long term care facilities receive quality of care and quality of life. The Division for Aging Services collaborates with the Health Division and has given feedback on a regular basis to the survey process. The Health Division has been responsive to all Aging Services referrals, and on many occasions the divisions have conducted joint investigations.

Ombudsman Program Data

During the last three years in Nevada, we have seen a 3% increase in the number of complaints in long term care facilities. 73% of the complaints received come from facility staff and administration. Based on the fact that the number of nursing facilities has not increased in the past three years, this high level of self-reporting shows a cooperative effort by the industry to coordinate complaint investigation and resolution.

Residential facilities for groups are rapidly growing in Nevada to meet the ever increasing demand for long term care alternatives. Inappropriate level of care complaints have increased by 22% in the last three years. Since this segment of the industry is relatively new, the self-reporting of incidents and complaints has not reached the same level as in nursing homes. There is much education to be done with this part of the continuum of care.

55% percent of the complaints investigated by the ombudsman were substantiated during the past year. The major complaint categories during this past year were:

1) care plan and assessment,
2) staff supervision,
3) accidents and improper handling,
4) abuse, neglect, and exploitation, and
5) dignity and respect, staff attitudes.

The ombudsman program in Nevada is one of the few nationally that does investigate complaints of abuse, neglect and exploitation. In a 1995 survey of ombudsmen programs by the Administration on Aging, Nevada was responsible for investigating 13% of abuse, neglect complaints reported nationally to ombudsman programs.

Recommendations for the Future of Quality Care

The Long Term Care Ombudsman Program's focus on expanding community presence into nursing homes and other residential care settings has become the most effective vehicle for combating the abuse and neglect of residents and promoting quality of care and quality of life. The program is unlike any other - its sole purpose is supporting and protecting the resident.

Ombudsmen provide a regular presence in long term care facilities. In doing so, they become familiar with the facility, the management, employees, residents, visitors and families. By regularly speaking with residents throughout the year, the Ombudsmen form a strong rapport with them, enabling the residents to develop skills that will allow them to have their viewpoint heard and respected and their needs met in a constructive and proactive manner.

Under the direction of the resident, Ombudsmen act on their concerns and any violations of the their rights. In addition to resolving individual problems, the work of the ombudsmen lays the foundation for systemic change within the long term care system.

The State of Nevada through Governor Bob Miller and the Legislature have been very supportive of the Ombudsman program. Title VI of the Federal Older Americans Act grant funds 38% of Nevada's Long Term Care Ombudsman Program. State funding of 62% of the Ombudsman Program expense allows the Division for Aging Services to provide professional service to the most vulnerable of our elderly population. Nevada's sincere commitment to patient safety, quality of care, and quality of life for elders in long term care residence is evident by its continual support of the Long Term Care Ombudsman Program.

As the patient advocacy demands of the senior population increase, the Division for Aging Services will seek continued and increased support from the U.S. Administration on Aging, the U.S. Congress, the State Legislature, and local community partners to preserve and expand ombudsman services.

Thank you for this opportunity to speak on behalf of the elders served by the Nevada Department of Human Resources Division for Aging Services. As the state with the fastest growing 65 and older population, we are pleased to offer our experience to the Senate Special Committee on Aging's effort to identify the strengths and weaknesses of national policy on long-term care. We pledge our continued partnership in seeking solutions and recommendations for future improvements.

Presented to the
United States Senate
Special Committee on Aging
Nevada Field Hearings
January 12 and 13, 1998

Senator REID. We will now hear from Rick Panelli who, as I have indicated, is the Chief of the Bureau of Licensure and Certification, Health Division, Department of Human Resources, State of Nevada. Mr. Panelli.

STATEMENT OF RICK PANELLI, CHIEF, BUREAU OF LICENSURE AND CERTIFICATION, NEVADA STATE HEALTH DIVISION

Mr. PANELLI. Senator Reid, thank you for this opportunity to be here today. The Bureau of Licensure and Certification is the regulatory agency that is responsible for certification and survey of all health care facilities in the State of Nevada and facilities for care of the dependent.

We would like to emphasize what Senator Reid has already brought forward today and that is that Nevada has a real crisis in terms of the number of facilities that are available, the number of beds that are available in long-term care. That includes homes for residential and group care facilities, skilled nursing facilities.

In 1991, we had 34 long-term care or skilled nursing facilities; in 1997, we have only 45. The number of individuals who are waiting to try and get into these facilities is increasing faster than the number of beds that are being provided. Over the next two to three years, we only anticipate or we have only been told to anticipate about 1,500 to 1,600 new beds coming on line in the State of Nevada.

The Bureau of Licensure and Certification annually conducts a survey or inspection of each long-term care facility in the state. The focus of these surveys are quality of life, quality of care, and residential behavior and facility practices. These are very large groups of areas that we look at.

I think the quality of life and quality of care are two of the main issues. When we find deficiencies in the facilities, the bureau and the Health Division encourages facilities to get into compliance by requesting that they submit a plan of correction for the deficiencies that are found.

In most cases, the bureau will partner with the facility to try and help them understand where their shortcomings are and then allow them to come back with a plan that would allow them to come into compliance and provide better care.

There are sanctions and remedies that are available. The sanctions extend all the way from a monetary penalty, which could be substantial, to a ban on admissions which the State of Nevada has, but the Federal Government does not have in place. We feel that that is a very substantial sanction because what it does is if a facility cannot take care of the people that it has in it, then we believe that they should not be admitting additional people until they get a handle on their ability to care for them.

We take care of, in this state, the 43 or 45 now long-term care facilities that are considered skilled nursing facilities. There are two main things that these facilities are cited or reported as. One is substantial compliance with regulations; the other one is called substandard quality of care.

The substantial compliance piece is probably not as good an indicator of what is going on in a facility as is the substandard quality of care. This one looks at actual outcome pieces, where the substantial compliance piece is looking more at what indicators might come and show us things in the future. So sometimes a facility might not be in substantial compliance, but still has a pretty good facility overall.

Nationwide, 75 percent of the facilities that are inspected the first time around are not in substantial compliance. In Nevada, we had no facilities that were in substantial compliance the very first time around. However, out of the 45 facilities over a two-year period, we only had 13 that were found to be in a substandard quality of care situation and that number has reduced now, through education and working with the industry, down to only five.

I think the negative issues with the present system would include the fact that it may produce a negative reaction to long-term care. It makes it difficult for individuals to choose what type of facility to go into because they may be looking at deficiencies that are not of substantial nature, and there is an increase in cost to the public for follow-up surveys.

The positive is that it helps to eliminate the catch-and-fix situation. If you have facilities out of compliance, back into compliance. Every time you catch them, they fix their problems. They are in for a while and then they are back out.

I think that in the future, we need to look at new regulations which will provide for allowing a continuum of care to go all the way from the group care setting last much longer before we get into a formal skilled nursing facility and allow people to stay there with heavier levels of care, providing more education and more training to the individuals who take care of those people.

Our largest increase in facilities is in what we call registered homes. These are homes, private homes that care for two or fewer people, and that industry is booming, but it is, at this time, unregulated and there is very little oversight.

I would like to thank you very much again for inviting me here and I will be glad to answer questions.

[The prepared statement of Mr. Panelli follows:]

UNITED STATES SENATE
SENATE SPECIAL COMMITTEE ON AGING
Field Hearings – January 12-13, 1998

Richard J. Panelli, Chief
Bureau of Licensure and Certification
Health Division
Department of Human Resources
State of Nevada

Bureau of Licensure and Certification (BLC) is responsible for statewide inspection surveys of Medical and Dependent Care Facilities for compliance with Federal certification regulations for Medicare and Medicaid and Nevada state licensure regulations

Code of Federal Regulations (42 CFR)
Nevada Revised Statutes Chapters (NRS 449)

1997	700 facilities	321	Homes for Individual Residential Care
		265	Residential Facilities for Groups
		45	Skilled Nursing Facilities/Nursing Facilities (SNF/NF)
1991	222 facilities	0	Homes for Individual Residential Care
		188	Residential Facilities for Groups
		34	SNF/NF
1997	pending facilities	29	Residential Facilities for Groups
		6	SNF/NF

BLC conducts annual on-site surveys of all health and care facilities to determine compliance with regulations

Annual on-site surveys focus on:

- Quality of Care
- Quality of Life
- Residential Behavior/Facility Practices

- Health Division encourages facility compliance through requiring a Plan of Correction (POC) for each deficiency found

Sanctions and Remedies:

- Directed POC
- Directed In-Service Training

47-539 98 - 3

- State Monitoring
- Monetary Fines (CMPs)
- Ban on Admissions
- Seriousness, frequency, pervasive nature
- Revoke, deny, suspend license, terminate Medicare/Medicaid reimbursement

The regulatory system not only establishes minimum standards for provision of Health Care it also:

- Educates providers
- Protects recipients - who are among our most vulnerable citizens.

<u>**43 SNFs / 2 NFs**</u>

Survey Activity July 1995 through October 1997

- No facility in substantial compliance on annual survey (75% the National Average).
- 13 facilities providing Substandard Quality of Care (5 in FY97).

"Substantial Compliance" - is not a good indicator of:

- Quality of Care
- Quality of Life
- Resident Behavior/Facility Practices

WHY?

- "Potential" for poor outcome
- 1 resident / pattern is not necessary

"Substandard Quality of Care" - is a good indicator of:

- Quality of Care
- Quality of Life
- Resident Behavior/Facility Practices

WHY?

- Actual harm or poor outcome has occurs
- Pattern/wide spread
- Major system failures

Negative Issues:

- Produces negative reaction to Long Term Care (LTC) industry as a whole
- Makes it more difficult for consumers to differentiate based on survey findings
- Increases costs – Follow-up survey process

Positive Issues:

- Helps to eliminate "catch and fix" compliance (only 2 repeat Substandard Quality of Care)
- Scope and Severity
- Remedies/Sanctions – CMP / Ban on Admissions

291 Residential Facilities for Groups
39 Residential Facilities for Alzheimer's and related Dementia

- 3 beds to 125+ beds
- 1 care level step above retirement/independent living
- Similar to "Assisted Living":

  Provide very "home-like" living conditions – many 6-bed facilities

  Limited Supervision

- New regulations:

  Allow for continuum of care where individuals remain in the same facility until they require daily skilled nursing

  Home Health may be utilized to meet care needs

  Less costly than a SNF/NF

359 Homes for Individual Residential Care:

2 or fewer residents

Complaint investigations is the only state oversight

Changes Resulting from the Regulation

- ❑ Eliminates the distinction between Level A and Level B participation requirements.
- ❑ Makes available to HCFA the full range of OBRA enforcement remedies. *§488.406*
- ❑ Codifies informal dispute resolution process (with no delay in enforcement) *§488.331*
- ❑ Offers one hearing — under either Federal or State procedures. *§488.330(e)*
- ❑ Classifies seriousness of deficiencies for the purpose of imposing a remedy through the use of scope and severity. *§488.408*
- ❑ Establishes and defines "substantial compliance" *§488.301*
- ❑ Defines "substandard quality of care" *§488.301*
- ❑ Establishes two civil money penalty ranges *§488.438*
- ❑ Explains "repeat deficiencies" for purposes of increasing a civil money penalty when deficiencies are found on a subsequent standard survey. *§488.438(d)*
- ❑ Establishes "tie breaker" rules which apply when there are disagreements between HCFA and the State about compliance, choice of remedies or timing of remedies. *§488.452*

Unchanged from Current Practice (Already Implemented)

- ❑ Survey frequency - no greater than 15 months between standard surveys and States cannot exceed a Statewide 12 month average. *§488.308*
- ❑ Unannounced surveys *§488.307*
- ❑ Mandatory imposition of Denial of Payment for New Admissions after three months of noncompliance. *§488.417(b)*

Background

- ❑ The Survey, Certification and Enforcement of SNFs and NFs was published as a Notice of Proposed Rulemaking (NPRM) in August 1992.
- ❑ HCFA received nearly 28,000 public comments in response to the NPRM.
- ❑ The final rule was published on November 10, 1994.
- ❑ This regulation becomes effective on July 1, 1995.

Health Care Financing Administration
Health Standards and Quality Bureau
Office of Survey & Certification
Division of Program Operations

6325 Security Boulevard, ME 2-D-2
Baltimore, Maryland 21207

A94-2355 f

SURVEY, CERTIFICATION AND ENFORCEMENT OF SKILLED NURSING FACILITIES AND NURSING FACILITIES

(HSQ-156-F)

POCKET REFERENCE GUIDE

Available Remedies

- ☐ Temporary Management *§488.415*
- ☐ Civil Money Penalties (CMPs) *§488.430 - 488.444*
- ☐ Denial of Payment for New Admissions *§488.417*
- ☐ Secretarial authority to deny all payments *§488.418*
- ☐ State Monitoring *§488.422*
- ☐ Directed Plan of Correction *§488.424*
- ☐ Directed In-service Training *§488.425*
- ☐ Closure of a facility or transfer of residents, or both *§488.426*
- ☐ Termination of Provider Agreement *§488.456*

Notice/Disclosure Requirements

Disclosure:

- ☐ Survey information may be disclosed to the public 14 calendar days after such information is made available to the facility. *§488.325 (a)*
- ☐ The State MUST disclose certain information to the State's long-term care ombudsman. *§488.325(f)*
- ☐ Substandard quality of care - The State must notify the State board for licensing nursing home administrators and the attending physician of residents. *§488.325(h)*

Notice:

- ☐ 15 days — non-immediate jeopardy for all remedies, except CMPs. *§488.402(f)*
- ☐ 2 days — immediate jeopardy for all remedies, except CMPs. *§488.402(f)*

	Isolated	Pattern	Widespread
Immediate Jeopardy to Resident Health or Safety	PoC Required: Cat. 3 Optional: Cat. 1 Optional: Cat. 2	PoC Required: Cat. 3 Optional: Cat. 1 Optional: Cat. 2	PoC Required: Cat. 3 Optional: Cat. 2 Optional: Cat. 1
Actual Harm that is not Immediate Jeopardy	PoC Required* Cat. 2 Optional: Cat. 1	PoC Required* Cat. 2 Optional: Cat. 1	PoC Required* Cat. 2 Optional: Cat. 1 Optional: Temporary Mgmt.
No Actual Harm with Potential for More than Minimal Harm that is not Immediate Jeopardy	PoC Required* Cat. 1 Optional: Cat. 2	PoC Required* Cat. 1 Optional: Cat. 2	PoC Required* Cat. 2 Optional: Cat. 1
No Actual Harm with Potential for Minimal Harm	No Remedies Commitment to Correct Not on HCFA-2567	PoC	PoC

Substandard quality of care: any deficiency in §483.13 Resident Behavior and Facility Practices, §483.15 Quality of Life, or in §483.25, Quality of Care that constitutes: immediate jeopardy to resident health or safety; or, a pattern of or widespread actual harm that is not immediate jeopardy; or, a widespread potential for more than minimal harm that is not immediate jeopardy, with no actual harm.

Substantial compliance

Remedy Categories

Category 1 (Cat. 1)	Category 2 (Cat. 2)	Category 3 (Cat. 3)
Directed Plan of Correction State Monitor; and/or Directed In-service Training	Denial of Payment for New Admissions; Denial of Payment for All Individuals, Imposed by HCFA; and/or Civil Money Penalties: $50 - $3,000 per day	Temporary Management Termination Optional: Civil Money Penalties: $3,050 - $10,000 per day

DENIAL OF PAYMENT FOR NEW ADMISSIONS **must be imposed when a facility is not in substantial compliance within three months after being found out of compliance.**

DENIAL OF PAYMENT AND STATE MONITORING **must be imposed when a facility has been found to have provided substandard quality of care on three consecutive standard surveys.**

Note: Termination may be imposed by the State or HCFA at any time when appropriate.

**** Required only when decision is made to impose alternate remedies instead of or in addition to termination.***

Senator REID. First of all, I would say to the Georges, again, appreciate very much your testimony. It certainly did not pass our ears here at this table, that in effect, you have given up most everything you have in an effort to help your mom. That happens often, but I think, and I will direct this question to Ms. Sloan, what about all the people that do not have a loving, caring daughter like Rose George? What happens to them?

Ms. SLOAN. The need for an advocate in dealing with the health care system throughout the continuum, I think, is critical. The ombudsman program assists families in the selection of community resources, helping them to understand how to access resources. Here in Nevada, we are very fortunate that our legislature has also funded a community ombudsman program.

Our community ombudsmen are available to assist families and individuals who are living in the community rather than those who may be institutionalized that are served by the long-term care ombudsmen program to access community resources.

There are also volunteer programs that will help to assist folks with respite services. You talked about that earlier. Our Catholic Charities program has an excellent respite program. Adult day care programs here in Nevada also offer respite services. As Dr. Bernick indicated, the need for payment for those services is critical.

But the need for an advocate navigating this system, you are right, there is a need for that.

Senator REID. We can talk about all these programs in Nevada. We are fortunate, we do have a number of these programs. We are fortunate that we have someone like you and the Attorney General caring about these programs.

But the fact of the matter is, we have here an intelligent, articulate woman who is trying to help her mother and she cannot get her into a facility. What do we do about that?

Ms. SLOAN. I think we continue to work together. It is my understanding that the family also has a preference for the facility in which Josephine would like to stay. She was offered a placement that the family refused. So we do need to continue to work together.

Senator REID. I would say that one of the things, and I direct this to Mr. Panelli. One of the things being done in Washington, the President has suggested legislation regarding managed care, that there be rules and regulations and programs established so that when an HMO or one of these other health care providers comes to a person, that person has some basis for selecting a health care provider. Right now there is not any.

I mean, you see an advertisement on television, that is about all you know. We need some information to determine how many deaths occurred in that facility, if any; how many cases of abuse were reported, some information so that someone like the Georges have information at their grasp that they can make that determination.

Mr. Panelli, is there anything at this stage to give them a basis for making that determination other than going in and talking to the personnel there?

Mr. PANELLI. Senator Reid, in Nevada, we have established a report card on long-term care. At this point in time, the report card is limited in that it only speaks to areas of deficiencies, deficient practices of the facility in the past. It talks about the number of complaints, the types of complaints.

Senator REID. Who is that available to, Mr. Panelli?

Mr. PANELLI. That is available to all the citizens in Nevada or anywhere else that is wishing to have it.

Senator REID. If I went to Rest Home X and said, "Give me this information from Mr. Panelli's office," would they be obligated to give it to me?

Mr. PANELLI. Yes. They would have that information available and they can contact our office to get that. They can contact any of the state offices to get that information. In addition, we will provide, out of our office, staff that is available at any time to sit down with people and talk to them about what they might find in a particular facility, the history on that facility.

Senator REID. Attorney General, is there anything in these real nice documents that you have put out to indicate that a person seeking admission to one of these facilities can ask for that information?

Ms. DEL PAPA. That is described in the long-term care——

Senator REID. Because that is very important.

Ms. DEL PAPA. It is. But, Senator, let me go one step further because the challenge in all of this, and Rick told you about it, too, because we cannot get these facilities fast enough, and even now the waiting list—and I can tell you even a challenge that we had and you mentioned it yourself when you were going to talk about the rural areas, because all of these problems become exacerbated when you then switch to the rural situation. We all know that.

We had, in one of our Medicaid fraud investigations, I hate to tell you, a situation where I wanted to close the facility. However, I could not because I would have put 300 people out on the street with no place to go. So, there is that time when you have to make that decision, and all of us here face that.

That is why we try to do everything that we can as far as working together, coming together with the protocols and the task forces, because there are really a lot of very dedicated and committed people who work in this area and we know the challenge we are facing because we cannot keep pace with the growth because it is occurring so quickly.

Senator REID. Mr. Panelli, based on the public data, the last data we have for 1996, Nevada's long-term care facilities have a much higher percentage of deficiencies for selected Medicare requirements than the national average. Is that a fair statement?

Mr. PANELLI. Yes, it is.

Senator REID. What does this really say about the quality of care in Nevada's long-term care facilities? Does it mean we are doing a better job of investigating or do we just have worse facilities?

Mr. PANELLI. Senator Reid, I believe there are many facets to that. One of them is that I think we do have a very dedicated group of people in Nevada to protect the health and safety of the individuals in long-term care. I think another thing is I think if you would look at the data, it was in 1996. Now looking at data that is coming through in the latter part of 1997, the numbers of deficiencies in our state is decreasing. We believe that is from education, training, partnering with the facilities.

Senator REID. You have given us that information?

Mr. PANELLI. Yes. And in HCFA, the National Restraint Reduction Initiative Report indicates that Nevada now has decreased the number of people that were in restraints. We were one of the highest in the nation. We believe that the industry, partnering with them, we have gotten to where we have decreased the number of people in restraints, which really says a lot for the industry.

Senator REID. The Attorney General will remember this. I held some hearings here in the State of Nevada a number of years ago on elder abuse. We had a very fine witness from the University of Nevada Medical School who talked about how much restraints were used here in Nevada and how unnecessary they were.

I think that was a step in the right direction, so I am very happy to hear that report because one of the easiest ways to take care of people who are placed in these extended care facilities is to put them in a bed and strap them down so they cannot move anyplace, and you can imagine yourself being placed in that situation.

Mr. PANELLI. Yes.

Senator REID. I am very, very happy to report that that is not happening very often. Is that a fair statement?

Mr. PANELLI. It is much reduced from what it was. It is still not where we want it.

Senator REID. The last question I want to ask, how about resources for you to do your job? Do you have enough resources to conduct this surveillance, these investigations, these surveys? Do you have enough people to do this?

Mr. PANELLI. At this time, we are understaffed, as I think many of the agencies are. We have a backlog, if someone wants to start a new long-term care facility, we are scheduled out several months before we can actually get in and do the survey. We try and partner with the people so that we can coordinate it as to when they are going to be ready, but you can see, we have not put on a new Federal long-term care surveyor in several years and it will be a while probably before we can do that.

Senator REID. Is that probably happening all over the country?

Mr. PANELLI. In the entire country, it is the same thing.

Senator REID. So that is something that we need to focus on. Ms. Sloan, I was impressed with the fact, and also learned something at this hearing which I am sure others did, that of the complaints you receive, almost three-quarters of them come from the facility itself, either staff or administration.

Give me an example of why a staff or the administration would complain about themselves.

Ms. SLOAN. That is an effort that was achieved through extensive education and working closely with the facilities for self-reporting to the division. It is a requirement that we have. An example might be if a patient had a fall. We need to know that the patient had a fall.

Senator REID. So now they are obligated to do that?

Ms. SLOAN. That is correct. So that we can then, on behalf of the patient, determine how that occurred. Was it because they were left alone when they should have been attended? Or was it because of an accidental fall that could not have been prevented by supervision or staffing?

Senator REID. Let me ask you, you heard the statistics of the study. The American Geriatrics conducted a study and said that about a third of people would rather die than go into an extended care facility. Why do people feel that way, and from your opinion, your experience, should they feel that way?

Ms. SLOAN. We are very sad that people feel that way. I think there are so many fears and myths as we grow older about a great many things, about what the future might hold for us. Dr. Takamura speaks of the gifts of longevity, trying to help us understand the positive aspects of aging.

Unfortunately, I think there has been attention on warehousing of elders in long-term care facilities, abuses in facilities that are not the norm. When a family needs the resource, and I think that the information that we see indicates that at some point in our lives, 43 percent of the population will require some time in a long-term care facility, perhaps for recuperation and rehabilitation, perhaps for a longer length of stay for the intensive service that is needed.

That should be an environment where the individual is a resident, not a patient; receives quality of care and quality of life; and that is what our ombudsmen program is for. We believe our Silver Striper program, our new initiative with volunteers will help bring eyes and ears into those facilities who will see and be able to take back to their community that there is quality of life, there is happiness, there is an opportunity for friendship and support in a long-term care facility.

The fears, I believe, have made us better consumers and that is extremely important. It has helped us to have family advocates and public advocates. But when a family or an individual needs that resource, they should be able to access it with confidence.

Senator REID. I guess I would ask you, you having been involved in this business for a long time, how do you feel personally? I mean, would you rather die than go into one of these facilities?

Ms. SLOAN. No, and if it were my parent or my loved one or myself, I know that there are very caring staff in the facilities and an environment in which I believe I could enjoy a quality of life.

Senator REID. Attorney General Del Papa, of the 130 complaints received by your Medicaid Fraud Control Unit, I am led to believe that only 20 criminal investigations were opened. What happened to the other 110 cases?

Ms. DEL PAPA. Senator, obviously you know you try to push these cases whenever you can make a case, but we work very closely with professional licensing facilities and that is one of the purposes, too, in entering into the protocols that I mentioned.

I mean, we will refer to a licensing bureau. There is a real good partnership that has developed over the years between these various agencies, and as I said earlier, sometimes you are faced with a decision that I mentioned, where it is a terrible choice that you have to make sometimes because sometimes you have no choice but to leave, as I said, a facility open and work with that facility when there have already been problems with it because there is just a lack of beds.

Senator REID. If you could dictate to Washington a couple things that they could do to help you in your work, what would that be?

Ms. DEL PAPA. Well, in this particular area, not speaking of other issues, Senator, but in all seriousness, I think really what I said earlier as far as the flexibility. Congress really needs to open up the flexibility on what Medicaid Fraud Control Units can do.

I say that to you very, very seriously because—particularly if we had some authority now because our funding is so restricted. You cannot step outside that area. We need to have the flexibility to go into Medicare, in particular, those facilities. That would be the number one thing that I would suggest.

And then, of course, number two, I think with reference to what we have to keep in mind, and I know you are painfully aware of it because I know how supportive you have been in this regard, but when you have a population that is growing as fast as this state's population, you really have to stay on the cutting edge as far as the funding formulas, those grants, and, of course, that is why our governor was so concerned when the Medicaid cuts were proposed at the national level.

It would have had a devastating impact, as you know, and I know you fought very hard in that regard as well. But again, I would like to applaud your efforts with reference to the National Registry to identify those people who have been convicted of patient abuse. I think that is a really good idea.

But my number one priority would be loosening up and letting those Medicaid Fraud Control Units have greater flexibility.

Senator REID. Rose George, again for the third time, I appreciate your being here. It is hard to get people who are in need to come forward. It is embarrassing for you to stand up here and tell everybody that you have sold your home and your resources. It is certainly not easy for your mother to be up here, kind of the focal point of everything that is going on.

But without the courage of people like you and your mom, though, we cannot do our job. We need real people that have real problems other than looking at some kind of a textbook trying to figure out how this happens. So again, we appreciate your being here and if there is anything that either of you would like to say after having listened to these two panels, feel free to do so.

Ms. GEORGE. I would just like to add, I know that Ms. Sloan said that we had the opportunity to put mom in a home. Well, we had one nursing home that we were going to place her in and they gave her bed away. We were ready to do it in three days. She was ready to go in and they called us and said they had given her bed away.

My feeling is they gave it to somebody that they could make more money off of. Also, there was another facility open, but I heard through the grapevine, do not put your mom in this facility because of abuse and neglect. I mean, how could I put my mother in a place like that? Is that my only alternative, to put her in one of those type of places?

I really think that if the government would consider caring for disabled in their homes, it is a lot cheaper than a nursing home. You pay a live-in $1,200 to $1,500 a month as opposed to $3,000 to $5,000 in a nursing home and it would provide jobs possibly for some of the Medicare recipients, too. It might be an answer for us.

Senator REID. Especially if we had some standards for people that did that so that you would not have to run an ad and get somebody that is homeless to come into your home.

Ms. GEORGE. Yes, right.

Senator REID. That is why this National Registry that we are trying to establish would also give people the peace of mind that if you do have to put someone in one of these convalescence facilities, that you will know that the person is not a criminal that is caring for your mom or dad or brother or sister, and that that person has not abused people in other such work opportunities.

Then dropping it down a little bit, I really think that we need some standards for people that care for those home health care facilities. More government involvement, maybe we can work with the state in doing that, but I think it is really necessary so that we do not have people stealing your jewelry, having nervous breakdowns during job responsibilities.

We appreciate very much the testimony from this panel. We will take this to Washington and hopefully arrive at some conclusions that will be satisfactory. Thank you very much.

While these panelists are leaving the state, we are going to be hearing from the next panel, Panel No. 3, which is entitled, "Tomorrow's Cure." As you will recall, the first panel dealt with state and national priorities and problems, the second panel dealt with the reality today, and this third panel is going to talk about what the future holds.

We are going to hear about ensuring available, affordable quality care for the future, long-term care in all its diverse forms, nursing homes, community care, home health care, hospice that has had a changing role in the spectrum of health care options in recent years. This role will continue to grow as the older population grows.

Specific issues such as financing options, health insurance coverage, and other new long-term care concepts all play a role in the formulation of national policy and we are going to talk about this in the third and final panel.

We are going to hear from Dr. Lawrence Weiss, Director of the Sanford Center for Aging, University of Nevada, Reno; Winthrop Cashdollar, Executive Director of the Nevada Health Care Association; Lea Mason, a registered nurse, who is the Secretary of the Home Health Care Association of Nevada; and Dr. Steven L. Phillips, who is a medical doctor and is the Medical Director, Social Health Maintenance Organization, Senior Dimensions, Sierra Health Services for the State of Nevada.

We also are going to hear from Margaret McConnell, also a registered nurse, who is the Administrator of the Charleston Retirement and Assisted Living Facility. We are first going to hear from Dr. Weiss.

STATEMENT OF LAWRENCE J. WEISS, PH.D., DIRECTOR, SANFORD CENTER FOR AGING, UNIVERSITY OF NEVADA, RENO

Mr. WEISS. Thank you, Senator, for allowing me to present testimony to this hearing today. I am representing the Sanford Center for Aging at the University of Nevada, Reno. Our center is dedicated to programs that benefit all older Nevadans and persons through a commitment to education, research, and community service.

Our faculty and staff and volunteers explore innovative ideas and aggressively seek new opportunities that enhance successful aging in the 21st century. The issue being addressed today, long-term care, if it does not impact you today, it will tomorrow. I will briefly convey to you not the problems, you have heard those; not some of the impact on tomorrow's seniors, you have heard some of that; but some of the suggestions on what we must do to assure that we as a nation can add quality of life to our remaining years even after chronic illness befalls us.

In order to deal with the tremendous imperatives that are haunting our personal health care, we as a nation must establish an affordable, accessible, quality care system that maximizes health, choice, and independence. I propose the establishment of an integrated delivery system.

To accomplish this, we have to think in terms of providing the full array of comprehensive services spanning the continuum, incorporating acute care services within a chronic care delivery system. The home is valuable. Home and community-based services are valuable. We need to enhance those services.

We need to pool our financing. We cannot have a Medicare system, Medicaid system, private insurance system. We need to pool it together and maybe come from those different sources that at least from the consumer perspective it has to be seamless, it has to be easy and user-friendly.

We have to focus on functioning. It has to be person-centered, a novel idea, the individually-tailored care that we need. We are not all the same. We need different things and it could be provided through that array of comprehensive services. We need to empower the consumer. How? Educate. We need to provide information. In this information age, it is much easier than it has been in the past to educate.

We have to empower the consumer to make decisions. What a novel idea to include the consumer in their own health care. But we must do it. We need to empower the family, provide the kinds of supportive services that we have heard to enhance that independence and autonomy. We must coordinate care.

We must provide some form of interdisciplinary, cross-discipline types of teams over time, through different settings. We must also utilize the kinds of technology that we have today, the automation. We are, as I mentioned, in the information age. Let's bring that. Let's make it paperless.

One of the worst things that people talk about in the Medicare system is the paper. That is changing because of the kind of automation that we have. We can employ that in all the settings or cross-settings with all the different services.

A way to accomplish this, we have a model program that you will hear about in a few minutes from Dr. Phillips called the social HMO. That is a demonstration. We have other demonstrations throughout the country that we can look to towards some of this. I implore that the committee consider more research demonstrations, practical, applied work.

In short, I request that the U.S. Senate Special Committee on Aging propose a national policy of long-term care that will prepare our country for the 21st century. We cannot continue down our current path. Certainly the baby boom generation will not tolerate it. The current non-system is too costly in terms of dollars and lacks the quality of life.

We must develop integrated delivery systems that are affordable, comprehensive, person-centered, empower the consumer, employ market forces, and incorporate integration techniques in a continuum of care concept. Thank you.

Senator REID. Thank you.

[The prepared statement of Mr. Weiss follows:]

TESTIMONY Presented to the U.S. Senate Special Committee on Aging Field Hearing, Reno and Las Vegas, Nevada, January 12 and 13, 1998

The Many Faces of Long-Term Care: Today's Bitter Pill or Tomorrow's Cure?

LAWRENCE J. WEISS, Ph.D.
Director, Sanford Center for Aging
University of Nevada, Reno
Reno, Nevada 89557-0133

Thank you Senator(s) for allowing me to present testimony at this hearing today. I am representing the Sanford Center for Aging at the University of Nevada, Reno. Our center is dedicated to programs that benefit all older persons through a commitment to education, research, and community outreach. Our faculty, staff, and volunteers explore innovative ideas and aggressively seek new opportunities that enhance successful aging in the 21st century.

The issue being addressed today is long-term care (LTC) and that its impact effects each and every one of us. If it does not effect us today, it will tomorrow. I will briefly convey to you what the problems are, their impact on tomorrow's seniors, and make some suggestions on what we must do to assure that we as a nation can add quality of life to our remaining years, even after chronic illness befalls us.

Establish an Integrated Delivery System: Tomorrow's Cure

In order to deal with the tremendous imperatives that are haunting our personal health care, we as a nation must establish an affordable, accessible, quality care system that maximizes health, choice, and independence. I propose to address these imperatives by discussing four major issues in the establishment of an integrated delivery system:

1) Expand the definition of LTC, incorporate the concept of the "continuum of care" which treats the person across settings and over time;
2) Enhance the role of the consumer and market forces to develop a new model of care;
3) Employ service integration techniques, especially focused on acute and chronic care;
4) Establish quality care outcomes through research.

First, let me define what LTC is or should be. LTC is not just nursing home care. LTC is any service, formal or informal, that addresses a person's level of functioning due to chronic disabling illnesses. Traditionally, our health care system only reimburses for "acute" care issues. Medicare only pays for care while the person is improving, not for on-going LTC services. Although in recent times, through the home health Part B benefit, some have argued that the tremendous increase in utilization has resulted in a more lenient view of Medicare Part B home care benefits to cover LTC services. The federal program has left the coverage of LTC services to the states through the Medicaid program. States only provide benefits for nursing home care for the Medicaid eligible persons. The eligibility requirements are very limiting, especially financially, resulting in the need to become impoverished before qualifying.

In addition, most states also provide very limited coverage under some Medicaid waivers to persons with moderate functional limitations of daily living activities through a home and community-based program. In Nevada that program is called CHIPS. Statistically only a small number of persons are served by these state programs. In

Nevada, only 1152 persons are served. The need is much greater. In short, for all practical purposes only the nursing home is an option for people in need of LTC. This limited definition of viable options for covered LTC services needs to change.

Our nation's health care system needs to define its service system along a continuum, not as isolated incidents that occur at a single point in time. The care system needs to be person-centered, across service settings, involve treatment of different conditions, different disciplines, and adjust to individuals changing needs over time. Lip service is paid to establishing the continuity of care. Only after preventive, primary, rehabilitation, and other long-term care services are a covered benefit will a continuum of care be effective. Form follows financing, so a system needs to pool its financial resources, extend the service options, and focus on the enhancement of individual functioning within a continuum of care.

Second, I support the enhancement of the consumer's role and market forces in developing a new model of care. We all value controlling our own destiny, having independence and autonomy, privacy, and some decision-making capability. The health care system is currently built on the medical model, which is not adequate to deal with the complexity of chronic illnesses and the lack of a "cure". Generally, the consumer or "patient" does not participate in his or her own health care decision-making process. Government is afraid to empower consumers, concerned that they will over-use services and therefore cost more. Some research activities that have studied the impact of the role of consumers do not display overuse and increased expenditures. When given a role in the decision process, consumers generally use less service. Increased participation by the consumer and their family should then increase the effectiveness of the care system by spreading of available resources and personal involvement. This collaborative model of care needs to be incorporated into LTC, acute care, and the continuum of care.

Most consumers and their families who have the resources to pay for services want to make decisions about which providers to use and most do. Unfortunately, those consumers who do not have their own resources do not make decisions. When it comes to LTC, we assume that the consumer can not make decisions, either about service type, provider, or day-to-day services. Therefore, public agencies go to great lengths to establish rules and regulations to try and ward off abuse, neglect, and try to assure some quality. Unfortunately, public agencies can not monitor care closely enough and the abuse continues. If caught in an infraction, public agencies do not have the clout or willingness to enforce the rules. When you have a service, such as nursing homes, in which one-third of the public would rather die before using, you have a problem. I maintain that if the consumer and their family were empowered, had the service options available, and the resources to make decisions, the quality of care across the industry would improve. Let market forces play a role, as they do in other industries.

Third, the whole array of services needs to be integrated into an easily accessible and appropriate system of care that centers on the person. Currently, a person gets lost in entitlements, eligibility requirements, and lack of communication between the many providers and service systems. Developing a truly seamless integrated delivery system is a critical feature in the establishment of effectiveness, efficiency, and quality in health care. Integrating LTC with acute care is especially needed given the incidence and cost of chronic conditions conveyed earlier.

One simple example of integrating acute and chronic care came out of a model program, Evercare, created by the United Health Care program in Minneapolis. This program provided a geriatric team, especially a geriatric nurse practitioner, to nursing home residents in order to provide primary care. Their results have shown a dramatic decrease in acute hospital admissions. Even though this model is limited in providing primary care only to the LTC nursing home residents, the benefits are obvious.

Other model demonstration programs that begin to develop integrated delivery systems are the Social Health Maintenance Organization and the Program for All-inclusive Care for the Elderly (PACE). Both of these models incorporate some of the integration techniques but are limited in scope or size.

Clearly, we as a nation need to learn from these models, develop variations on the theme, and employ service integration within our delivery of health and LTC care. In order to accomplish this, we need to utilize integration techniques. One important integration technique is the use of automated technology that provides a person-centered health data and communication system. Such a system can track all health related issues, communicate that information to all providers, and aid in the coordination of services, while simultaneously comparing the care with standards or benchmarks. Other integration techniques that need to be considered in designing a system of care include:

- Pooled financing or a single payor method;
- Individually tailored plans of care;
- Interdisciplinary clinical care coordination; and
- The full array of services (including low cost housing, assisted living, transportation, social, mental health, personal care, home and community-based services, and other services that provide functional enhancement, prevention or primary care).

The fourth and final imperative in developing the future integrated delivery system is the need to establish quality care outcomes through research. We certainly have reached a level of sophistication in our health service research that we can employ scientific techniques in trying to determine what works and what does not work.

Experimentation with different techniques in the provision of care is essential in determining what is most effective and efficient. The allocation of limited health care resources depends on determining what works from an economic perspective and what works from a quality of life perspective. Research demonstrations are essential in that quest for the ideal model of care.

The Case for a Long-Term Care System

Why should I make the above recommendations and why should we be concerned about LTC? There are many reasons why we should focus on LTC and shape a national policy, which currently does not exist. First, the major cause of illness, disability, and death are chronic conditions. The number of chronic health conditions has increased dramatically since the turn of the century. Those persons who have a chronic condition live longer today, especially with cancer and cardiovascular diseases, and are most likely to require LTC services. This is especially true for those 65+. Today, there are 100 million persons who have a chronic condition. By the year 2040, the number will increase to 160 million. Of those who are disabled, 20% need help with basic daily activities and 60% of those are 65+ years. Please note that most of the figures reported are taken from a very excellent publication, Chronic Care in America: A 21st Century Challenge, produced by the Robert Wood Johnson Foundation and authored by Dr.'s Catherine Hoffman and Dorothy Rice.

Second, we are living longer. Since 1900, life expectancy has increased about 30 years, to where people now routinely live into their 70's and 80's. Today, there are 33 million persons 65+ or about 13% of the total population. The net increase in growth of 65+ persons, is one per minute, according to the 1993 census. By the year 2040, there will be 87 million persons 65+ or 21% of the population. Nevada's 65+ population is growing in faster due to the in-migration of retirees. But more devastating to LTC services is the tremendous growth in 85+ persons. Currently, we have about 3-4 million persons 85+ or 1% of the 65+ population. By the year 2040, the 85+ population will grow to 4% or greater of the 65+ population, totaling 12-23 million people. This is the fastest growing age group of any in the population. Life expectancy demographic research predicts that by the year 2040, males will reach 75-86 years and females will reach 83-92 years of age.

Third, the incidence of disability and chronic conditions increase with age. It is well known to seniors and service providers alike that with increasing age, disability and chronic conditions increase. A study by the Scripps Gerontology Center, Miami University, found that both moderate and severe disability increase with age. Based on an Ohio sample of seniors that were representative of the nation, those that were 65-69 years of age had 10% incidence of disability, those 85-89 years of age were 44% moderately or severely disabled, and those 95+ had 74% incidence of disability. Admissions to nursing home level of care correspond to these figures. In addition, those persons with more than one chronic condition increase with age. In other words, two-thirds of those who have a chronic condition and are 65+ years, have more than one chronic condition.

Fourth, those who have chronic conditions account for 70% of the national expenditures on personal health care. The direct medical care costs for persons with a chronic condition account for $425 billion. If you add indirect costs for morbidity and mortality, the total becomes $659 billion annually. As expected, hospital care and physician services account for two-thirds of the total personal health care dollars, whereas 12% is spent on nursing home care. Medical care costs more for people with chronic conditions. In fact, having more than one chronic condition dramatically increases the total health care cost by six-fold over those with only acute care conditions. These figures are overpowering. We need to focus on these financial issues, change our methods and incentives of reimbursement, and develop integrated systems of care.

Fifth, chronic care is financed primarily by individual out of pocket expenses and public sources. If you exclude acute care expenses, the individual accounts for 33% or $23 billion of nursing home care expenses nationally, Medicaid accounts for 52% or $36 billion, Medicare accounts for 9% or $6 billion, and private insurance 2% or $2 billion annually. Long-term care costs for home health primarily come from Medicare, 39% or $8 billion, individual expenses account for 21% or $4 billion, Medicaid 16% or $3 billion, and private insurance accounts for 12% or $3 billion annually. None of these figures calculate the economic value of informal care. Informal care is estimated to be 75-80% of the total expenditures.

So if it is estimated that $100 billion was spent on formal services, then it could be estimated that $400-500 billion is spent on informal care of chronic conditions. The impact on individuals and their families as well as public sources, especially state governments, is enormous. The economics of LTC demand a national policy.

In summary, I request that the U.S. Senate Special Committee on Aging propose a national policy of LTC that will prepare our country for the 21st century. We can not continue down our current path, certainly the baby boom generation will not tolerate it. The current "non-system" is too costly in terms of dollars and lacks quality of life. We must develop integrated delivery systems that are affordable, comprehensive, person-centered, empower the consumer, employ market forces, and incorporate integration techniques and a continuum of care concept.

Senator REID. We will now hear from Margaret McConnell.

STATEMENT OF MARGARET McCONNELL, R.N., ADMINISTRATOR, CHARLESTON RETIREMENT AND ASSISTED LIVING

Ms. MCCONNELL. Good morning, Senator Reid, members of the committee, ladies and gentlemen. I would like to thank you for the opportunity to be here this morning and testify.

I am struck by what a difference a few years make. When I entered this field in 1980, just a few years ago, the topics we are discussing today were not of such major import. However, with the staggering growth of our elderly population, long-term care has now become a major national issue.

In this decade alone, as we have been discussing, since 1990 to the year 2000, our elderly population is going to increase by more than 40 percent, and with this incredible increase comes the challenge to all of us to offer a quality lifestyle to our seniors while not over-burdening the taxpayer with the associated costs.

Research now shows that the greatest demand for long-term care is going to be for those seniors whose incomes are less than $20,000 a year. To meet these challenges with which we are now faced, we have to be creative, innovative, and open-minded. I would like to ask us to think of a long-term continuum of care without walls.

Let's look at expanding, as we have been discussing this morning, our in-home care options. Let's look at expanding retirement, residential, and assisted living options. And yet, let's maintain those valuable nursing home beds for our most compromised seniors. Expanding the alternatives to skilled nursing facilities is appropriate and it is necessary because more and more seniors today, and their families, are demanding less institutionalized, more individualized, more non-medical long-term care.

So as we acknowledge what our seniors are asking for and what their families are demanding, let's expand in-home care and assisted living. And as well as doing that, let's look at some considerable cost savings. I would like to briefly mention four cost-saving measures I believe we could implement.

We can look at expanding our Medicaid waiver program, which is now serving effectively 22 states. Let's encourage the expansion of long-term care policies to offer more alternatives to skilled nursing facilities so that more people can be served in their homes, and in assisted living.

Third, let's study the SSI reimbursement program for our nation's indigent and possibly expand this funding alternative, again for more in-home and assisted living programs. And fourth, let's encourage managed care to expand reimbursement to treat people in more non-institutionalized settings.

Besides funding and cost issues for long-term care, I encourage you to allow regulations to remain with the states as much as possible. In turn, we can have more autonomy depending on the demographics of our individual States. In addition to these funding and regulatory issues, I would like to last address the issue of training to long-term care providers.

Let's consider offering incentives to encourage more people to enter this rapidly-growing field and let's encourage partnerships with programs such as the Sanford Center on Aging with Sierra Health Services so that we can train more people to enter this field and increase the quality of our care providers in the field.

I realize these brief comments merely scratch the surface of this complex and vital issue. In closing, I would like to commend this committee for holding this special hearing on this increasingly important topic. Through fact-finding, planning, and openness to new ideas, I believe we can together find answers to the compelling issues of long-term care today and in the future. Thank you.

[The prepared statement of Ms. McConnell follows:]

FIELD HEARING OF THE

U.S. SENATE SPECIAL COMMITTEE ON AGING

"The Many Faces of Long Term Care: Today's Bitter Pill or Tomorrow's Cure"

Las Vegas, NV – January 12, 1997
Presentation by:

Margaret McConnell, R.N., M.A.

Owner/Administrator
The Charleston Retirement and Assisted Living

Reno, NV – January 13, 1997
Presentation by:

Wendy V.C. Simons

Administrator/Partner
Park Place Assisted Living Residential Neighborhood for Seniors

The Charleston
Retirement & Assisted Living Center

BIOGRAPHY

Margaret McConnell

Margaret McConnell is a native Nevadan, born, raised and educated in Reno, Nevada.

Margaret is a Registered Nurse with a Bachelor's Degree in Nursing from the University of Nevada, Reno, and a Master's Degree in Marriage and Family Counseling from UNR.

She worked for 17 years as a psychiatric nurse and psychologist for the State of Nevada's Mental Health programs in both Northern and Southern Nevada.

About 13 years ago, Margaret and her husband entered the private industry through the purchase of The Charleston Retirement and Assisted Living facility. Margaret is the Administrator of The Charleston.

Margaret is Chairperson of Governor Miller's Board of Examiners for Long Term Care Administrators, Co-Chair of the National Board of Examiners Residential Care/Assisted Living Examination Committee. Margaret is also active in her professional work association and seniors abuse prevention work, is on the Nevada Geriatric Education Advisory Board, and is Vice President of the Nevada Tennis Association. Margaret is both an avid golf and tennis player.

47-539 133

2121 W. Charleston, Las Vegas, Nevada 89102 • Fax (702) 382-8407 • (702) 382-7746

FIELD HEARING OF THE U.S. SENATE SPECIAL COMMITTEE ON AGING

LAS VEGAS NV – JANUARY 12, 1997

The Many Faces of Long Term Care: Today's Bitter Pill or Tomorrow's Cure

BY

Margaret A. McConnell, R.N., M.A.
Owner/Administrator : The Charleston Retirement and Assisted Living

A VISION FOR THE FUTURE
OF
LONG TERM CARE

The statistics relating to the care of the elderly are reviewed daily and are absolutely staggering. As has already been discussed numerous times today, we must acknowledge our rapidly growing elderly population. In this decade alone, from 1990 to the year 2000, the elderly population is projected to grow by more than 40%. Along with this incredible increase comes the challenge of offering a quality lifestyle to our elderly, without overburdening taxpayers with the costs. To meet the demands of our elderly, we must work together nationwide to offer services that are creative and cost-effective, while meeting each individual's needs.

Turning to the future of long term care and its problems, I will discuss several steps that I believe must be taken to ensure quality of life for residents of long-term care facilities. In discussing this topic, I think it useful to refer to the Assisted Living Facilities Association of America's outline of future trends in long term care.

- **The general public and health care professionals must increasingly recognize and accept the assisted living residence as an appropriate and viable long-term care alternative.**

Once a senior is no longer able to function at home, we must make services available to deal with their changing lifestyle. Assisted living is the next step in the evolution of housing and health care as an option for those who cannot live alone, but do not need the twenty-four hour supervision of a nursing home.

At this time, there is no question that assisted living is the fastest growing segment of health care. Assisted living is a "special model" of care for our elderly, where the resident comes first. This philosophy of responding to the individual needs of each resident has resulted in a dramatic increase of assisted living facilities across the United States. Since the late 1970's, when professionally managed assisted living was first introduced, the industry has grown to over 30,000 licensed residences. These residences house an estimated one million individuals.

There are several characteristics which distinguish assisted living from other forms of long-term care and lend to its growing popularity. These characteristics include: independence, privacy, increased choices, and a nurturing spirit. As Americans live longer, more individuals and their families are seeking compassionate, low-cost care in non-institutional environments with a high quality of life. These people are increasingly turning to assisted living facilities as a solution to their housing problems.

- **Many nursing homes will convert into assisted living residences and states will begin to increase the regulation of assisted living residences as more companies enter into this market.**

In the past decade, there has been a gradual shift away from nursing homes, as people have increasingly recognized the limitations of this restricted, but most necessary level of care. Throughout the country, regulations have become increasingly stringent on nursing homes. Most significantly, this has included heightened demand on care takers for documentation and accountability. Unfortunately, in spite of these efforts, we continue to hear of quality of care problems in our nursing homes. Let us learn from the nursing home experience and not repeat the same mistakes in retirement and assisted living centers. Although legislation and regulation is essential to a smooth running, organized country, it is essential that we not over regulate retirement and assisted living facilities. Instead, we must allow individual states to oversee and regulate the assisted living industry. In most states there are significant differences in the needs of elderly. It is important to recognize these differences and allow flexibility at the state level to monitor assisted living facilities. In addition, we should encourage professional organizations in assisted living to support, educate, counsel, and nurture private care facility operators. This peer monitoring could provide checks and balances to assure quality care in the assisted living environment.

- **States should increase the use of public funds to support low-income persons in assisted living residences in lieu of nursing homes.**

As I said earlier, assisted living is the fastest growing segment of health care, allowing our seniors to reside in a less restrictive setting than a nursing home. However, most of the new construction currently being done is aimed at the senior who can afford $1,500.00 to $3,000.00 per month in rent. This leaves over 80% of our nation's population who are not able to afford this monthly fee. Since approximately 90% of assisted living costs are paid privately and since the costs of most assisted living residences are too high for most seniors to be able to afford, it is essential that alternatives be developed to enhance and expand payment mechanisms for assisted living.

One alternative for enhanced reimbursement is the Medicaid Waiver Program. As most of you are aware, Medicaid is the primary payment mechanism for nursing home residents. The reimbursement rate in a nursing home is approximately twice the monthly cost of assisted living, on a monthly basis. It has been estimated that as much as 50% of today's national nursing home population could be served in assisted living residences. The dollar cost savings could be astronomical if thousands of appropriate seniors were moved to assisted living residences from nursing homes with Medicaid Waiver reimbursement as the payment mechanism.

More than twenty states nationwide are now implementing the Medicaid Waiver Program as State officials realize that they can not only save money but also serve people more appropriately in assisted living residences. These officials state they were driven in this direction by the concepts behind assisted living—the privacy, the maximized independence, and the dignity for each resident. In Nevada, the Medicaid Waiver Program is relatively small at this time, due primarily to budget constraints, and has an extensive waiting list of several months.

Another manner in which states can increase the use of public funds to support assisted living is by augmenting the Supplemental Security Income (SSI) program. SSI financially supplements our nation's neediest seniors. The monetary reimbursement per month for retirement and assisted living centers needs to be increased as this would allow seniors more choices in quality care living arrangements. The current SSI reimbursement rate is so low, about $750.00 per month in Nevada, that most facilities are unable to offer services to the SSI recipient. The trend over the past few years has been that fewer and fewer assisted living operators can accommodate these seniors. I am unaware of any new facility coming on line in Nevada, that will be able accept SSI recipients. Since SSI recipients comprise a significant percentage of our consumers, we have a serious issue confronting us.

- **Partnerships will be developed to better offer services to residents as they age in place.**

In Nevada, our Licensing Board for Long Term Care Administrators is actively working with the Sanford Center for Aging to offer continuing education to our long-term care administrators.

These efforts are aimed at insuring that administrators are up to date and working with Nevada's elderly population in the most innovative and practical ways. Caring for Nevada's frail elderly is a huge responsibility and it is imperative that this work be carried out by qualified, well-informed caregivers.

To further insure quality care for our seniors, programs, courses and curriculum could be added to our colleges and universities nationwide to prepare administrators, supervisors and caretakers to work with the frail elderly in the community, in assisted living, or in the nursing home setting. Curriculum should include subjects such as fiscal, organizational, and dietary management, along with resident care.

Long-term care industry workers must understand the whole person, not just the person's medical, dietary, or daily hygiene needs. These workers must embrace the importance of encouraging each resident to be as independent as possible.

In closing I'd like to commend the committee today for holding this special hearing. It is through fact gathering, planning, and openness to new ideas that we can together find an answer for the compelling issues of long term care today. In establishing a national policy on long term care, I encourage you to include consumers, families, long term care representatives, and educational and policy makers from throughout the United States.

Thank you,

Margaret McConnell
1-12-97

Wendy V.C. Simons
Consultant
1530 Pass Dr. • Reno, NV 89509
(702) 323-7706 • (702) 323-3102 Fax

December 30, 1997

Honorable Charles E. Grassley
Chairman
United States Senate
Special Committee on Aging
Dirksen Senate Office building
Room G-31
Washington, D.C. 20510

Dear Senator Grassley and Senate Committee Members:

Thank you for the opportunity to participate as a panelist in your Senate Special Committee on Aging field hearing on Tuesday, January 13, 1997 in Reno, Nevada. The topics to be discussed are of great importance and the course of future planning needs to be progressive and innovative.

Through my presentation I hope to cite the exceptional communication that has developed within our state and identify how this communication has allowed Nevada to step beyond the traditional patterns of thinking into a potential blending and multi-dimensional track of service to our seniors. We are just beginning to feel the great influx of the over 65 population and the many providers of services to them are identifying similar needs. The public and private sector must partner to develop flexible solutions to future challenges.

I am grateful to be considered for your panel and remain deeply committed to charting new pathways of service to this senior population whom I have spent my whole life with.

I remain,

Sincerely,

Wendy V.C. Simons

FIELD HEARING OF THE U.S. SENATE SPECIAL COMMITTEE ON AGING

In

RENO, NEVADA – JANUARY 13, 1998

"The Many Faces of Long Term Care: Today's Bitter Pill or Tomorrow's Cure"

Presentation by:

Wendy V.C. Simons

Park Place Assisted Living Residential Neighborhood for seniors

FIELD HEARING OF THE U.S. SENATE SPECIAL COMMITTEE ON AGING

Reno, Nevada – January 13, 1998

TESTIMONY OUTLINE

SECTION I

SECTION II

SECTION I

DESIGN TO FUNCTION: MULTI-DIMENTIONAL THINKING

In 1953 I had the honor and pleasure of sitting in the lap of an elderly gentleman, William Cornwall, who happened to be a senior engineer on the Oakland/Bay Bridge in California. I was 3 years old at the time and he would tell me fabulous stories about creatures beyond the imagination. I asked him one day, how he built the bridge. He replied, "Design to function in multi-dimensions."

As our country is being challenged to think outside of the norm with regard to long term care options, this elderly man's statements come back to mind. It is a time for us to think beyond the linear black and white we are so familiar with and move into more creative systems of long term care.

Nationwide, we are seeing one creative approach, the trend of "assisted living" explode. The residential style, social model of care has been in existence since the 1940's known formerly as residential care homes. The current mass development of assisted living is being dictated by the consumers of health care who do not consider skilled nursing facilities as an option of choice. The trend of assisted living is still being generated and supported by private sector dollars. It is growing through market demand and with the creative designs of the individuals developing this housing and health care alternative combining independence with personal care in a warm, dignified, community setting. To date, assisted living is recognizing individuality and choice and due to the fact that no significant reimbursement is available from the federal level and no federal regulations have been generated to cripple the creation of this option in the long term care continuum.

Nevada has been a leading state in pioneering regulatory guidelines. Regulations have been in place since 1955, with multiple revisions and evolutions. During the past 5 years, dramatic changes have occurred. Administrators must be licensed and certified, caregivers must be fingerprinted and undergo continuing education criteria, facilities must be bonded as well as licensed, and in 1998, new Administrator's will be required to pass a national standardized test. The most significant item to note is that the assisted living/residential care industry in Nevada and the regulatory agency, Bureau of Health Facilities, worked in a public/private sector relationship to write the regulations and laws governing the industry. This demonstrates the value of a state recognizing it's own regulatory needs, consumer desires and industry input to create a system of aging in place.

It is important not to fall into the traps of the traditional past, but to forge a strong pro-active relationship will all the providers of service to our seniors, consumers of long term care components and governmental entities. It is further important to think beyond what we are familiar with and enter the multi-dimensional thought process for solutions in the future.

Had Steven Spielberg limited himself to traditional thinking, Jurassic Park would not have been created to be the spectacular product it became. We too, must continue a course of thinking outside the lines to generate long term care solutions for change, and we must be willing to risk a bit as well.

Wendy Simons 1/98

(2)

ITEMS TO CONSIDER

- **REGULATIONS SHOULD REMAIN WITH THE STATES.**

Each part of the country has it's own particular demographics and profiles. A federal standard would repeat the mistakes of previous long term care entities. Consumer choice and quality business practices will dictate success and failure.

- **INCENTIVES FOR CREATING TRAINING PROGRAMS FOR EMPLOYEES OF LONG TERM CARE PROGRAMS SHOULD BE CONSIDERED.**

1. There is a national shortage of workers for long term care settings. Just as we are considering educational incentives for our children's education, we should consider incentives for the late life worker re-entering employment in the health care industry.
2. A new commitment to training and education of future health care workers needs to come from the industry as well. Partnering with educational institutions for program and curriculum development for caregivers and other allied fields must be a priority for all in the long term care industry.
3. Community based workshops offering educational opportunities for individuals to understand aging issues and preventative health must be encouraged.

- **A REVIEW OF THE EXPENDITURES OF FEDERAL DOLLARS FOR INDIGENT CARE IN SKILLED NURSING FACILITIES SHOULD BE CONDUCTED.**

1. While the private sector is choosing Assisted living or home based care as an alternative, State and Federal dollars continue to be spent in skilled nursing facilities for individuals who would be appropriate in an assisted living setting. Some attention has been given to this area, and by no means are the Medicaid clients a source of great revenue to the skilled facilities, however many individuals are forced to "spend down" to be eligible for Medicaid assistance in a skilled setting. If slightly supplemented in an assisted living setting, some individuals would have resources last longer resulting in savings to the Medicaid program.
2. Individuals who would choose to be in an assisted living facility and who are on the SSI/Medicaid program are unable to be supplemented above the base rate without penalty. Families should be allowed to contribute without fear of deduction from the Medicaid dollars. (Nevada has just initiated this program.)

Wendy Simons 1/98

(3)

- **LONG TERM CARE INSURANCE POLICIES ARE RECOGNIZING THE DOLLARS SAVED IN ASSISTED LIVING.**
  Many Long Term Care insurance policies are now reimbursing for Assisted Living as an alternative to skilled nursing facilities. This should be encouraged when appropriate.

- **MANAGED CARE AND MEDICARE MANAGED CARE NEED TO RECOGNIZE ASSISTED LIVING AS A COST SAVING.**
  1. Often times, an individual in an Assisted living facility undergoing a health crisis can be maintained for a brief period of time through supportive services coming to the facility. Currently, some managed care and Medicare managed care programs require hospitalization for services to continue. This is not a good use of dollars if the alternative is appropriate.
  2. Community based "house call" programs should be considered in assisted living facilities. This would reduce the cost of some medical offices and allow physicians and nurse practitioners to evaluate their patients in their own setting.

- **SAFETY NETS NEED TO BE ENCOURAGED, BUT INDIVIDUALS SHOULD NOT BE IN A COCOON.**
  1. Continued communication between all the components of the health care continuum needs to be encouraged. No one agency should have complete control, power or turf over another. When considering financial reimbursement for programs, "funding formulas" often slant service away from those most in need.
  2. Financial incentives should be considered for community based care programs that allow a multi-dimensional flow. Sometimes an individual needs a Band-Aid other times a meal or a hug, but rarely a "mummy wrap" of services.
  3. If all the funds are wrapped up in one agency there is a tendency for that agency to spend on it's own special interests. We need to consider a blending of services.

- **ASSISTED LIVING, AS A COMPONENT OF THE MULTI-DEMENSIONAL CARE SYSTEM MUST BE ENCOURAGED.**
  1. Creative designs must be allowed and no one facility should be required to be like another. (Just as we choose car types, home types and store types, consumers should be allowed to choose the type of assisted living design they find appropriate.)
  2. With the increasing numbers of aging individuals and the projected numbers of individuals with probable Alzheimer's dementia, flexibility in design and housing as well as personal care options will be critical to best save health care dollars. As was cited in JAMA, October 22/29, 1997- Vol 278, No.16, "Alzheimer disease costs (medical, Long term care, home care, and lost productivity for caregivers totals a direct and indirect dollar expenditure approaches $100 billion each year. This figure will increase in the future and truly challenge our creativity and resources.

- **ADDITIONAL RESEARCH DOLLARS NEED TO BE DIRECTED TO THE STUDY OF ALZHEIMERS DISEASE AND RELATED AGING ISSUES.**
  To effectively plan and implement care options, strategies must be based on anticipation of effective care systems in this, the greatest component need.

Wendy Simons 1/98

SECTION II

AN OVERVIEW OF ASSISTED LIVING/RESIDENTIAL CARE HOMES IN NEVADA

By
WENDY V.C. SIMONS

I. **BRIEF HISTORY OF THE EVOLUTION OF RESIDENTIAL CARE**

History in Nevada
Changes and National trends

II. **CLARIFICATION AND TERMINOLOGY**

Board and Care, Adult Group Care, Residential Care, Foster Care, Domicilliary Homes, Rest Homes, Assisted Living Facilities

III. **WHERE DOES IT FIT IN THE OVERVIEW OF OPTIONS?**

Retirement Communities, Home Based Care, Skilled Nursing Facilities
Licensure Requirements, Inspecting Agencies, Etc.

IV. **WHAT SERVICES ARE PROVIDED?**
WHAT ARE THE REIMBURSEMENT RATES?

Room and board, assistance with personal hygiene, personal laundry, medication supervision, socialization, activities, heath care co-ordination, other activities of daily living assistance

V. **FUTURE DIRECTIONS**

New designs and interest in alternative living
In home support agencies
New levels of professionalism, yet home environment

Wendy V.C. Simons 1/98

RESIDENTIAL CARE HOMES / ASSISTED LIVING IN NEVADA

By Wendy V.C. Simons

BRIEF HISTORY

Residential Care Homes have been in Nevada since the 1940's. During the early years they were actually more boarding home type facilities, created in existing residences in local communities and usually by an individual who had some nursing background. In fact, Margaret Von Fluee (my mother) opened the first such facility in downtown Reno at 315 Hill Street in response to several agencies stating they had no place to locate "old folks" in a safe environment outside of a hospital setting.

The following years saw the creation of Skilled Nursing Facilities as we know them today, when reimbursement became available from Medicare/Medicaid programs. Yet during the expansion of long term health care options, residential care homes (board and care homes) maintained their existence and evolved as non-medical models of care; providing room, board and some personal care assistance. The majority of these early homes housed from 10-20 individuals and would expand through additions to accommodate more clients. In the ensuing years, a few larger complexes were built in the Reno and Las Vegas areas.

Initially, group care homes were licensed by the Nevada State Welfare division and the early regulations to govern them were created around 1955. In 1974 the Nevada State Health Division took over the responsibility of licensure and inspection of larger facilities. Stricter life safety codes were enacted and many facilities were retrofitted with sprinkler systems. There were about 11 such facilities in the state at this time. Nevada State welfare continued to license "Family Care Homes" caring for 3 or fewer residents.

The most significant transition occurred in 1986 when the Bureau of Health Facilities became responsible for regulations and licensure for the smaller care homes. Categories and regulations were created for facilities caring for "six or less" and "seven or more" individuals. The state licensure list jumped from (15) fifteen facilities to over three hundred (300) statewide.

It is interesting to note that during my affiliation as a Director with the National Association of Residential Care Facilities (NARCF) I discovered that Nevada's regulation of facilities was years ahead of many states, and that in 1990, only twenty-one (21) states had regulations in place for these facilities!

(2)

During the past three years, Nevada has undergone a dramatic change and evolution in the regulations of residential care/ assisted living. Through a significant joint venture effort among facility providers and the state regulatory agency, Bureau of Licensure and Certification, a complete revision of the standards and regulations governing residential care facilities was adopted in December 1997. The new regulations allow for more of an aging in place philosophy of care providing certain conditions and standards of care are established. The blending of a standard created by regulators and the provision for **consumer choice** in residential care options would have never occurred if not for the visionary thinking of the Chief of the Bureau of Licensure and Certification, Sharon Ezell, and the leaders of the residential care/ assisted living industry gathering together to discuss and create the current regulatory document.

Since 1955 Nevada has remained pro-active in charting the future course of residential care/assisted living. The newest regulations are evidence of that as well as the requirement in 1994 that administrators of facilities have certification and licensure in addition to the facility license. In 1998, Nevada's Board of Examiners for Long Term Care (BLECA) will adopt a new national exam for administrators thanks to the efforts of longtime Nevada provider, Margaret McConnell. The 1997 Legislature adopted the requirement for fingerprinting of caregivers and bonding of facilities. Nevada has remained in the forefront as a leader in collaborative efforts between agencies and providers in the residential care industry and has demonstrated that a State can direct its needs better than a federal entity. In this manner, Nevada can serve as a model for others to follow.

The massive growth in assisted living/residential care facilities has been created by a consumer interest and desire for increased options in long term care. This social model of care has evolved not by the availability of federal dollars creating physical plants, but by individuals seeking a less institutional standard of service.

The future of residential care and the newly developing assisted living care system should be dictated by individual states. Each section of the country has specific demographics and human profiles that are best controlled by the individual areas. It is predictable that most aging individuals and their families will choose the setting they are most comfortable with, both esthetically and financially. Ultimately, as we anticipate the future history of this type of care system, consumer choice and individual preferences will write the text.

Wendy Simons 1/98

(3)

CLARIFICATION OF TERMINOLOGY

In Federal studies this industry is termed "Board and Care Homes". Nevada refers to them as "Residential Care Facilities for Groups" or "Adult Group Care Homes". The V.A. system used the term "Domicillary Care homes". Some states call smaller homes "Foster Care Homes for the Elderly", and sometimes they are called "custodial care" and the newest term for recently designed facilities is "Assisted Living Facilities".

Ultimately, all these titles and names apply to a non-medical model of care, unlike skilled nursing facilities which fall into the category of medical models of care.

WHERE DO RESIDENTIAL CARE/ ASSISTED LIVING FACILITIES FIT

One must clearly understand the spectrum of elderly housing options to understand where Residential Care/Assisted Living homes fit in the continuum of care.

Ideally, everyone would prefer to age in place in his or her own home. However, when an individual no longer has sufficient physical or mental abilities to prepare meals, handle financial affairs, manage medications, attend to personal hygiene and daily living necessities then it is time to research and engage support systems and alternatives. These may include:

1. Home based support- usually the first choice, such as caregivers, home health services, etc.
2. Community living complexes- (Retirement communities) which provide shelter and meals for those not in need of supervision and assistance.
3. Residential Care/ Assisted Living facilities- which provide meals, lodging, activities of daily living (ADL's) assistance, and medication supervision.
4. Extended Care Facilities- which provide residence and skilled nursing services in a medical setting.

It is easy to see that Residential Care/ Assisted living is between home and nursing home.

It is also prudent to note that individuals may move in and out and between any of the above systems of service.

Wendy Simons 1/98

(4)

SERVICES PROVIDED IN RESIDENTAL CARE/ ASSISTED LIVING

Residential Care/ Assisted Living facilities provide twenty-four hour supervised living, meals, laundry, medication supervision and assistance, socialization, activities and health care co-ordination in a non-medical residential group living environment. The design and types of homes are unique to each operator.

Keep in mind these are not medical facilities, but residential style environments, many managed by the owner/operator in the case of the smaller homes. Some facilities operate with managers and other staff, depending on the size of the home and the number of clients. Eighty-five (85%) percent of the licensed facilities in Nevada are small facilities of 6 or fewer residents. The owners are usually individuals who have been involved in the health care field and have an entrepreneurial spirit. The reason for the success of these homes is due to the fact that many families prefer a home-style setting for their aging relative and want to avoid the nursing home setting.

Currently we are seeing a dramatic increase in the number of newer Assisted Living Complexes. Their focus remains the same as the smaller setting, a non-medical, social model of care allowing consumer choice of services and care needs.

WHAT TYPE OF CLIENT IS APPROPRIATE

The residents of these facilities must be ambulatory, or if in a wheelchair, able to transfer independently. Residents must be mentally and physically able to evacuate the facility with or without assistance in case of an emergency. Residents must be free of communicable disease. Residents must be able to self-medicate with supervision and should have some capacity for self care. If a resident is accepted with one of the new "allowable conditions" as stated in regulations, provisions must be made to provide supervision by an appropriately skilled medical person for the allowed conditions. Incontinence is allowed and is managed according to each facilities philosophy.

The typical resident is an individual who living alone would not eat properly or care for himself/herself properly. The individual may or may not need assistance with one or more activity of daily living (ADL). The usual assisted living individual is a widow about 85 years of age who was in a subtle state of decline in an independent living setting. It is not uncommon for couples to move in to an assisted living setting due to the care needs of one of the individuals. Residents in assisted living may come as a result of caregiver burnout, lack of community resources and/or relocation by a family member living in the area.

Wendy Simons 1/98

(5)

Most recently we have seen the increase of facilities who are willing to take what might have been considered and ICF I or II (Intermediate care) level client that would been normally place in a skilled nursing facility. Curiously enough, many of these clients do well in a small residential setting and it is not uncommon for an individual who needed a wheel chair in a larger building to be walking in a residential home setting. Individuals that might seem quite confused in large living environments often do better in a home-like setting as well. Behavioral issues often disappear in a more residential setting.

CHARGES AND REIMBURSEMENT SOURCES

At this writing, the cost of placement in residential care/ assisted living facility in Nevada ranges between $ 748.66 (for the state assisted/ SSI client) and $3000.00 per month. Private pay facilities usually scale their rates based on the services needed by the resident. Unfortunately there is a decline in the number of available placements for the state assisted client and no new facilities have been built in the last ten (10) years that accommodate the SSI client. The newly built assisted living facilities accept only private pay individuals. Some low income individuals have qualified for the Medicaid waiver program while placed in residential care settings which increases the rate of reimbursement to the $900.00 range. However, this is still not an incentive to accommodate the SSI subsidized client when the private pay market is strong.

FUTURE DIRECTIONS

The growing **consumer interest** with regard to long term care options will impact this industry greatly in the future. Already we are seeing larger corporations such as Mariott, Kennsington, Sunrise, Manor Care, Standish, Alternative Living Services, ARV and numerous others developing "assisted living" facilities across the nation. Many of these corporations have recognized the **consumer demand** for non-medical care options for their loved ones. The "assisted living" trend is being dictated by the **interest of the public** in this alternative level of care. It is evident that our country and our state must pay attention to this **expressed choice of individuals** and break away from the limited options of the past and allow for a multi-dimensional care system.

Our challenge is to think much as Steven Spielberg did when he created "Jurassic Park". We must evolve beyond lateral flat-screened thinking in care options and allow for the development of new creatures. Computer technology and the willing to risk allowed Spielberg to develop what could not exist before.

Creative thinking in health care options must allow us to develop what has not existed before. This is what we are seeing in the development of "assisted living" as an entity to itself. It is an industry with multiple designs and multiple personalities. Assisted living remains aware of the need for "high touch" service and not just high tech documentation.

The creative challenge continues. To individuals, to states and to future economic decisions of the government.

Wendy Simons 1/98

(6)

BOB MILLER
Governor

STATE OF NEVADA

CHARLOTTE CRAWFORD
Director

MYLA C. FLORENCE
Administrator

DEPARTMENT OF HUMAN RESOURCES
WELFARE DIVISION
2527 N. Carson Street
Carson City, Nevada 89706-0113
(702) 687-4770

November 20, 1997

WENETTE VAN CUREN-SIMONS
PARK PLACE
2305 IVES CT
RENO NV 89503

This letter informs all Adult Group Care Facilities (AGCFs) of the upcoming increase in Supplemental Security Income (SSI) payments.

Beginning January 1, 1998, the federal SSI payment will increase 2.1 percent. In addition, the state supplement for aged and blind individuals will increase 6 percent effective January 1, 1998 from $311 to $329.66. Due to systems requirements, this increase will be delayed approximately six weeks. Retroactive payments for January and February 1998 will be sent by the Social Security Administration around the second week of February. The new schedule of payments for aged and blind individuals will be as follows:

Federal Payment	State Payment	Total Payment
$494.00	$329.66	$823.66

A disabled individual's federal payment is $494 with no state supplement.

Welfare Division policy requires each client in an AGCF receive a personal needs allowance. For 1998, the personal needs allowance is increased to $75 per month. The balance of the combined federal/state SSI payment is available for room and board costs.

Should you have any questions, please contact Jeanette Hills, Chief, Eligibility and Payments, at (702) 687-4386.

Sincerely,

Myla C. Florence

Myla C. Florence
Administrator

MCF:CR/saL1.11

pc: Division for Aging Services
Mental Health/Mental Retardation
Washoe County Social Services
Clark County Social Service

Working for the Welfare of ALL Nevadans

O-1563B

WENDY V.C. SIMONS

INTRODUCTORY SUMMARY

Wendy is a native Nevadan, born and raised in the "old folks" home, as her mother opened the first senior care home in the state in the late 1940's. She has been considered a senior advocate for many years through numerous affiliations and dedications to senior care issues. She is the creator of a unique design in assisted living called Park Place, and has gained the reputation of being proactive in legislative and regulatory issues in Nevada.

WENETTE (WENDY) V.C. SIMONS
1530 Pass Drive
Reno, Nevada 89509
(702) 323-7706 (H) * (702) 323-3102 (FAX)
(702) 746-1188 (W) * (702) 746-1189 (FAX)

BIOGRAPHICAL SKETCH

- **Second generation care provider –Margaret Von Fluee (mother) developed the first residential care home in the state of Nevada in 1948. Born and raised in the "old folks home", have been active participant since childhood; eventually taking over as administrator in 1992 upon graduating from University of Nevada at Reno.**
- **Developed and operate Park Place Assisted Living Facility in Reno, a 60 resident assisted living neighborhood: a unique design concept still unduplicated.**
- **Professional reputation for being "the person to contact" with regard to care choices and counsels families on the multitude of options available in the state of Nevada.**
- **Have presented in numerous provider workshops and seminars for Washoe Medical Center and Saint Mary's Hospital personnel, created a joint venture seminar with the Bureau of Licensure and Certification on the new state regulations adopted in 1997 with a emphasis on admission assessment and regulatory compliance.**
- **Made presentations nationally for the Assisted Living Federation of America Institute and the American Association for Homebuilders as well as the National Association of Residential Care Facilities. (1984 in Minnesota, 1989 in Boston, 1990 in Tulsa, 1990 Washington, D.C., 1996 in Nevada ALFA Institute)**
- **Presenter in the V.A./ U.N.R. Conference in 1992 on Alternatives to Long Term Care.**
- **Subject of cover story on Residential Care in 1991 October issue of Senior Spectrum.**
- **Expert witness, 7th Judicial Court, State of Nevada, in client assessment for alternative placement from a long term care facility.**
- **Presenter before numerous State legislative committees since 1976.**
- **Co-producer and Host of the "Senior Scope" television show for KOLO Channel 8 for 10 years. Topics of the program have included: Care options for families; Senior abuse, neglect, exploitation; Medications and the elderly; Health and cost containment issues; Managed care; Late life romances; Sanford Center for Aging; etc.**
- **Member of the NAAB "Pass Point" Committee for the National Exam for Residential Care Administrators, 1997**

CURRENT PROFESSIONAL AFFILIATIONS

- Member of the Founders Council of the Assisted Living Federation of America
- Member and past Vice Chairman of the Sanford Center for Aging Studies, Community Advisory Board at University of Nevada, Reno.
- Member of the Nevada Adult Care Association and past President.
- Past President and member of the Executives Association of Reno
- Member of the Sierra Continuity of Care Association
- Member of the Senior Coalition of Northern Nevada

OTHER ORGANIZATIONS AND AFFILIATIONS AND HIGHLIGHTS

- Member of the Executive Committee of the Assisted Living Federation of America 1991-1993
- Past member of the Washoe Zephyrs Toastmasters and Evaluator of the Year 1991
- Past Chairman for Nevada ALFAA Council of States
- Past President of the Older American's Advisory Council of Northern Nevada by Governor appointment for 1990-1992
- Selected one of Reno's "10 Most Watchable Women" 1992
- Past member of the Nevada Junior Livestock Show Board by Governor Appointment, 1987-1991
- Past President of the Swope Middle School Parent's Group.
- Past Secretary of the Reno High School AAA Parent's Group
- Coordinator and Commentator of the Governor's Conference on Aging Fashion show 1990
- Lecturer at UNR Animal Science Department 1976-1982
- Miss Reno Rodeo 1970
- Judge of Horse Shows, Drill Team Competitions and Parades for over 30 years.

EDUCATION

- B.S. in Education from the University of Nevada, Reno
- Licensed Residential Care Facility Administrator, RCFA 5611

Senator REID. Mr. Cashdollar.

STATEMENT OF WINTHROP CASHDOLLAR, EXECUTIVE DIRECTOR OF THE NEVADA HEALTH CARE ASSOCIATION

Mr. CASHDOLLAR. Good morning, Senator Reid, and representatives of the Senate Aging Committee. I am Winthrop Cashdollar, Executive Director of the Nevada Health Care Association, an association of Nevada's long-term care providers. The Nevada Health Care Association is affiliated with the American Health Care Association, a federation of 50 state health care organizations which represents more than 11,000 nursing facilities, sub-acute care, and assisted living long-term care providers nationwide.

Senator, thank you very much for the opportunity to be a part of this proceeding and to be with so many distinguished and informative speakers and for this opportunity to look forward and to discuss ways in which lawmakers, the public, government, and caregivers can work together to reach tomorrow's cure.

I do not think that we can reach tomorrow cure's merely by tweaking or tinkering with our current long-term care system. Rather, we must show the courage, imagination, and resolve to build something better. In the next few minutes, I would like to touch upon long-term care issues of access, quality, and financing.

With regard to access, Senator, in your opening statement, you expressed the need for a long-term care system that places people on the requirements of their condition rather than on the requirements of programs. I think that we saw a very clear demonstration with Josephine George, that that is not occurring under the current system.

The nation invented Social Security and Medicare so that a person would not have to sell her house or her daughter would not have to sell her house in order to pay for health care. Social Security was designed for income security; Medicare was designed for health care security.

But because we did not address long-term care when we invented those programs, the long-term care component leaves people vulnerable to just exactly what we do not want to happen, which is for them to either lose all their wealth or assets and go on welfare in order to receive long-term care. I would like to suggest, as many other people here today have, that what we need is integration.

People have spoken on this panel and earlier panels of the need for an integrated service delivery system. I would like to suggest that we need to integrate the government programs for acute care and long-term care and income security. In a few minutes, I will get to principles for doing so that are espoused in this SecureCare proposal by the American Health Care Association.

I also would like to take just a moment to touch on one of the most promising services that has come about through the evolution of long-term care and that is assisted living. In Nevada's communities and in communities all across the nation, assisted living facilities are meeting the long-term care needs of a growing number of elderly.

Our public policy should foster the continued growth of assisted living and must not stifle this positive approach. With your permission, Senator, I would like to submit for the record materials from the American Health Care Association's National Center for Assisted Living, which provide detailed information about assisted living and about measuring and improving what people living in these facilities believe are important factors in long-term care quality.

Senator REID. That will be done.

Mr. CASHDOLLAR. Thank you, sir.

[The information follows.]

ncal

NATIONAL CENTER FOR ASSISTED LIVING

1201 L Street, NW
Washington, DC 20005-4014
Phone: 202-842-4444
FAX: 202-842-3860

ASSISTED LIVING

MEETING THE NEEDS OF A GROWING ELDERLY POPULATION

Fact: *The average ancient Greek lived until 18. The median life span of a Puritan was 33.*[1] *In 1991, the average life expectancy of an American male was 71.8 years and 78.9 years for females.*[2]

Fact: *In 1994, about one in eight Americans was age 65 and older. By 2030, one in five Americans will be a senior citizen.*[3]

Fact: *In 1994, 7.3 million Americans needed long term care services. By 2000, this number will rise to 9 million, and skyrocket to as many as 24 million by 2060.*[4]

INTRODUCTION

A combination of extended life expectancy and the graying of America is resulting in an unprecedented demand for a variety of long term care services.

A rapidly growing industry known as "assisted living" has emerged on the long term care spectrum between boarding houses for the elderly (where services are limited to housing) and skilled nursing facilities (which offer complex medical care).

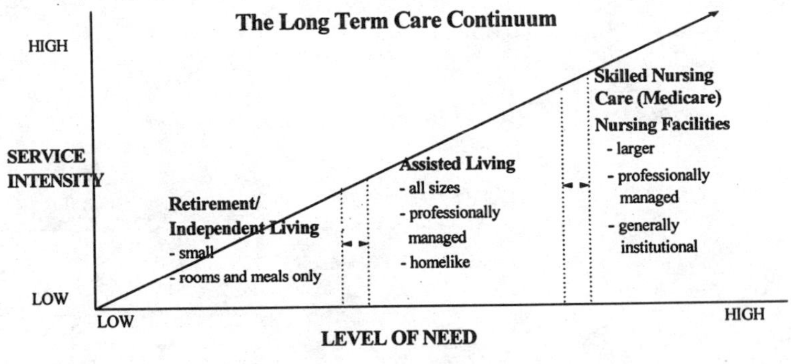

© 1997 by the National Center for Assisted Living

NCAL is the assisted living arm of the American Health Care Association, a federation of 50 affiliated associations representing more than 11,000 non-profit and for-profit assisted living, nursing facility and subacute providers nationally.

Based on a Scandinavian model for senior living, assisted living first emerged in America during the mid-1980s. The concept of assisted living is still so new that the businesses that offer it and the states that license it do not agree on a precise definition or name for assisted living.

Throughout the United States, assisted living is known by as many as 26 different names. Some of the most common are "residential care," "personal care," "congregate care" and "board and care."

In general, assisted living is not a substitute for, but a complement to, nursing facility care. Assisted living combines housing, personal services and light medical or nursing care in an environment that promotes maximum individual independence, privacy and choice. While assisted living residents may be too frail to live alone, they are too healthy to need most of the nursing services provided in a nursing facility. Assisted living residents share the risks and responsibilities for their daily activities and well-being with a residence staff geared to helping them enjoy the freedom and independence of private living.

Assisted living residences are not bound by federal regulation, which helps to keep costs down, as does the fact that assisted living residences generally do not offer the high-tech medical services available in nursing facilities. Whether proprietary or non-profit, assisted living residences serve mostly a private-pay clientele; therefore, consumer demand, not government mandate, is driving the industry's development in America.[5]

THE ASSISTED LIVING PHILOSOPHY

The philosophy of assisted living is to provide or arrange for supervision, assistance and limited health care services to relatively healthy senior citizens when needed. Residents can receive help with an array of personal activities, including: eating, dressing, bathing, transferring and toiletting, as well as meal preparation, laundry, housekeeping, recreation and transportation. While assisted living residences typically do not provide 24-hour skilled nursing care, help with daily tasks may include the supervision of medication by a qualified staff person.

The philosophy also emphasizes the right of the individual to choose the setting for care and services. The American Health Care Association's National Center for Assisted Living (NCAL) believes residents' rights should include the right to:

- Privacy
- Be treated at all times with dignity and respect
- Control personal finances
- Retain and have use of personal possessions
- Interact freely with others both within the home and in the community
- Practice religion or abstain from religious practice
- Control receipt of health-related services
- Be free from abuse and neglect

In the *1997 Facts and Trends: Assisted Living Sourcebook*, results of a NCAL national survey found residences had adopted policies addressing specific issues that many residents view as personal rights. Most residences placed no restrictions on visitors during the day, while 47 percent of the facilities allowed residents to have overnight guests.[6]

© 1997 by the National Center for Assisted Living

The survey also found that a majority of residences (70 percent) allowed the use of tobacco and (47 percent) the consumption of alcohol.

Consistent with the varying policies found in apartment living, the NCAL survey found 33 percent of residences allowed residents to keep small pets. Another 37 percent provided residence-owned pets for all residents to enjoy.

ASSISTED LIVING FACTS

- **Number of Residences** -- The absence of a common definition for assisted living makes it difficult to pinpoint the number of residences in the United States. Past studies put the range between 40,000 and 65,000 residences, housing up to one million people.[(7)] However, recent analyses by NCAL indicate that the number of assisted living residences is probably closer to 25,000, and that there are approximately 800,000 people living in those residences.

- **Resident Profile** -- The "typical" assisted living resident is an 82-year-old woman who is mobile, but needs assistance with one or two personal activities. Although most elderly assisted living residents are female, due to women's longer life expectancies, 29 percent are male. The "average" age of elderly residents, women and men combined, is 82 years according to NCAL's survey.

  The survey also found that while nearly one-third (31 percent) of all residents needed no help taking care of their own personal activities, others did in varying degrees. On average, assisted living residents needed help with 1.6 common personal activities.

Personal Activities	Independent	Some Help	Dependent
Bathing	34%	49%	17%
Dressing	58%	30%	12%
Transferring	78%	15%	7%
Toiletting	84%	10%	6%
Eating	88%	8%	4%

NCAL's survey also found a full 65 percent of assisted living residents needed or accepted help with housework, while 49 percent needed or accepted help with their daily medication.

Residents stay in assisted living residences an average of 3.3 years, and arrive from a variety of settings, according to the NCAL survey.

- 59 percent moved from their homes
- 14 percent came from a nursing facility
- 11 percent came from another assisted living residence
- 11 percent came from hospitals
- 5 percent came from other settings

© 1997 by the National Center for Assisted Living

Conversely, as needs change, elderly people leave assisted living residences. The NCAL survey found that a majority of residents left their assisted living homes because they needed a higher level of medical care.

- 14 percent returned to their homes
- 45 percent went to a nursing facility
- 12 percent went to another assisted living residence
- 11 percent went to a hospital
- 16 percent died
- 3 percent went to other settings

- **Costs** -- Costs for assisted living residences vary greatly and depend on the size of units, services provided and location. The NCAL survey found that 52 percent of all assisted living facilities charge between $1,001 and $2,000 in average monthly rent and fees. Another 20 percent charge between $2,001 and $3,000 and 4 percent charge more than $3,000 each month. A full 24 percent charge less than $1,000, with less than 1 percent charging under $500 per month.

DESIGN AND SERVICES

Assisted living services can be provided in free-standing facilities, near to or integrated with skilled nursing facilities, as components of continuing care retirement communities, or at independent housing complexes.

The NCAL survey found that residents typically can choose furnished or unfurnished studio or one-bedroom units with a private bathroom, though shared bathrooms are quite common. Living units can be shared with another individual. Assisted living residences can range from a high-rise apartment building to a three-story home.

The average size of an assisted living residence is 32 units. NCAL's survey found that 27 percent of residences had kitchenettes and another 14 percent offered full kitchens. Expansive common areas are typical of assisted living residences.

Because assisted living is an evolving long term care industry, the range of services offered by residences is wide. However, some generalizations can be made. Assisted living residences typically offer:

- 24-hour protective oversight and emergency response system
- Three meals a day plus snacks in a group dining room
- The provision and/or coordination of a range of services that promote resident quality of life, including:
    - Personal care, such as help with eating, bathing, dressing, and toiletting
    - Limited health care
    - Provision and/or coordination of required social services
    - Supervision and oversight for persons with cognitive disabilities
    - Social and religious activities

© 1997 by the National Center for Assisted Living

- Exercise and educational activities
- Transportation
- Laundry and linen service
- Housekeeping and maintenance

Assisted living residences generally offer more than basic services. Popular amenities can be available on site, particularly in larger assisted living residences. According to American Association of Retired Persons, a sampling of the various amenities offered includes: libraries; recreation rooms, sometimes with exercise equipment or pool table; cafes and shops; beauty parlors; and chapels.[8]

SERVICE AND STAFFING

When first arriving at an assisted living residence, each resident receives an individualized assessment to determine how the residence's services best can serve his/her needs. This service plan includes an assessment of the individual's physical and psychosocial capabilities. The individual, family, or a responsible party usually assists with the development of the service plan, which is reviewed and updated as needed.

Assisted living residences offer supervision and oversight of individuals with physical and mental impairments. Generally, assisted living residences adopt a philosophy of "aging in place" that allows individuals to remain at the residence as long as they are able to be supervised and maintained by the residence's staff.

The number and type of staff employed by assisted living residences varies greatly and depends on a number of factors, including state regulations, the number of people living in the residence and residents' service requirements.

Assisted living residences employ staff members directly or contract for services with outside providers. A residence staff may include: personal care attendants, nurses, activities coordinators, food service managers, administrators and maintenance personnel. Contract services frequently include: podiatrists, nutritionists, physical therapists, beauticians and physicians.[9]

LICENSURE AND REGULATION

Assisted living residences are not defined or regulated by the federal government. In the absence of federal regulations, most providers are subject to state and local laws. The NCAL survey found most assisted living residences (96 percent) were licensed by the states in which they operate. Residential care is the most common licensure term, followed by assisted living. But regulations between states vary regardless of the licensure term. As a result, competition between providers has become the catalyst for establishing levels of service, controlling costs, and maintaining a high quality of care.

WHO PAYS?

About 90 percent of assisted living services are paid for with private funds, making this market highly sensitive to economic forces.

© 1997 by the National Center for Assisted Living

The Supplementary Security Income, Older Americans Act, and Social Services Block Grant programs pay for some assisted living services, while about 22 states allow the federal Medicaid program to pay for some service components. States have the option to pay for assisted living under the Medicaid program by:

Including the services in the state's Medicaid plan. The Health Care Financing Administration (HCFA) has proposed expanding the Medicaid program to allow states to reimburse for personal care services in a variety of settings, other than the home, which may include assisted living residences.

Petitioning the Department of Health and Human Services for a home- and community-based services waiver under Medicaid. Several states are experimenting with expanding the availability of assisted living services through these waivers.

Other important funding facts to consider:

Assisted living is covered as an "alternative care benefit" in a growing number of long term care insurance policies. Since most elderly Americans do not carry long term care insurance, the majority of people in assisted living residences and/or their families still pay for the care themselves.[10]

Medicare does not pay for assisted living services under any circumstance. Medicare is limited to the provision of short-term, acute care for the elderly.

Managed care is not a significant factor in assisted living currently. According to the 1996 NCAL survey, 5 percent of assisted living residents pay for their care through a managed care program. However, as managed care grows and searches for lower cost alternatives, it is likely to play an increasing role in assisted living.

CONCLUSION

The scope of long term care services offered to the growing number of elderly Americans is ever-expanding. Assisted living, a relatively new and widely popular phenomenon, is on the forefront of this expansion, offering elderly clientele an attractive mixture of independence and personal care.

October 1997

© 1997 by the National Center for Assisted Living

SOURCES

(1) Williams, Doris K. Residential Care Services for the Elderly: Business Guide for Home-Based Eldercare 1991; 1.

(2) Frank B. Hobbs and Bonnie L. Damon. 65+ in the United States. U.S. Bureau of the Census. Current Population Reports, Special Studies, 3-1

(3) Ibid., 2-2

(4) U. S. Bureau of the Census. Statistical Abstract of the United States: 1995

(5) Kane, Rosalie A. and Karen Brown Wilson. Assisted Living in the United States: A New Paradigm for Residential Care for Frail Older Persons? 1993; preface.

(6) American Health Care Association's National Center for Assisted Living. 1997 Facts and Trends: The Assisted Living Sourcebook

(7) Lewin-ICF, Inc. Policy Synthesis on Assisted Living for the Frail Elderly November 9, 1992, II-2.

(8) Assisted Living in the United States, 21.

(9) Ibid., 30.

(10) "Assisted Living: New Thinking, New Model for Frail Elderly" Report on Long Term Care February 23, 1994.

© 1997 by the National Center for Assisted Living

Mr. CASHDOLLAR. Senator, also in your questions to Panel 2, you expressed the need for practical and user-friendly information that would give consumers an idea of how they could pursue quality long-term care. I believe that consumers should have some choice and some exercise of choice in long-term care settings, as Ms. George indicated.

I think that Mr. Panelli's testimony made it clear that we have got kind of a complicated system for telling the public about quality in long-term care. I believe he said that 75 percent of facilities were not in substantial compliance. I think I would just like to make a plea at this point for a system that the public can readily understand.

All that the system now is measuring is deficiencies. We have a system that is all stick and no carrot. I think what we need is a system that focuses on appropriate measures of quality, allows a facility to compare itself to itself over time and to compare itself to other facilities. I see the yellow light is on. I am just going to bolt forward and talk about SecureCare a little bit.

Members of the audience should all have a copy of this in the packet they received when they came here. I would encourage members of the Senate Aging Committee and others to contact the American Health Care Association or me for more information about this. I also urge the Senate Aging Committee seriously to consider proposing an integrated system, a system that protects people against impoverishment such as Dr. Weiss had expressed.

Briefly, the principles of SecureCare are one, transferring long-term care from a welfare program to a health care program. What this means is that America's elderly should not have to go on welfare to receive long-term care services.

Two, coordinate long-term care private resources with Medicare and Social Security. What I mean by this is to finally realize the promise of Social Security and Medicare in terms of securing the financial and health care security for all of America's elderly.

Three, encourage personal and family responsibility for long-term care. The heart of this principle is that in order to make sure that we are going to be able to meet the long-term care needs of America's elderly, we have to re-integrate and assign a primary role to family and personal responsibility and private resources.

Four, maximize quality and control costs through market competition and consumer choice. I think we have got to integrate into our system the kind of incentives that we know can work to improve long-term care through the market and through incentives. I will stop now.

Senator REID. Thank you very much for your very good testimony.

[The prepared statement of Mr. Cashdollar follows:]

Mailing address; PO Box 3226
Carson City, Nevada 89702
(702) 885 - 1006

Statement
of
Winthrop Cashdollar, Executive Director

Nevada Health Care Association

The Many Faces of Long-Term Care: Today's Bitter Pill or Tomorrow's Cure?

Hearings of the

United States Senate
Special Committee on Aging

January 12 & 13,1998

NEVADA HEALTH CARE ASSOCIATION

Good morning, Senator Reid, and representatives of the Special Committee on Aging. I am Winthrop Cashdollar, Executive Director of the Nevada Health Care Association (NHCA), an association of Nevada's long term care providers. NHCA is affiliated with the American Health Care Association (AHCA), a federation of 50 state health care organizations which represents more than 11,000 assisted living, nursing facility, and subacute long term care providers nationwide. Thank you for the opportunity to speak to the U.S. Senate Special Committee on Aging on behalf of long term caregivers and those for whom we care. In my testimony at these hearings, I would like to combine a Nevada perspective with a national perspective and, in so doing, to draw upon some forward-looking work and ideas of the AHCA.

The Nevada Perspective: Challenges We Face May Make Our State a Bellwether

Nevada is unique in many respects. Our state's population growth is the fastest in the nation. The state's economy has developed around a booming gaming industry and rich mineral wealth. Our intergovernmental arrangements are also unique. When it comes to long term care, however, Nevada faces the same challenges as the rest of the nation – only in more concentrated form. Nevada's unique demographics, fiscal circumstances, and state and local government roles can make it a bellwether – or a canary in a silver mine – for the nation's long term care policy.

Demographic Factors

According to information recently publicized by the State of Nevada, our state continues to have the fastest rate of population growth in the nation. With statewide population growth now at 5.5 % annually (6.8% in Clark County), Nevada's population is projected to top two million in 1999. Nevada's elderly population is also growing rapidly, driven not only by overall population growth, but also because the state's beauty, climate, recreational opportunities, and tax structure make it a desirable state in which to retire. U.S. Census data from the 1990 census indicate that Nevada had the greatest percentage growth in population over age 65 between 1980 and 1990 (94%). This continuing growth in the state's elderly population will require a very substantial increase in long term care capacity, workforce, and spending in the coming years.

Fiscal Factors

Nevada levies no state income tax. The state and its counties rely heavily on revenue from gaming and mining. Although these are generally rich sources of government revenue, they leave state and local treasuries subject to boom and bust. Indeed, gaming tax receipts are currently lagging state projections and the price of gold has fallen below $300 an ounce. The rapid growth and development of the state also brings intensified competition for public funds for education, infrastructure, and other needs. Although all states should anticipate an increased fiscal burden for long term care, changing fiscal circumstances in Nevada could intensify budget problems in relatively short order.

Leading the Way to Tomorrow's Cure?

If necessity is the mother of invention, then Nevada must become inventive – and soon. The state's demographic, fiscal, and intergovernmental circumstances are likely to test the limits of the current long term care system sooner and more severely than other parts of the nation. This means that Nevada may need to address access to services, long term care workforce, and financing issues very soon. Although I believe that the nation as a whole needs to move faster on real long term care reform, I would also suggest that Nevada could take a leading role as a site for demonstrating the national reform proposals that follow in this testimony.

The Need for Change in Access to Long Term Care Services

The current governmental division of responsibility for acute health care and long term care for the nation's senior citizens is confusing; places beneficiaries more according to program rigidities than clinical needs; and causes too many of our frail elderly to fall between the cracks of the system. One of the most common complaints about our current government long term care system is that it steers the vast majority of beneficiaries and resources to institutional long term care.

The differences between Medicare and Medicaid are confusing to elderly Americans. Most Americans do not make the distinction between acute care and long term care that our government programs do – an accident of legislative evolution. In order to rationalize access to the full continuum of acute care/long term care services, it is time that we better integrate acute care and long term care for America's senior citizens. This will require a restructuring of the current division of labor between the federal government and the states.

The Need for Change in How We Pursue Quality in Long Term Care

Our long term care system has evolved a very extensive and complicated regulatory apparatus to pursue the safety and well-being of the nation's long term care residents. Ten years after the enactment of the Nursing Home Reforms of the Omnibus Budget Reconciliation Act of 1987 (OBRA '87), however, there remain serious misgivings about the quality of care in the nation's long term care facilities. Long term caregivers have gotten scant credit for their efforts to realize the promise of the OBRA '87 reforms. Many in the Congress, the state legislatures, and the public want to apply still stronger doses of the same medicine.

However, more of the same – pushing still harder on the current regulatory apparatus – can only yield marginal benefits at best. It is time for the nation to try a new approach to long term care quality improvement.

The current regulatory approach to quality is all stick and no carrot. The current system registers only "deficiencies" and offers no recognition or rewards for improvement. We all know from personal experience, and from what we have heard about other industries and endeavors, that such a negative approach is not the best way to pursue quality. Indeed, the current regulatory system has serious negative consequences for the morale, motivation, and retention of long term caregiver staff.

Long term care residents would be better served by an approach that focuses on improving key measures of well-being and satisfaction over time. Appropriate and consistent quality measurement is crucial to the ability of long term care providers to understand central quality issues; to learn from mistakes; and to improve. If quality measurement is not consistent; if it dwells too much on factors not relevant to resident well-being; if it focuses on fault-finding rather than improvement; then it is not conducive to enhancing quality of care.

The state of South Dakota has asked HCFA for a waiver to demonstrate an alternative system for measuring and improving quality in the state's long term care facilities. This system, which would run parallel to the current regulatory system, would facilitate the comparison between nursing facilities on key measures of resident well-being and satisfaction. It would also, of course, allow a facility to compare its performance on key measures of quality over time. The NHCA and AHCA strongly urge Nevada's Senators and Members of the Senate Aging Committee to take an active role in helping such a demonstration to go forward in South Dakota – or even in Nevada.

The Need for Change in How We Pay for Long Term Care

Our society has not made adequate provision for financing the costs of long term care. Individuals and families are not saving for, or insuring themselves against, the costs of long term care. The demographic tidal wave of Americans who will be elderly in the coming decades will stretch Medicaid beyond its capacity.

Most elderly Americans are unaware of the magnitude of long term care costs and of the limits of government assistance. Most Americans do not foresee needing long term care. Most do not realize how costly months or years of long term care can be. Many Americans wrongly assume that government programs or their general health insurance will cover the costs of any long term care services they might need. For all these reasons, individuals and families face long term care costs for which they have not planned and which they cannot afford.

The costs of long term care can quickly wipe out the assets even of those who have worked and saved for a lifetime. The average cost of nursing home care is now approximately $41,000 per year (according to the AHCA). While the single greatest risk of catastrophic health care cost facing the elderly is the cost of nursing home care, the nation's current long term care policy does not promote personal planning, saving, or the purchase of insurance against the risk of long term care costs. Nor does the nation's government sector provide comprehensive social insurance against the financial catastrophe of long term care costs. Only after a long term care recipient has been impoverished does government assistance become available through Medicaid – a welfare program.

In recent decades, total Medicaid payments (state and federal) have seen tremendous growth. Although Medicaid spending growth has leveled off in the very recent past, total Medicaid spending tripled during the first half of this decade -- from $54.5 billion in federal fiscal year 1989 to almost $160 billion in fiscal year 1995 (HCFA data). Under current policies, demographic certainties -- with or without an economic downturn – will bring a return of rampant Medicaid growth in the years to come.

Without fundamental long term care financing reform, our growing elderly population will come to rely much more heavily on Medicaid to pay for long term care. According to the Health Care Financing Administration (HCFA), Medicaid was the source of payment for more than two-thirds (68.3%) of nursing facility residents in 1996. U.S. Census Bureau projections show that the fastest growing segment of our population is people age 85 and older – the age group which needs long term care the most. Today's long term care financing system cannot meet tomorrow's long term care needs.

An Alternative: Integrate Acute Care and Long Term Care for the Elderly

The nation created Social Security and Medicare because Americans did not feel it was right to let old age, disability, or the costs of health care bankrupt senior citizens after a lifetime of work, taxpaying, and self-sufficiency. Yet Medicaid requires that those who have worked and paid their own way for the whole of their adult lives must lose everything (or legally hide everything) before they can get help with long term care. It is a welfare program. It is time to change this – time to move long term care from welfare to health care. Congress should transform government programs to make a federal long term care program – along with Social Security and Medicare – the third pillar of security for America's senior citizens.

Many reject the idea of "federalizing" long term care out of hand because they believe it would inevitably cost incalculable sums of taxpayer money. A new federal entitlement would indeed cost untold billions if it were developed as an entirely federal benefit merely added to Medicare coverage. The new benefit can be made quite fiscally responsible, however, if it is conditioned on a prior exercise of responsibility by beneficiaries. For example, government long term care coverage could be extended only after an individual purchases an appropriate long term care insurance policy.

This is not a new idea. Rather, it is a combination of several ideas already proposed or in practice. The idea of federalizing Medicaid long term care can be credited largely to former Senator Nancy Kassebaum (R-KS). During the 104th Congress, Senator Kassebaum introduced legislation that proposed dividing the Medicaid program. Her legislation would have sent the component of Medicaid that provides acute care to the poor (along with Food Stamps, AFDC, and the Supplemental Feeding Program for Women, Infants, and Children) to the states and would have sent responsibility for long term care for the elderly to the federal government. Such an arrangement would allow states to take undivided responsibility for the welfare population, which would facilitate consolidation and coordination of all the various programs that serve this population. Meanwhile, the federal government would have sole responsibility for the elderly, facilitating the integration of acute health care, long term care, and income security programs.

The idea of establishing federal long term care coverage that follows a period of personal responsibility dates back almost ten years to legislation introduced by then Senator George Mitchell (D-Maine). Senator Mitchell's "Long Term Care Assistance Act of 1988" would have put in place federal long term care coverage beginning after a two-year period, during which an individual would have been responsible for his or her own long term care. Individuals would have been expected to cover themselves during this period of personal responsibility with savings or long term care insurance if they could afford it.

A variation of this proposal is already in practice in New York State. New York currently extends Medicaid long term care coverage to those who purchase qualified long term care insurance policies even if they have considerable assets. Under this program, designed and supported with the help of the Robert Wood Johnson Foundation, an individual who purchases a policy that meets all the requirements of the program qualifies for New York's relatively generous Medicaid long term care coverage when the benefits of the private insurance policy are exhausted. (Connecticut, Indiana, and California have similar programs.) Such a program offers a responsible alternative to the practice of using legal loopholes to qualify for Medicaid coverage by hiding assets. This same approach could be adopted nationwide and linked to the Medicare program.

SecureCare: Principles for Long Term Care Reform

The American Health Care Association is working to move forward with reforms to address the long term care access, quality, and financing needs of America's senior citizens. As the nation's largest association of long term care providers, AHCA is committed to leading efforts to bring about progressive and compassionate reforms that will enable our nation to address the problems of the current health care system for those in need of long term care services and to meet the demographic, political, and fiscal challenges on the horizon. I would like to take this opportunity to present to the Senate Aging Committee AHCA's SecureCare principles for long term care reform.

- **Transform long term care from a welfare program to a health care program.**

  Fundamental compassion and fairness demand that we end a policy that requires Americans to bankrupt themselves and become welfare recipients in order to receive needed long term care services.

- **Coordinate long term care private resources with Medicare and Social Security.**

  Health care policy should support the integration of physician, hospital, and long term care into a seamless system that provides Americans with the health care, long term care, and financial security they need and deserve.

- **Encourage personal and family responsibility for long term care.**

  The government sector should not be expected to – and will not be able to – pay for all the long term care that a growing population of elderly will need. Families and individuals must have the information and tools they need in order to plan for their long term care needs. Consumers need to learn about and use new resources such as private long term care insurance.

- **Maximize quality and control costs through market competition and consumer choice.**

  To provide Americans with care that is efficient and cost effective, the federal program for acute and long term care coverage must be funded through a consumer-driven, competitive insurance market. Insurers and providers must be held accountable for the quality of the care they provide. Consumers and their families should be free to choose where they receive their care.

AHCA is working to turn its SecureCare principles into a more detailed proposal for long term care reform. I invite Members of the Senate Aging Committee and other interested parties to contact the AHCA – or me – for more information on the SecureCare proposal.

Conclusion

Although the nation's demographics and fiscal forecasts make long term care a daunting issue, lawmakers dare not shy away from it. If neglected or mishandled, the long term care issue could haunt us for a very long time. Only if we take timely steps on a path that will lead long term care policy in a new direction will we avoid the problems that plague current entitlement programs for the elderly. The Nevada Health Care Association commends Senator Harry Reid for holding these hearings and for his work to address long term care issues.

SECURECARE

Secure Care

MEETING

THE NEEDS

OF AN

AGING NATION

FACT: The average Ancient Greek livec until age 18. The median life span of a Puritan was 33 years. In 1991, the averag American life expectancy was about 72 years for men 79 years for women. ■ FACT: In 1994, about one in eight Americans was age 65 or older. By 2030, one in five Americans will be a senior citizen. ■ FACT: In 1994, 7.3 million Americans needed long term care services. By 2000, this number will rise to 9 million, and by 2060 it will skyrocket to about 24 million.

Society Is Changing And So Must Our Long Term Care System

Americans are living longer and healthier lives, thanks to better diet, better medical care, and safer living and working environments. But no one is immune from the effects of aging that far too often result in chronic illness and reduced physical or mental ability. *Consider one more fact: two out of every five Americans will require nursing home care at some point in their lives.*

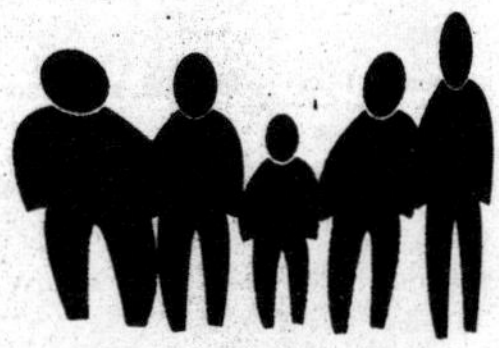

Two out of five Americans will be cared for in a nursing home at some point in their lives.

SOURCE: *New England Journal of Medicine*

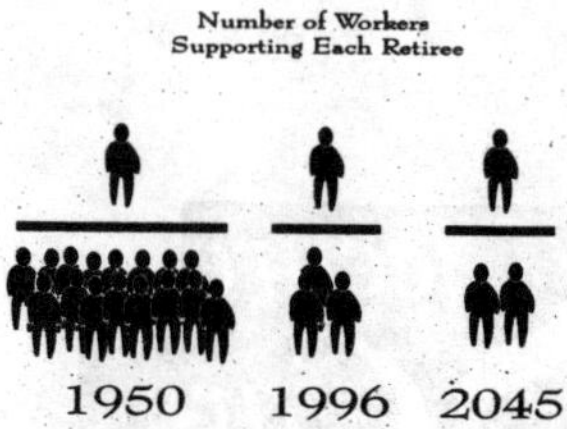

Ratio of Retirees to Workers

In 1950, there were 16 workers to every retiree. Today there are three. By 2045, there will only be two workers to support each retiree.

SOURCE: *New York Times*

Our population and our lifestyles are changing in ways that significantly affect how we provide for those in need of long term care.

Change is everywhere:

In the workplace—The number of workers to support each retiree is declining.

In our families—Our mobile society means that sons and daughters liv farther from their parent than ever before.

In our homes—The num ber of single-parent an two-working-parent house holds continues to grow.

All these changes mean greater burden for ou families and our society i providing and paying fo the long term care that growing number of ou citizens will require.

THE CURRENT LONG TERM CARE SYSTEM IS BROKEN

Problem: Long term care is costly, and older people are not financially prepared to pay the $41,000 annual cost for a nursing home stay or the average $89 per visit fee by a home care registered nurse.

Problem: Most people mistakenly believe that Medicare will cover the cost of long term care. The reality is that Medicare only covers nursing home costs for a short period of time following a hospital stay to recuperate from an acute illness or injury.

Problem: Two out of three nursing home residents are forced onto Medicaid to pay for their care. Medicaid is a federal-state program that provides health care to people who are impoverished. Medicaid was designed to help the poor, not the elderly. But Medicaid has become our nation's long term care system by default.

Problem: Millions of people who worked all their lives and paid taxes have been impoverished because they got sick and needed long term care. Millions more face the same fate unless the system changes. For the elderly to qualify for Medicaid, they must spend all of their life savings until they meet the state-determined poverty level. Thus, the need for long term care forces the middle-class elderly onto welfare to receive care.

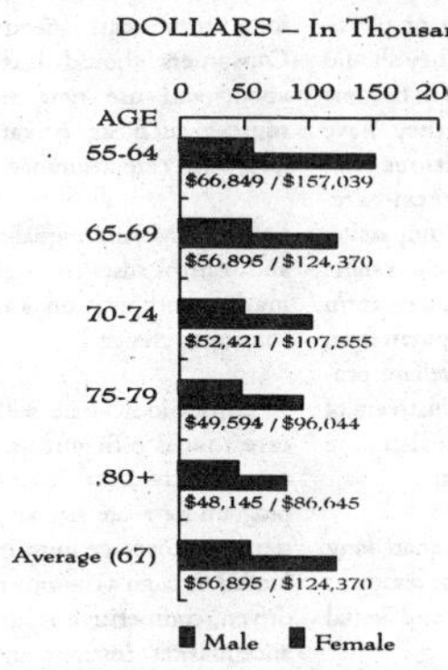

Long Term Care Costs – 1995

The average American man can expect to spend $56,895 on long term care. The average woman will spend $124,370.

SOURCE: Lifeplans Inc.

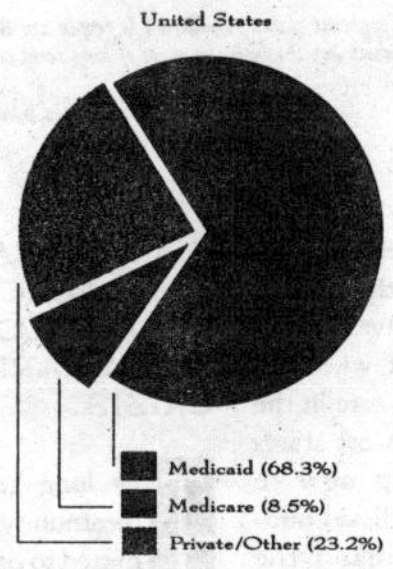

Residents by Primary Payer Source – 1996

More than 1 million people rely on Medicaid to pay for their nursing home care.

SOURCE: Health Care Financing Administration

POPULATION – In Millions

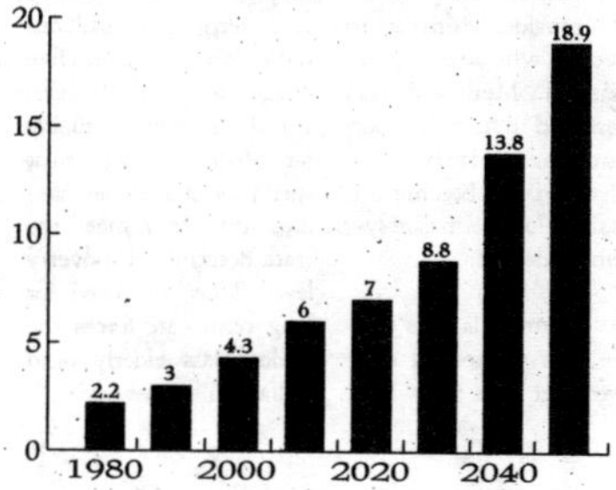

85-and-Older Growth Chart

The fastest growing segment of our population is people age 85 and older. People in that age group are the heaviest users of long term care services.

SOURCE: U.S. Bureau of the Census

Problem: Medicaid cannot support the demographic tidal wave of aging baby boomers who will need long term care in the next century. Most states are struggling now to meet their Medicaid budgets. The demand the elderly will place on Medicaid soon will outweigh Medicaid's ability to meet the elderly's long term care needs.

SECURE CARE: A SOLUTION TO THE LONG TERM CARE CRISIS

The long term care community is committed to progressive and compassionate reforms that will enable our nation to meet the long term care needs of all Americans.

We call our approach *SecureCare*. It is built on four principles designed to solve our nation's long term care crisis while preserving the safety net for America's poor elderly and disabled.

Solution: Transform long term care from a welfare program to a health care program.

The elderly are not forced to impoverish themselves to get hospital or physician services. They should not be required to become poor because they have medical conditions that require long term care. Fundamental compassion and fairness demand shifting our nation's long term care financing system from the Medicaid welfare program to the mainstream of our nation's health care financing system.

Solution: Coordinate long term care private resources with Medicare and Social Security.

Health care policy should support integration of hospital, physician, and long term care into a seamless system that provides all Americans with the personal security, health, and long term care services they need and deserve.

Solution: Encourage personal and family responsibility for long term care.

The government's capacity to pay for long term care is decreasing. Families and individuals must have the information and tools they need to plan for their long term care needs. Consumers should learn about and use new resources such as private long term care insurance.

Solution: Maximize quality and control costs through market competition and consumer choice.

To provide individuals with care that is efficient and cost effective, the federal program for acute and long term care coverage must be funded through a consumer-driven, competitive insurance market. Insurers and providers must be held accountable for the quality of the care they provide. Consumers and their families should be free to choose where they receive their care.

THE TIME FOR CHANGE IS NOW

Our nation is not prepared to care for its aging population. We must replace the existing long term care system with a new system that is designed to meet the long term care needs of our grandparents, our parents, and ourselves before the current system collapses.

Elderly and disabled Americans deserve quality long term care. It is what each of us wants for our loved ones and ourselves. If we are to ensure that quality long term care is available to all who need it, the nation must work together for change. *SecureCare* is that change.

Senator REID. Lea Mason, will you please proceed?

STATEMENT OF LEA MASON, R.N., SECRETARY, HOME HEALTH CARE ASSOCIATION OF NEVADA

Ms. MASON. Thank you, Senator. Senator Reid, Mr. Chairman, and everyone in the room, thank you so much for having the Home Health Care Association of Nevada, which we affectionately call HHCAN, participate on this very prestigious panel. We are honored and pleased that you have invited our views on this complex and challenging issue.

There are about 105 licensed and certified home health agencies in Nevada and about 60 percent belong to our association. The leadership of HHCAN and all Nevada home care providers share Senator Reid's concern for the elderly citizens of Nevada and the nation.

Not much information has surfaced in the national media describing the massive cuts to home health care reimbursement enacted by the passage of the Balanced Budget Act of 1997. Nevada citizens, however, will soon face the devastating effects of that legislation.

For decades, home health and hospice care have supported the young, the disabled, the chronically ill, the elderly, and the dying in their homes. We have fostered independence, promoted health, and given comfort. We have educated, treated, provided personal care and therapy, and come to care for millions of patients and their families.

We have seen care in the home progress from simple dressing and catheter changes to high tech intravenous therapy and ventilators. We now provide care at home that as recently as five years ago was considered unsafe in the home and safe only in acute care, sub-acute care, or skilled nursing facilities.

Home health and hospice care have saved millions by enabling patients to recover in the most comfortable and cost-effective environment, their own homes. Every week we receive thank yous and letters of satisfaction from patients, families, and the community. But in January 1998, many elderly Nevadans will lose their current home health services, and as the year passes, many other Nevadans may find they are unable to get the services that they need.

It has been estimated that more than 16 billion will be deleted from projected Medicare home health and hospice expenditures over the next five years. What does this mean to Nevada? It means a shift from Medicare to Medicaid, Nevada's medical program for the poor. This shift could spell disaster for Nevada, the state with the fastest growing 65 and older population, as cited by Senator Reid in December of last year.

So Congress, albeit with good intentions, obvious concern, and a genuine desire to help, appears to have passed the buck from the Federal to the State Government. The multitude of changes in Medicare, as included in the Balanced Budget Act of 1997, herald the demise of desperately needed home care services.

We have provided a growing amount of evidence concerning these changes and we do not need to discuss them here, but we would like to point out that by shedding its responsibility to the elderly, the Federal Government has put at risk those older patients who need home care services in order to continue to live independently at home.

While we understand Congress faced enormous challenges and difficult decisions, the saddest part of this scenario will be the effect on elderly Nevadans who have thus far been able to retain their pride and independence with the help of home care.

Let me give you a real life example. One of our Nevada home health agencies received a call from the daughter of a 96-year-old woman who resides in an assisted living facility. The daughter was told by their current home care provider that beginning in February, Medicare would not pay for the daily care her mother received for a draining hip wound because it was chronic.

Her mother is unable to do the care, but is independent enough to live away from a nursing home. While the daughter is willing to learn the care, she is unable to provide it every day and has not found anyone willing to assume that responsibility. The mother and daughter cannot afford to pay an agency to do the care, but have too many assets to qualify for Medicaid. The daughter said she was given until the middle of January to find an answer for her dilemma.

What will Nevadans face in similar situations? In order to receive care, elderly patients will be forced into nursing homes. Emergency room visits and hospital stays will increase as elderly patients bounce in and out of facilities because diabetic, cardiac, and other conditions have begun to deteriorate, and elderly patients and their families will be forced to "spend down" assets in order to remain at home but still qualify for Medicaid.

It has been well-demonstrated that acute, sub-acute, and skilled nursing care are more expensive than home care and all of the described scenarios are much less desirable than quality care at home. Quality care will be more difficult to provide, however, as costs escalate.

But the most troubling aspect of the Medicare cuts is that Nevada's taxpayers will be paying for the changes in home care, not only through increased costs, but also through the pain of watching friends and loved ones lose their dignity and independence.

We in Nevada must ensure that home health care for our elderly is available, affordable, and accessible. I see I have already hit the red light, so I would just like to say that we in home care appreciate and care for our elders and that we share Senator Reid's concern, and we would like to move forward to a satisfactory solution.

[The prepared statement of Ms. Mason follows:]

SENATE SPECIAL COMMITTEE ON AGING
FIELD HEARING
THE MANY FACES OF LONG TERM CARE:
TODAY'S BITTER PILL OR TOMORROW'S CURE?
CHAIR: SENATOR HARRY REID
JANUARY 12, 1998
9:00 - 11:30 A.M.
WEST CHARLESTON LIBRARY
6301 WEST CHARLESTON
LAS VEGAS, NEVADA

Senate Special Hearing on Aging
Field Hearing
January 12, 1998
Las Vegas, Nevada
Prepared by Lea A. Mason, R.N., B.S.N.
Director, Barton Memorial Hospital Home Health and
Hospice of the Lake/Valley
South Lake Tahoe, CA
Gardnerville, NV

Honorable Senator Harry Reid:
Mr. Chairman:
Distinguished Panel Members and Guests:

Thank you for inviting the Home Health Care Association of Nevada (HHCAN) to participate on this most prestigious panel. We are honored and pleased that you have invited our views on this most complex and challenging issue. There are about 105 licensed/certified home health agencies in Nevada, about 60% of which belong to our association. The leadership of HHCAN, and all Nevada home care providers, share Senator Reid's concern for the elderly citizens of Nevada and the nation.

Not much information has surfaced in the national media describing the massive cuts to home health care reimbursement enacted by the passage of the Balanced Budget Act of 1997. Nevada's citizens, however, will soon face the devastating effects of that legislation.

For decades, home health and hospice care have supported the young, the disabled, the chronically ill, the elderly and the dying in their homes. We have fostered independence, promoted health and given comfort. We have educated, treated, provided personal care and therapy, and come to care for millions of patients and their families. We have seen care in the home progress from simple dressing and catheter changes to high tech intravenous therapy and ventilators. We now provide care at home that as recently as five years ago was considered safe only in an acute care hospital, a subacute unit, or a skilled nursing facility. Home health and hospice care have saved millions of dollars by enabling patients to recover in the most cost-effective and comfortable location - their homes. Every week we receive thank yous and letters of satisfaction from patients, families and the community.

But in January, 1998, many elderly Nevadans will lose their current home health services. And as the year passes, many other Nevadans may find they are unable to get the home care services they need. It has been estimated that more than $16 billion will be deleted from projected Medicare home health and hospice expenditures over the next five years. What does this mean to Nevada? It means a shift from Medicare to Medicaid - Nevada's medical program for the poor. This shift could spell disaster for Nevada, the state with "the fastest growing 65 and older population" (Senator Harry Reid, December, 1997). So Congress, albeit with good intentions, obvious concern, and a genuine desire to help, appears to have passed the buck from the federal to the state government.

The multitude of changes in Medicare included in the Balanced Budget Act of 1997, herald the demise of desperately needed home care services. The stacks of evidence we have provided concerning these changes need not be discussed here, but we would like to point out that by shedding its responsibility to the elderly, the federal government has put at risk those older patients who need home care services in order to continue to live independently at home.

While we understand Congress faced enormous challenges and difficult decisions, the saddest part of this scenario will be the effect on elderly Nevadans, who have thus far been able to retain their pride and independence with the help of home care. Let me give you a real life example. One of our Nevada home health agencies received a call from the daughter of a 96 year old woman who resides in an assisted living facility. The daughter was told by their current home health care provider that beginning in February, Medicare would not pay for the daily care her mother received for a draining hip wound, because it was chronic. Her mother is unable to do the care, but is independent enough to live away from a nursing home. While the daughter is willing to learn the care, she is unable to provide it every day, and has not found anyone willing to assume the care. The mother and daughter can not afford to pay an agency to do the daily care, but have too many assets to qualify for Medicaid. The daughter stated she had until the middle of January to find a solution for her dilemma.

What will Nevadans face in similar situations? In order to receive care:

1. Elderly patients will be forced into nursing homes.
2. Emergency Room visits and hospital stays will increase as elderly patients bounce in and out of facilities because diabetic, cardiac and other conditions have begun to deteriorate.
3. Elderly patients and their families will be forced to "spend down" assets in order to remain at home, but still qualify for Medicaid.

It has been well demonstrated that acute, subacute, and skilled nursing care are more expensive than home care, and all of the described scenarios are much less desirable than quality care at home. Quality care will be more difficult to provide, however, as costs escalate. But, the most troubling aspect of the Medicare cuts is that Nevada taxpayers will be paying for the changes in home care, not only through increased state taxes to fund Medicaid, but also through the pain of watching friends and loved ones lose their dignity and independence. We in Nevada must ensure that home health care for our elderly is available, affordable, and accessible.

I know our time is brief, so I would just like to say that we care for our elderly and thank the Senator for allowing us to share our concerns. We will be happy to provide any and all information that will help Senator Reid and his colleagues to arrive at a satisfactory solution. Our recommendations will be submitted before February 2, 1998, and let me repeat, we very much appreciate being allowed to participate on this important issue and we look forward to being called upon in the future.

Questions:

1. Why should home health care be considered as an alternative to the use of long term care facilities?

   While long term care facilities provide quality care, there are not enough beds in Nevada, especially in rural areas. Waiting lists are weeks to months long. In order to be placed in long term care facilities, many rural residents would have to relocate to areas outside their communities. This removes them from their support systems, both emotionally and physically. A home care option provides many levels of care, from simple case management to high tech services. Home care can also bring in community resources, reducing the cost to state and federal programs, and improving the patient's quality of life.

2. How can we control costs in the home care industry?

   Any program that is cost reimbursed, as home care is now, will never be cost-effective. I can briefly share with you that the Prospective Payment System, which utilizes a flat rate per illness episode, would be the best possible option for cost savings. It requires health care providers to be efficient, effective, and prudent in their care delivery - without sacrificing elderly citizens on the altar of cost cutting.

   HCFA has been working on this alternative for nearly five years, and in spite of enormous input and involvement from providers and state associations across the nation, has not been able to arrive at a workable solution. Instead, home care is looking at changes to Medicare that while they were supposed to improve the system, have had the unintended consequences of being punitive, unproductive, and the cause of the closure of many home health agencies. The cost savings identified by regulators will result in less care, higher costs in the long run, and most of all, increase the burden on Nevada; which will have to jump into the breach and pick up where Medicare leaves off.

HOME HEALTH CARE ASSOCIATION OF NEVADA
P.O. BOX 12190 RENO, NV 89510-2190 702-323-6003 FAX 702-853-2166

Ruth Jagodzinski, President
Roberta Skelton, Vice President
Lea Mason, Secretary
Richard Hodges, Treasurer
John Busse, Exec. Director

TO: SENATOR RAY RAWSON, CHAIR
MEMBERS, LEGISLATIVE COMMITTEE ON HEALTH CARE

FROM: JOHN D. BUSSE, Executive Director,
Home Health Care Association of Nevada

DATE: November 17, 1997

RE: December 1, 1997, Report on Home Health Care Issues

Introduction

The Home Health Care Association of Nevada appreciates the opportunity to participate in the study as outlined in the Assembly Concurrent Resolution No. 28, and assist you in our area of expertise.

There are 105 licensed/certified home health care agencies in Nevada — about 60 percent belong to HHCAN — the growth of home health in the past 5-7 years is in part due to the health care industry and payers (private and government) recognizing that home health can deliver quality care at a lower cost. For appropriate clients home health can mean quicker recovery, less institutional care, and lower cost for all of us.

General

The Federal Regulatory changes contained in the Balanced Budget Act of 1997 (BBA 1997) will be felt far beyond the agencies and clients. Attached is a summary providing specifics on curtailment of payment and services under Medicare. The details for many of these federal cutbacks have not yet been published.

The total impact will not be known for some time, however, we can anticipate a cost shift from the federal to the state and local level, including Medicaid. We may experience shortages in services due to underfunding and smaller providers leaving the field or going out of business. One way or the other, we will feel this shift ··· most likely through higher insurance premiums and higher taxes.

The new financial "beneficiary cap" per 60 day period for Medicare will effect from 20—30 percent of current home health clients including the long-term heavy care clients, some of whom have been cared for by their family with home health support for 10 years. We will see cost shifting to Medicaid; more placement and more Medicaid applicants, as families are forced to "spend down" to keep a mother, father, child, etc. at home.

continued . . .

Other BBA Federal Regulation also include a $50,000 bond be posted by each agency, and criminal background check and fingerprinting of all Certified Nurse Assistants (CNAs). Nevada's AB 155 makes fingerprinting and FBI background checks mandatory for all owners and employees of SNF's ICF's HHA's and group care homes.

Other Federal cuts that will affect Medicare clients include reduced O_2 and DME, drugs, and increased documentation for allowable DME.

Mandates for a Prospective Pay System for home health care by 10/1/98 OR a reduction of payments of another 15 percent.

Shift of the home health care benefit from Part A to Part B of Medicare will be completed by 2002. For Medicare recipients without Part B, there will no longer be any home health care benefit, and premiums will be over $100 a month for Part B.

1997 Balanced Budget Act (Medicare changes for home health care)

The following is an outline of key elements that will have considerable impact on Medicare beneficiaries and subsequently, to providers and payers.

Specifics for many of these listed categories have not yet been provided.

Budget Provision	Important Dates
Interim payments: The cost limits for FY's 1998 and 1999 must be based on 105% of median and a per-patient cap based on 1994 costs	Affects cost reporting periods on or after *October 1, 1997.* HCFA must release cost limit numbers *January 1, 1997* and disclose per-patient caps by *April 1, 1997.*
Location of services: HHAs and hospices are paid based on the location of the patient's home, not the provider's office.	Affects cost report periods that start on or after *October 1, 1997.*
Part B shift: Shifts home health visits to Part B, except the first 100 following a three-day hospital stay.	Affects visits made on or after *January 1, 1998.*
Venipuncture: Medicare no longer covers as a home health qualifying service.	Budget mandates that this provision must take effect six months after the budget's enactment (August 5, 1997). HCFA officials are still working out the details but estimate this could effect patient certifications after **February 5, 1998.**

A prospective payment system for home health agencies.	If HCFA doesn't have PPS in place for HHAs by *October 1, 1998*, payments must be reduced for HHAs by another 15%.
Home oxygen reimbursement cuts: Compounding a phased-in 30% fee cut will be a freeze on consumer price index updates for the next five years.	On *January 1, 1998*, there will be a 25% reduction from the 1997 fee schedule. On *January 1, 1999*, another 5% will be cut.
New Inherent Reasonableness (IR) regulations: HCFA has received carte blanche to determine how it will use IR authority to process cuts of 15% or less.	HCFA expects to write new regulations as soon as possible. The IR authority previously given HCFA expired on *August 5*.
Competitive bidding demonstration: HCFA must establish five projects at three locations each. At least one site must test competitive bidding on O_2.	The budget requires these projects be in place by *January 1998*, though a HCFA official stated that it is more realistic to look for the projects to begin *January 1, 1999*.
Reimbursement cut for Part B prescription drugs: Payments on such DME drugs as albuteral will be reduced from 100% to 95% of the average wholesale price.	The cuts will affect all services provided on and after *January 1, 1998*.
Blood glucose monitoring strips cut by 10%: On the plus side, coverage will be expanded to include Type II diabetics.	The budget requires all of these changes to be in effect by *January 1, 1998*.
Early hospital transfers: HCFA must select 10 DRGs for which payments will be reduced to hospitals when patients are transferred too early to HHAs and skilled nursing facilities. HHAs can expect a drop-off in referrals of sickly patients.	Payments will be reduced to hospitals beginning *October 1, 1998*.
Hospice: The two biggest changes involve patient benefit periods (after first six months, there will be recertification every 60 days) and the ability to use contract physicians.	Affects all services provided after *August 1, 1997*.

Surety bonds: All HHAs and HME suppliers must post security bonds of at least $50,000 and up to $3 Million to continue participating in Medicare program. Midicaid will require a separate bond.	Budget requires this to be in effect by *January 1, 1998*. HCFA is expected to issue its requirements in *October 1997*.
Consumer Price Index Update: Orthotic and prosthetic payments increase 1% annually. Increases on all other DME and PEN will be frozen	The CPI increase for orthotic and prosthetic payments kicks in *January 1, 1998*.
Apply fee schedules to parenteral and enteral nutrition (PEN), home dialysis equipment and supplies: These items are currently paid using a "reasonable charge" method.	A fee schedule must be in place by *January 1, 1998*. However, the changes must not result in higher or lower reimbursement in its first year.

Example: Venipuncture—A seemingly innocuous curtailment of coverage is the disallowance of venipuncture (blood drawing). This is a service needed to monitor the laboratory results for patients with strokes, heart attacks, and other conditions requiring ongoing control and oversight through lab test.

SUMMARY

The concerns for availability and continued appropriate home health services are shared by all home health providers. The BBA of 1997 will, without a doubt, reduce payments and the access to care in the home. Unfortunately, the real impact on providers and consumers will not be felt until much later because many regulatory details are still being worked on by HHS and HCFA, with yet unknown consequences. Two separate letters of concerns from two agencies who serve large rural populations are attached.

Availability, access and funding concerns have to be addressed in collaboration with health care providers and regulators which hopefully we can achieve at the state and local level since the federal involvements were almost exclusively driven by budget savings concerns.

HHCAN pledges continued involvement and interaction with those seeking solutions and answers to the problems, concerns and issues involving home health.✦

MacKelvie & Associates, P.C.
Attorneys at Law
333 West Wacker Drive
Suite 950
Chicago, Illinois 60606-1218
(312) 332-0533

FAX (312) 332-0547

MEMORANDUM

TO: Our Clients & Friends

RE: Balanced Budget Act of 1997
The Home Health Benefit

As you may know, the Balanced Budget Act of 1997 ("BBA") created dramatic changes for Medicare home health and hospice benefits. Among the major changes included a new interim reimbursement system, payment based upon location of service, nondiscrimination in post-hospital referrals, a shift to Part B, a new statutory definition of "part-time or intermittent care", a "homebound" definition and the elimination of venipuncture as a qualifying skilled nursing service. The BBA also established normative standards for clinical claims, eliminated PIP, reduced Diagnostic Relatd Groups ("DRG") payments to hospitals for "early" home health discharges, and instituted the development of a Prospective Payment System ("PPS"). I am general counsel for the American Federation of Home Health Agencies ("AFHHA"). AFHHA and the home care industry are concerned about the impact of onerous provisions of the BBA on home health beneficiaries and on the home health industry. Below is an analysis of the BBA as it impacts the financial aspects of home health.

The constriction of the home health benefit as directed by the BBA contradicts the Health Care Financing Administration's ("HCFA") vision statement, which would guarantee access to quality health care to patients regardless of where or who provided the care. The entire Medicare Program should be focused on the beneficiaries who paid their tax dollars with the anticipation of receiving a benefit in the future.

Unfortunately, the BBA poses the threat of significantly limiting the availability of home health to Medicare beneficiaries, while ultimately replacing home health with services rendered in hospitals or skilled nursing facilities, at a higher cost to the Medicare Program.

Current statistics indicate that, on average, a day's treatment received by a Medicare beneficiary from home health is $1,784 less expensive than a day's care in the hospital (based on the current Medicare reimbursement for hospitals). The statistics also show that home health is $246 per day less expensive than care rendered in skilled nursing facilities (based on skilled nursing facilities average per diem payments). ***(Source: Hospital and skilled nursing facilities data from Social Security Bulletin, Annual Statistical Supplement, 1994 and 1995. Home care information is from HCFA, Bureau of Data Management.)***

Home Health Care in the 90s and Beyond

The home health industry is the future of health care, because of the level of care that can be rendered in the patient's own home, without compromising standards of care provided. The government is concerned over the growth in the home health industry, growing from 4% to 10.5% of the Medicare expenditures from 1986 to 1993, per testimony before Congress on July 23, 1997 by Dr. Bruce Vladeck, then the Administrator of HCFA.

When you consider the cost-effective nature of home health, who is to say that it should not be 25% of the Medicare benefit, if similar care can be provided at a lower cost?

Many individual providers of Medicare home health services are now faced with very onerous changes in their operations as a result of the passage of the BBA. If there is not a change in the legislation as it was passed, many such providers could be faced with cutting over 50% of its operations in order to meet the cost restrictions imposed by the BBA. The BBA will result in services to patients being cut in order to meet the per beneficiary cost limits in the BBA. This reduction of costs would affect the employment of many individuals, and could result in the closure of branch offices in rural areas.

Scoring of the Home Health Provision

In looking at the scoring of the savings projected from the home health benefit by the Congressional Budget Office (CBO), it would appear that Congress was provided incorrect information by either the CBO or by HCFA. It also appears that the scoring of the savings from the home health industry is incorrect.

Congress was told that the home health provisions of the BBA would lead to a ***reduction in the rate of growth of the Medicare home health benefit.*** HCFA said that it **sought $16.1 billion in such reductions** in growth over the five-year period from fiscal year 1998 through fiscal year 2002. However, as shown below, HCFA's own **budget projections had earlier shown a growth of only $11.3 billion** over that same five-year period.

Page 3

Fiscal Year	Initial HCFA Budget for Home Health from Office of Actuary	Budgeted Growth in Home Health Expenditures per HCFA	Projected Scoring by Congressional Budget Office by Year	Difference Between HCFA Budgeted Growth versus CBO Projected Cuts
1997	$ 20,429,000,000			
1998	22,680,000,000	$ 2,251,000,000	$ 1,100,000,000	$ 1,151,000,000
1999	25,097,000,000	2,417,000,000	2,000,000,000	417,000,000
2000	27,466,000,000	2,369,000,000	4,100,000,000	(1,731,000,000)
2001	29,691,000,000	2,225,000,000	4,200,000,000	(1,975,000,000)
2002	31,704,000,000	2,013,000,000	4,700,000,000	(2,687,000,000)
Total	$136,638,000,000	$11,275,000,000	$16,100,000,000.00	($4,825,000,000)

Source: HCFA, Office of the Actuary, February 14, 1996 for FY 1997 budget.

Clearly, HCFA sought ***not to constrain growth*** in the industry, ***but to cut back the level of services currently available to Medicare beneficiaries***. The net overall cutback in benefits available to the Medicare beneficiaries, based on the CBO scoring, for the five-year period would be $4.8 billion, as shown above. These cuts in expenditures take into account that HCFA projects an additional million beneficiaries entering into the system during the five-year period, resulting in a disproportionately higher per beneficiary reduction in cost.

However, when reviewing the changes mandated by the BBA, the cuts go significantly deeper. In the worst case scenario, cuts of **$54.7 billion** in Medicare home health benefits would be made for the same representative group discussed above and on the five-year budget **of $136 billion or 40% of the benefit**. A summary of cuts affecting the Medicare home health benefit available to Medicare beneficiaries through the application of the various provisions of the BBA is presented as follows:

Summary of Cuts Through Application of Provisions of BBA of 1997

Fiscal Year Using Federal Government FYE September 30,	Cuts Through Using FY 1994 Base Year for Per Beneficiary Cost Limits	Cuts From Changing Rates from 112% of Mean to 105% of Median	Required 15% Cut at End of Fiscal 1999 if HCFA Doesn't Implement PPS	Summary of Total Cuts Allowed For Under CBO Scored Legislative Act
1998	($ 4,940,550,758)	($ 2,660,917,386)		($ 7,601,468,144)
1999	(5,464,655,872)	(2,944,851,619)		(8,409,507,491)
2000	(5,984,310,031)	(3,222,253,495)	($2,738,915,471)	(11,945,478,997)
2001	(6,467,780,447)	(3,483,482,932)	(2,960,960,492)	(12,912,223,871)
2002	(6,904,495,114)	(3,719,925,732)	(3,161,936,872)	(13,786,357,728)
Total	($29,761,792,222)	($16,031,431,164)	($8,861,812,835)	($54,655,036,221)

Source: AFHHA computations of BBA 1997 provisions. Computations available upon request.

The error of the scoring appears in comparing the information in the two tables above. CBO scored the net "reductions in growth" at $16.1 billion, but Congress in fact included language in the BBA that could potentially cut $54.7 billion from the Medicare home health budget over the five year period.

There was much discrepancy in the scoring of the home health savings as those pointed out Congress in these analyses.

Use of FY 1994 as Base Year for Computing Per Beneficiary Cost Limit

As the above table presents, solely applying the computations to roll back utilization to the fiscal year ended September 30, 1994, utilization rates would result in cost cuts of $4.9 billion in the initial year, due to cutting the number of visits per beneficiary by an average of 16.44 visits. The five year aggregation of cuts from this provision would be $29.8 billion.

Change in Cost Limit Computation from 112% of mean to 105% of Median

Home health care experts believe that a 15% "reductions in growth" (a/k/a cut) would occur from changing the cost limit calculation from 112% of the mean to 105% of the median. This change would result in approximately $2.7 billion in cuts in the first year and $16.0 billion for the five year period.

Failure on HCFA's Part to Implement a Prospective Payment System by 1999

After the end of fiscal year 1999, assuming that HCFA has not implemented a PPS (which it has failed to do on a number of occasions), the BBA calls for an additional 15% reduction in rates. The effect on spending in 2000 through 2002 will approximate $8.8 billion in additional cost cuts from this provision alone.

Forecasted cuts for the ensuing years are similarly appalling. Such deep cuts most certainly endanger the Medicare beneficiaries by restricting their access to care in their homes. Budgeted cuts to the home health benefit also endangers the solvency of the Medicare Program, as more expensive care such as emergency room visits, hospital stays or nursing home care, will replace the services previously provided by home care.

Venipuncture

Another provision of the Balanced Budget Act also cuts Medicare home health spending, but its impact is not as easily measured. HCFA has identified a perceived overuse of the home health benefit by those individuals receiving venipuncture services as their primary diagnosis. These patients are normally on a drug regime to maintain a certain blood clotting factor to reduce the risk of stroke, heart attack or other serious conditions. Pursuant to the HCFA plan, venipuncture patients would not qualify for the home health benefit, but, although homebound they would have to travel to the physician's office or lab to have venipuncture procedures done. HCFA has indicated that contract phlebotomists could travel to the patient's home and draw the blood at a lower cost to the Program. That proposal may be fine in metropolitan areas, but it is impractical in rural areas of the South and West.

What HCFA obviously fails to consider is the skilled assessment of the patient that takes place during a home health visit by the nurse. Because these patients are homebound, their only medical contact may be with the nurse. The assessment and monitoring of the patient is vital in reporting changing health status, monitoring high risk potential, and perhaps alleviating higher cost care by greatly reducing patients visiting the emergency room or being admitted to the hospital. Removing venipuncture coverage places such patients at an extremely high risk of deteriorating health status and subsequently utilizing higher cost Medicare services.

HCFA does not deny that venipuncture patients are homebound, but rather argues that venipuncture service is not a changing health status for the patient. However, current HCFA regulations state that high-risk patients to be provided the home health benefit. The Home Health Agency Manual (HIM-11), Section 234.9 A1, states:

> **"Include all skilled observation of the patient where the physician determines that the patient's condition is such that a reasonable probability exists that significant changes may occur which require the skills of a licensed nurse to supplement the physician's personal contacts with the patient."**

Elimination of venipuncture as a qualifying skilled nursing service in the BBA is shortsighted, and has a high potential that the higher utilization patients who cannot obtain further home health benefits will almost surely be institutionalized.

Why Has the Home Health Industry Grown?

There has been significant growth in the home health industry. The former Administrator of HCFA, Dr. Bruce Vladeck, testified before Congress, explaining that the growth was attributed to the popularity of the services with physicians, their patients and the patients' families, the increase in the high-tech services that could be provided in the patients' homes, and hospitals discharging their patients quicker. There are other more global reasons why the home care benefit has grown including demographic trends, market reasons and government tinkering with the health care delivery system.

The Facts About Home Health Reimbursement

Home health is one of the few Medicare components that remains cost reimbursed, with no provision for profit from its operations with the Medicare Program. Home health agencies are reimbursed, normally up to sixty (60) days after the service is rendered, the lesser of their reasonable costs or a maximum aggregate per visit limit. Providers normally "carry" the government between the time that the service is rendered and when payment is received.

What the Home Health Industry Should Request

AFHHA has asked several Congressmen to introduce a technical correction's bill to resolve the problem caused by incorrect scoring of the home health provisions of the BBA. There is a need for swift action since those providers, whose fiscal years started on or after October 1, 1997, already have had to operate under the provisions of the BBA. They are reducing staff and services to come under the revised cost limits and to comply with the restrictions on the delivery of services. These onerous provisions of BBA must be corrected before too much damage is done.

AFHHA has drafted proposed language for a technical correction. Your support would be invaluable. CBO refused to score the home health industry-initiated proposal to implement a PPS designed to attain savings in the home health benefit and to increase efficiencies in the provision of care. Evidentially, CBO refused to score the industry proposal because HCFA indicated that it could not implement the PPS plan in the time frame necessary.

The overriding concern of both HCFA and the homecare industry should be for the Medicare patients who face significant cuts in their access to home health services, and also for home health agency employees who will be terminated if the BBA draconian reductions are not redressed.

Your review of these matters and your assistance would be greatly appreciated.

<u>Overall Assumptions Used in Testing CBO Scoring</u>

To test the theory that the BBA as written would cut much deeper than the expected savings, statistics generated from HCFA's Office of the Actuary related to its forecasts of growth in the home health industry. These HCFA forecasts were made during the summer of 1997 prior to the initiation of the legislation.

Per Beneficiary Cost Limits 42 USC 1395x(v)(1)(L), Balanced Budget Act, Section 4602(c)(v), Section 1861(v)(1)(L)

Page 7

Using HCFA's own data, AFHHA attempted to correlate the monetary effect of reducing the average number of visits per beneficiary from their projected 1998 level of 75.5 visits to the 1993 level of 59.06 visits; that is a reduction of 16.44 visits per beneficiary. This reduction in available services to Medicare beneficiaries by itself, in the first year of implementation, would have resulted in cost cuts of $4.9 billion. For subsequent years, AFHHA applied the percentage growth in average visits per beneficiary as contained in HCFA's actuarial report to the base year figure of 59.06 visits, while using HCFA's estimated cost per visit for each of the ensuing years. The following represents the yearly cost reductions by cutting the available benefits to the home health beneficiary:

1998	$ 4,940,550,758
1999	5,464.855.872
2000	5,984,310,031
2001	6,467,780,448
2002	6,904,495,115
	$ 29,761,792,224

Clearly, there had to be some error in the calculations of the savings when the CBO scored the savings from the Medicare Home Health Benefit. However, the above calculation only takes into account the cuts in Medicare spending as a result of establishing a per beneficiary visit limit at the fiscal 1994 level.

Reduction of Cost Limits from 112% of the Mean to 105% of the Median 42 USC 1395x(v)(1)(L), Balanced Budget Act, Section 4602(a)(5), Section 1861(v)(1)(L)

Also implemented by the legislation was a reduction in the cost limits to be implemented in fiscal year 1998 HCFA will determine the cost limits based on 105% of the median instead of 112% of the mean. Industry analysts have equated this reduction to equal an approximate 15% cut in the cost limits.

In an attempt to quantify the monetary effect of these reductions in reimbursement rates, AFHHA multiplied the reduced number of visits per beneficiary (as established with fiscal year 1994 as the base year) times the number of unduplicated census as identified by HCFA of projected Medicare home health recipients. This number was then multiplied by the estimated cost per visit established by HCFA, and then multiplied by 15%, representing the reduction in the per visit cost limits from the mean to median shift.

Following these assumptions, the forecasted reductions in costs to the Medicare home health benefit during fiscal 1998 would have been $2.7 billion. The following reflects the total saving projected over the five-year period:

Page 8

1998	$ 2,660,917,386
1999	2,944,851,619
2000	3,222,253,495
2001	3,483,482,933
2002	3,719,925,733
	$ 16,031,431,166

Failure on HCFA's Part to Implement a Prospective Payment System by 1999 42 USC 1395 et seq; 42 USC 1895(e); Balanced Budget Act; Section 4603 (adding 42 USC Section 1895); Section 1861(v)(1)(L)

After the end of fiscal year 1999, assuming that HCFA has not implemented a PPS(which it has failed to do on a number of occasions). the BBA calls for an additional 15% reduction in rates. That 15% reduction will result in $8.8 billion in additional cost cuts through 2002.

On a combined basis, the total cuts in Medicare spending resulting in the reduction in cost limits and if the 15% reduction of PPS is not implemented will total $54.7 billion over the five year period. Consequently, there will be a reduction in total forecasted expenditures for the Medicare home health benefit of 40%, rather than 11.8% as HCFA has stated.

Page 9

As Required by the Balance Budget Act of 1997
--Roll Utilization Back to 1993 Levels (Fiscal Year 94)
--15% Reduction in Cost Limits from Shift of Limits from 112% of Mean to 105% of Median
--15% Rate Cut in 1999 if PPS is Not Implemented

	1998 Projected	1999 Projected	2000 Projected
HCFA Data from Office of Actuary:			
Total Medicare Home Health expenditures	22,680,000,000	25,097,000,000	27,466,000,000
Total Projected Home Health visits	320,792,079	340,344,453	357,397,528
Average cost per visit	70.70	73.74	76.85
Total Unduplicated Census	4,250,000	4,425,000	4,590,000
Visits per Beneficiary	75.50	76.90	77.90
Savings achieved through using Fiscal Year 1994 per beneficiary limits:			
Projected visits per beneficiary per HCFA	75.50	76.90	77.90
1993 average visits per beneficiary	(59.06)	(60.15)	(60.93)
Reduction in number of visits per beneficiary	16.44	16.75	16.97
Total cut in visits (Unduplicated census x visits per	69,880,492	74,107,077	77,870,007
Medicare Home Health expenditures, HCFA Office of Actuary	22,680,000,000	25,097,000,000	27,466,000,000
Total reduction in cost limits (reduction in visits x cost per visit)	(4,940,550,758)	(5,464,655,872)	(5,984,310,031)
	17,739,449,242	19,632,344,128	21,481,689,969
Reduction in cost per visit based upon changing rates from 112% of mean to 105% of median (estimated at 15% by industry)	(2,660,917,386)	(2,944,851,619)	(3,222,253,495)
	15,078,531,856	16,687,492,509	18,259,436,473
15% Reductions in costs if HCFA does not implement PPS system as Required by the Balanced Budget Act of 1997			(2,738,915,471)
Net Medicare Home Health Expenditures after BBA cuts	15,078,531,855	16,687,492,509	15,520,521,002
Budget Cuts from Balanced Budget Act of 1997	(7,601,468,145)	(8,409,507,491)	(11,945,478,998)

Page 10

As Required by the Balance Budget Act of 1997
–Roll Utilization Back to 1993 Levels (Fiscal Year 94)
–15% Reduction in Cost Limits from Shift of Limits from 112% of Mean to 105% of Median
–15% Rate Cut in 1999 if PPS is Not Implemented

	2001 Projected	2002 Projected	Five year total
HCFA Data from Office of Actuary:			
Total Medicare Home Health expenditures	29,691,000,000	31,704,000,000	136,638,000,000
Total Projected Home Health visits	371,369,606	381,745,936	1,771,649,603
Average cost per visit	79.95	83.05	
Total Unduplicated Census	4,720,000	4,820,000	
Visits per Beneficiary	78.70	79.20	
Savings achieved through using Fiscal Year 1994 per beneficiary limits:			
Projected visits per beneficiary per HCFA	78.70	79.20	
1993 average visits per beneficiary	(61.56)	(61.95)	
Reduction in number of visits per beneficiary	17.14	17.25	
Total cut in visits (Unduplicated census x visits/ beneficiary)	80,897,817	83,136,606	385,891,998
Medicare Home Health expenditures, HCFA Office of	29,691,000,000	31,704,000,000	136,638,000,000
Total reduction in cost limits (reduction in visits x cost per	(6,467,780,448)	(6,904,495,115)	(29,761,792,224)
	23,223,219,552	24,799,504,885	106,876,207,776
Reduction in cost per visit based upon changing rates from 112% of mean to 105% of median (estimated at 15% by industry)	(3,483,482,933)	(3,719,925,733)	(16,031,431,166)
	19,739,736,620	21,079,579,153	90,844,776,610
15% Reductions in costs if HCFA does not implement PPS system as Required by the Balanced Budget Act of 1997	(2,960,960,493)	(3,161,936,873)	(8,861,812,837)
Net Medicare Home Health Expenditures after BBA cuts	16,778,776,127	17,917,642,280	81,982,963,773
Budget Cuts from Balanced Budget Act of 1997	(12,912,223,873)	(13,786,357,720	(54,655,036,227)

47-539 98 - 6

Senator REID. We appreciate your traveling these 450 miles to be here today. She is based in Douglas County and it is not convenient, but we appreciate your being here today. Your testimony is very probative. We will now hear from Dr. Steven Phillips, who is the Medical Director of Social Health Maintenance Organization, Senior Dimensions.

STATEMENT OF STEVEN L. PHILLIPS, M.D., C.M.D., MEDICAL DIRECTOR, SOCIAL HEALTH MAINTENANCE ORGANIZATION, SENIOR DIMENSIONS, SIERRA HEALTH SERVICES, INC.

Dr. PHILLIPS. Senator Reid and members of the field hearing committee, thank you for this opportunity. As a geriatrician who is actively involved in both clinical and administrative roles of health care for older Nevadans, I truly am honored to have this opportunity to address the future of long-term care and hopefully provide some potential remedies for its current ailments.

The field of long-term care must no longer be held synonymous with institutional care and/or spending one's final days, months or years in a nursing home setting. The warehousing of those no longer capable of caring for themselves or who are without the necessary family and social support to remain in the community at large has resulted in today's bitter pill of long-term care.

This may have been the case in the past, but does not reflect the current and future direction of health care needs in the United States of America. The nursing facility represents only one discrete part within the continuum of care. A continuum of care is intended to unite all areas of health care into an integrated delivery system.

The discrete parts within the health care delivery system are the various levels of care that meet an individual's needs, not necessarily an institution's needs or a payer's needs. These include independent living, group care, assisted living, rehabilitation, extended care, skilled nursing, hospice, home health care, and yes, acute care as well.

The common characteristic that unites these parts into a continuum of care is the primary care physician or equivalents. A continuum of care requires that a component management system be replaced by a more systematic approach. Component management focuses on only one aspect of the health care system at a time.

Inherent problems of component management include not recognizing health care as interrelated, all diseases tend to be treated the same, factoring treatment over prevention, leading to an uncoordinated delivery system without continuity of care, paying primarily for the most expensive services in the most expensive setting, weakening of the patient/physician relationship, and finally, placing clinicians and administrators at odds with one another.

The discrete parts within the health care delivery model have become very focused on what they do and how to maintain financial solvency. This has created barriers that must be appreciated and sensitively addressed in order that everyone feels comfortable working within an integrated system.

I feel that without integration, the provision of the most cost-efficient and quality-based services cannot occur. One way to look at value within any health care model is value equals quality over cost, that formula means sometimes we pay more at times for quality and therefore better value.

Traditional Medicare, fee-for-service provides greater incentives for a component management approach to health care delivery. This has created an emphasis on acute care intervention rather than prevention. The Senator has already mentioned, under traditional Medicare, mandatory three-day approved stay in a hospital before going to a skilled facility. That has caused a "gaming" in the system, if you will.

This system of care prevents health care providers from proactively meeting the needs of those they serve in the most appropriate care setting. Managed care, under Medicare Risk HMOs is being paid up front for services. They have been able to develop some preventive care models, but to this date, I am sad to report that few Medicare Risk HMOs have truly been successful in aligning the health care delivery elements with those financial aspects required to maintain those they serve in the most appropriate setting, based upon the true need of the patient.

I want to spend a little time on the Social Health Maintenance Organization II, otherwise affectionately known as SHMO II. It is a designated Health Care Financing Administration (HCFA) demonstration project that is funded through a risk-adjusted payment mechanism. This is a major step in financing for health care by HCFA and Medicare, that payments are based upon actual risk from screening that is done on a health plan's membership.

The components of the Social HMO include care coordination, extended care benefits, and a geriatric resource team. In my testimony, I have further explained what care coordination and extended care benefits are. They include such things as respite for caregivers, for both group home placement, short-term, and institutional placement of loved ones so that someone can go away for the weekend.

The only approved functioning Social HMO actually is right here in Nevada. It puts Nevada squarely in the forefront of the future for health care delivery. Finally, some quick recommendations for long-term care policy.

I believe that we must emphasize the entire continuum of care in all current and future Federal and state initiatives. I also feel that schools of medicine, nursing, and other allied health care professionals must develop curricula that foster an understanding and willingness to work within the continuum of care.

Finally, there should be requirements for all of us who require continuing education units, continuing medical education credits, that it include the continuum of care. Thank you very much.

Senator REID. Doctor, thank you very much.

[The prepared statement of Dr. Phillips follows:]

"The Many Faces of Long-Term Care: Today's Bitter Pill or Tomorrow's Cure?"

Testimony before the

Senate Special Committee on Aging
Field Hearing

12 January 1998
West Charleston Library
Las Vegas, Nevada

13 January 1998
Washoe Medical Center Auditorium
Reno, Nevada

Presented by
Steven L. Phillips, MD, CMD

Senator Reid and members of the field hearing committee. I am Steven L. Phillips, Medical Director of Senior Dimensions Extended Care a HCFA designated Social HMO demonstration project based out of Las Vegas, Nevada. As a Geriatrician who is actively involved in both the clinical and administrative roles of health care for older Nevadans I am truly honored to have this opportunity to address the future of long-term care and potential remedies for its current ailments.

The field of long-term care must no longer be held synonymous with institutional care and/or spending one's final days, months or years in a nursing home setting. The ware housing of those no longer capable of caring for themselves or without the necessary family and social support to remain in the community at large has resulted in today's bitter pill of long-term care. This may have been the case in the past but does not reflect the current and future direction of health care needs in the United States of America. The nursing facility represents only one discrete part within the Continuum of Care. A Continuum of Care is intended to unite all areas of health care into an integrated delivery system. The discrete parts within the health care delivery system are the various levels of care that meet an individuals needs. These include independent living, group care, assisted living, rehabilitation, extended care, skilled nursing, hospice, home health care, and acute care. The common characteristic that unites these parts into a Continuum of Care is the primary-care physician or equivalent.

A Continuum of Care requires that a component management system be replaced by a more systematic approach. Component management focuses on only one aspect of the health care system at a time. Inherent problems of component management include:

- -not recognizing health care is interrelated;
- -all diseases tend to be treated the same;
- -factoring treatment over prevention;
- -leading to an uncoordinated delivery system without continuity of care;
- -paying primarily for the most expensive services in the most expensive setting;
- -weakening of the patient-physician relationship; and
- -placing clinicians and administrators at odds with one another.

The discrete parts within a health care delivery model have become very focused on what they do and how to maintain financial solvency. This has created barriers that must be appreciated and sensitively addressed in order that everyone feels comfortable working within an integrated system. Without integration the provision of the most cost-efficient and quality-based services cannot occur.

Traditional Medicare fee-for-service provides greater incentives for a component management approach to health care delivery. This has created an emphasis on acute care intervention rather than prevention. For those clinicians that have identified someone that requires skilled nursing and/or rehabilitative services not available or reasonable to provide in the home or outpatient setting they must place this person in an acute care hospital. This is frequently an unjustified use of acute care services and exposes that patient to an environment which may lead to adverse outcomes. This system of care prevents health care providers from proactively meeting the needs of those they serve in the most appropriate care setting.

Medicare Risk HMOs have been given more flexibility in the manner in which health care is delivered to those they serve. These HMOs are paid a fixed amount per enrolled member per month (PMPM) that is a calculation that reflects the average adjusted per capita cost (AAPCC) of a traditional Medicare recipient within a specific county or region served. The AAPCC varies significantly from state to state and even county by county. By receiving payment in an up front manner the HMO can theoretically allocate resources to preventative care activities and allow for the movement of patients to the most appropriate level of care. This requires the development of an integrated delivery model that supports the Continuum of Care. Few Medicare Risk HMOs have truly been successful in aligning the health care delivery elements with those financial aspects required to maintain those they serve in the most appropriate setting, based upon true need.

The Program for All-Inclusive Care for the Elderly (PACE) has recently been moved from demonstration status to programmatic status. The PACE model allows for the blending of Medicare and Medicaid dollars for those individuals that are found to be eligible for placement within a nursing facility setting. The objective is to provide all needed services that will allow the PACE members to remain in the most independent setting possible. This model relies upon the creation of health care teams that assess and manage member needs in a coordinated fashion relying heavily upon an interdisciplinary team approach.

The Social Health Maintenance Organization II (SHMO II) is a designated Health Care Financing Administration (HCFA) demonstration project that is funded through a risk adjusted payment mechanism. The intent of SHMO II is to address medical, psychological, functional, and social needs of seniors in a coordinated manner. There are three components within the SHMO II demonstration: Care Coordination; Extended Care Benefits; and a Geriatric Resource Team.

Care Coordination is based upon the elements of:

-screening for risk;
-assessment of those identified to be at-risk;
-development of a plan of care based upon identified risks;
-implementation of the plan of care;
-monitoring the plan of care;
-reassessment of the patient;
-evaluation of the plan of care; and
-reporting of the outcomes.

Each element is critical to the overall success of adequately addressing the medical, psychological, functional, and social needs of the senior population that is being served.

The Extended Care Benefits are designed specifically to augment the health plan's existing benefits and community based-services. They are made available through the Care Coordination process and are not an entitlement, rather they are determined by established criteria. These benefits include:

-counseling for situational disorders;
-nutritional services;
-transportation;
-personal care;
-homemaker services;
-adult day care;
-in-home companion;
-short-term institutional care;
-short-term group home care;
-maintenance therapy;
-home safety; and

-a personal emergency response system.

The rationale behind the use of these services is to reduce the burden of disease while maintaining the member's health in the safest and most independent environment possible.

The final component of the SHMO II demonstration project is the Geriatric Resource Team (GRT). The GRT is represented by multiple health care disciplines that assist in further clarification of the needs of high-risk member's. The GRT provides intervention recommendations and assists the primary care providers with reassessment and evaluation as needed. In addition to its clinical role the GRT serves as an educational resource for the entire health care delivery system. A core knowledge of geriatric expertise is often lacking with both traditional Medicare and Medicare Risk HMO delivery settings. For this reason the SHMO II demonstration incorporated the development of a GRT into the study design.

Presently there are a total of six (6) Medicare HMOs that have been selected by HCFA to participate in the SHMO II demonstration. Due to the complexity of this program only one (1) of the selected participants is operational at this time. That HMO is Health Plan of Nevada and has truly placed the state of Nevada squarely in the forefront of senior health care in the United States. The SHMO II demonstration is available through Senior Dimensions Extended Care (SDEC). SDEC began on November 1 ,1996 in Las Vegas, Nevada and is scheduled to be offered in the Reno/Sparks area by March 1, 1998. Over the next several years, Care Coordination, Extended Care Benefits and a Geriatric Resource Team or their equivalents are likely to become a standard of practice within all Medicare Risk HMOs. This demonstration has allowed for the creation of a true Continuum of Care directed and coordinated through a long-term care initiative that ensures the appropriate utilization of resources based principally upon the needs of the members served. At the end of our first twelve months, we have been successful in maintaining 85 percent of our at risk members for nursing home placement in a less restrictive environment. As an advocate for improving senior health care the SHMO II demonstration truly enhances my ability to address the medical, psychological, functional, and social needs of those patients I serve.

Recommendations for Long-Term Care Policy

1. Emphasize the entire Continuum of Care in all current and future Federal and State initiatives.
2. Schools of Medicine, Nursing and other Allied Health Care Professionals will develop curricula that foster an understanding and willingness to work within the Continuum of Care.
3. Institute requirements that all health care professionals have a specified number of CME, CEU or other equivalent continuing education credits which pertain to the Continuum of Care.

4. Eliminate impediments that inhibit health care professionals and organizations/institutions within the Continuum of Care to deliver the most appropriate care based upon an individuals needs and personal desires.
5. Create a demonstration program that fosters the partnering of the multiple components of the Continuum of Care into a model program that incorporates all of the discrete parts into a united project with a common goal of maximizing the care of those they serve.

Senator REID. You are aware of the legislation that I am pushing that would, in effect, give medical schools more direction as far as training people in geriatrics. All medical schools now have mandatory courses in pediatrics, but only a handful have mandatory courses in geriatrics and that is simply wrong. Medical schools have not maintained contact with reality in that regard. So we need to do better in that regard.

Before we get to the questions of the panel, I have a series of questions here from the audience that we will answer before the day is out, but here is an interesting statement made by Stephen Walker, and we got this comment this morning. The only reason I mention his name is if I did not mention his name, someone would think I made this up.

"I live in a group home. It's the happiest I've been in years. They're wonderful. Is there help for the good people to expand and spread the kindness that I have felt?" So that is really interesting. That is from someone here in the audience.

Dr. Phillips, you talk about continuum of care. What I assume you mean—why don't you put that in lay terms so that we all understand what you are talking about?

Dr. PHILLIPS. Continuum of care is an approach to bring together all of the disparate parties, if you will, such as care in a nursing home, nursing facility, care in a hospital, hospice programs, home health care, that they truly become continuous.

One way I heard last night, and I am going to recognize Jerry Reed for his way of simplifying this, and if you look at it, it is an ability to align all services. It kind of looks like an assembly line where you start at one end, you just move right on through. It is aligning all services, recognizing that it is not that simple in health care just to align things like that, but it becomes, if you will, virtually integrated.

In other words, everyone has the ability to communicate with one another in a systematic manner. So if my mother goes to the hospital and needs short-term rehabilitation in a nursing facility, the hospital and that facility talk with one another. When my mom goes back to her home in Sonoma, CA, someone talks so that when she goes back to her primary care physician, that person knows what has occurred.

Senator REID. And it is not that way now?

Dr. PHILLIPS. That is correct, sir, for the most part.

Senator REID. Also, give us the benefit of your experience with Nevada being one of the SHMOs. These are not Little Abner SHMOs.

Dr. PHILLIPS. No, sir. This has truly become the most exciting thing I have done in my ten years of geriatric program development. We have been operational since November 1, 1996 in Las Vegas, have approximately 26,000 members under the Social HMO. We will be in Reno by March 1 of this year.

We have successfully maintained, if you will, being able to allow our members who were in need of placement in nursing facilities, 85 percent are still at home because of the extended benefits we are able to provide. We do not have to meet requirements of Medicare or Medicaid for criteria to provide a home health attendant, to provide personal emergency response system. It is actually our charge over our next four-year demonstration. We will come to close December 31, 2000.

Senator REID. How do you think it is working?

Dr. PHILLIPS. So far, sir, it looks very, very successful.

Senator REID. What would you change if you could to make it better?

Dr. PHILLIPS. It would be real helpful if we had more physicians and other health care providers who have training through their graduate schools before they got to this demonstration. That has been probably our biggest task, is to bring physicians and other health care providers on board.

Senator REID. Doctor, we have a question from the audience that fits right into that. The person writes about like I do and I cannot read the name very well. The question is—we have talked about medical school training for physicians and we know what a shortage we have now and if we do not do something, what a shortage we are going to have in the future. It is going to be even more dramatic.

But they also, I think, bring out what you have stated. "How about some type of training for people who work in geriatrics, for allied health providers?" We really need to have some programs in that regard so that people are better trained to do all the things we have heard from the witnesses today.

I do not know how we are going to do that, but at the Community College in Elko, we had a tremendous need filled in Nevada for the last 30 years. We have been mining above-ground, open pit mines where you need truck drivers and shovel operators and those kinds of people who can be trained in big cities.

All of a sudden, there is a tremendous need in Nevada for underground miners and we do not have any that are trained to do that anymore. So Elko Community College has a program now that will train you to be an underground miner. You will get a degree in underground mining. It takes less than a year to get that and there are jobs that are guaranteed.

My point is, if the health care field provided good jobs for these people, there would be a way of training them. Dr. Moore would do it out here at the Community College and other places and I think this is something we need to focus on because everybody today, in one way or another, has talked about the lack of qualified personnel to take care of these facilities.

In Reno, one of the concerns that we had, and we are going to have some testimony on tomorrow, some of the testimony is going to talk about similar to the Georges, but a little different. They went into a facility, were glad to get there, but were kind of flabbergasted about how the people did not know how to take care of them, as soon as they got there.

By that, I do not mean medical care, but just simple counseling and talking to them, making them feel good about being there. So this was a very good question.

Ms. Mason, as you may know, I voted against the original budget bill, where I was one of 27 that voted against it for the reasons that you have outlined, I think, quite clearly. But in spite of that, we now have the laws that exist. You heard me say earlier that we do not do a good job of reviewing home health care claims.

I can remember ten years or so before home health care came into being going with a doctor here in Las Vegas who was a physician who specialized in infectious disease. Most of his patients will get well, but it took a long time. They needed a long-term infusion of drugs and he took me to the hospital saying there is no reason for these people to be in the hospital. They can be taken care of at home. Think of the cost to society for their being here.

Well, we now have home health care. These same patients, a lot of them, if not most of them, would be taken care of at home. But, Ms. Mason, how can we control the costs of the home health care industry? That was the concern of Congress. These costs did not gradually go up; they skyrocketed up. How can we control these costs?

Ms. MASON. Well, Senator, right now, home care is cost-reimbursed, and it does not take a rocket scientist to figure out that if you get reimbursed whatever you say your costs are, it is not very cost-effective.

Senator REID. That is the way Medicare used to be.

Ms. MASON. Exactly. We in the home care industry have recognized this for years. The hospice program, which is paid on a per diem basis, is probably the original capitated program or the original managed care program in the country. What you are is reimbursed for a certain amount of money and you have to spread that money over quality care.

Home care needs to be not cost-reimbursed. Right now, our best hope for that is what is called the prospective payment system. We have been working for about five years with HCFA, the Health Care Finance Administration to try to get a prospective payment system in place.

Unfortunately, even with the involvement of home care and a huge amount of input, they just have, for whatever reason, not moved forward with that prospective payment. Instead, we have got the Balanced Budget Act, most of which is very punitive, counter-productive, and in the long run is going to cost us more money.

Senator REID. You say that because people that we can keep out of convalescence centers, we have talked about that all day today, saves money. So what you are saying we can keep people in homes through home health care?

Ms. MASON. Correct.

Senator REID. We save money?

Ms. MASON. Yes. But unfortunately, some of the requirements of the Balanced Budget Act are going to force home health agencies out of existence because they are going to be unable to continue to incur the costs that the new regulations have put into being. I think the biggest example of that is probably the surety bond.

The surety bond was put into place because there were agencies after Operation Restore Trust, every industry has agencies that do not do a very good job and home care is no different from any other industry. Unfortunately, because of some of the findings of Operation Restore Trust, the surety bond was put into place so that should an agency go out of business, Medicare would not be left holding the bag, so to speak, to pay for the money that they could not recover from that agency.

Senator REID. Bonds are very expensive.

Ms. MASON. They are very expensive and the regulations, the way they are now, there are no companies out there who want to do it. So home health agencies are not going to be able to comply with that requirement, which means they are going to go out of business.

I happen to serve a 1,700-square-mile area of northern Nevada and northern California whose population density is probably about one person every 5,000 miles. So it is very difficult for us to be able to service that population and those people are going to go wanting because there is just no one to service them. We are the only agency in the vast majority of our geographic territory.

Senator REID. And you have done a good job in your testimony indicating that unless we do something quickly, the elderly patients will be forced into nursing homes when they could stay at home and could cut down on hospital stays and emergency room visits because of chronic disease that they have, diabetes, et cetera.

Elderly patients and their families will be forced to spend down, meaning deplete their assets, in order to remain at home but still qualify for Medicaid.

Ms. MASON. As the Georges we talked about earlier.

Senator REID. As the Georges did. Mr. Cashdollar, this SecureCare sounds like it could be a very expensive program to the taxpayers. Do you have any ideas how much a program like this would cost?

Mr. CASHDOLLAR. Well, Senator, as you well know, the United States is already spending hundreds of billions of dollars on acute care and——

Senator REID. And you said hundreds of billions?

Mr. CASHDOLLAR. Hundreds of billions of dollars for the acute care and long-term care of elderly Americans. What SecureCare would try to do is structure an integrated system to provide acute care and long-term care under a single program, but put in place an appropriate and primary role for private resources, be it savings, be it long-term care insurance, be it something such as a reverse home equity.

Without even attempting to answer the question of what it would cost, I would like to suggest that with the help of the Senate Aging Committee and Nevada senators and the U.S. Senate, that we could structure a program that would be more efficient with the current resources that we already have, as Dr. Weiss has suggested, and with the right kind of incentives to encourage people to look ahead, to plan ahead, and to save or to ensure for long-term care.

Senator REID. Mr. Cashdollar, are there programs that you are aware of where insurance funds are adequate for extended care, convalescence care?

Mr. CASHDOLLAR. As everyone was, I was shocked to hear the story that you told of people who had a long-term care insurance policy that paid $280 a month. That clearly is not adequate. As you also know, the Congress passed into law the Kassebaum-Kennedy legislation, the Health Insurance Accountability and Portability Act.

That introduced Federal standards for long-term care insurance, and I think that is a very positive step because tied to the favorable tax treatment of long-term care insurance are these standards. As I am sure you can understand, insurance companies will make use of these standards because they will have to because of competitive pressures to offer better and better products.

I know the products are already much better than the one you discussed. So long-term care insurance products have gotten better and better, they have evolved over recent years because of competition and market innovation, and yes indeed, long-term care insurance policies are working.

As you said, they only pay for a very small share of long-term care. That is because they are relatively new. But for instance, there are several states around the nation that have coupled their Medicaid program to long-term care insurance in a way that is very useful. New York is a good example, California also has a program.

If an individual buys a long-term care insurance program that is approved by the state, then that individual gets favorable consideration under Medicaid when the insurance policy is used up. In other words, if they buy good insurance and use it up, they get to hold on to more of their assets under Medicaid than they otherwise would. In other words, they do not have to bankrupt themselves.

Senator REID. Ms. McConnell, tell me why you believe that assisted living, which is the new hot topic and I think a good one that we should talk about, why, if at all, do you feel it is in need of Federal regulation.

Ms. MCCONNELL. I think we should guard against too much Federal regulation in this industry.

Senator REID. I heard you mention that.

Ms. MCCONNELL. The reason I say that is looking at the demographics and the differences throughout our country, if we can allow assisted living to be driven by consumer needs within a demographic area, driven by the needs of the people and regulated by the states in which the people are being served, I think we will be better served than some of the lessons we have seen and learned with Federal regulations for nursing homes, the industry, and trying to adapt or provide the same regulations for everyone throughout the country.

Sometimes it does not work when you are in Iowa and have special needs compared to someone living in the metropolitan area of Los Angeles. So I would encourage some autonomy in this area.

Senator REID. And, of course, other needs vary based upon climatic conditions.

Ms. MCCONNELL. Absolutely.

Senator REID. Dr. Weiss, without exception, seniors are confused about Medicare HMOs, Medicare choice options, and health care generally. Now, you have talked about this integrated delivery system and you have heard Dr. Phillips' statements. Are we going to just confuse people more with this so-called integrated delivery system, or is there a way that we can make it so that it is more understandable to the public, the consumer?

Mr. WEISS. I think it is just the opposite. The whole idea is to make it more friendly, more consumer-sensitive, rather than confused more. I think when you eliminate a lot of the eligibility requirements needed by every distinct service and try to group that together and determine that, and I support certainly all the public and private initiatives on that level, that it will be easier to the consumer.

Senator REID. You also have talked more than anyone else today about the enhancement of the consumer's role in these new models. Tell us some of your ideas about enhancing the role of the consumer.

Mr. WEISS. Well, I think in part, our systems have developed with a model, a medical model primarily, which does not really enable the person to participate. The people are not necessarily treated with respect when they go in and work with health professionals on many levels, whether it is waiting for an hour-and-a-half or two hours for a service in a physician's office, or it is not asking the person themselves about what the issues are.

I think incorporating that person and have it be centered around that person rather than a particular service and have reimbursement reflect that, then I think you are going to see more efficiency within the system.

When people are given choices, when they are given the capability of participating and collaborating in their own health care, the concern always has been that they use more; that if there is flexibility in what those services are, that they are going to go out and come out of the woodwork and use all those services and that just has not been the case.

Just the opposite is seen in the consumer-directed movement, particularly with the younger disabled.

Senator REID. And the fact that some of the people needing information have cognitive problems, it is even more important that there be adequate information for not only those that have less ability to consume this information, those around them also need the information.

So it is not as easy as a lot of programs where you are trying to figure out what is the best TV set to buy when you are dealing with people's health, and sometimes the people that need the help are not prepared to make those decisions themselves. So that is another problem we have.

Mr. WEISS. I think that is where education and information accessibility comes in really well.

Senator REID. If you do not mind staying there for a little while, you might be able to help me answer some of these questions that we have from the audience, and if you cannot, we have got people who have testified previously that can help. I want to answer as many of these as we can. If you would be patient with me, I would appreciate it.

We have a question here for Frankie Sue Del Papa and we will make sure she gets that. Carla Sloan was here. Did she leave? Maybe we can get Carla here because she has been given a number of questions. Here is one for me that I will probably ask for some help on.

"Can the government work together with private insurance to enhance long-term care benefits such as providing more exposure, credibility, and reduced costs for much-needed product?" This is from a registered nurse, Margaret Carpiner.

Mr. COOPER. Senator, may I interrupt for one minute? I do not understand picking up these cards? We do not have all the cards.

Senator REID. We will get them, though. You just be patient.

I think we have answered this question quite well. We have talked a lot today about the need to have private insurance. I think we would all acknowledge that we are not going to solve our problems with extended care in the out years by having the government assume all the responsibility. We are going to have to develop a partnership with the private and public sector.

And so, I would say to Margaret that that is what I have learned here today, is that the problem is not nearly close to being solved, but with some of the legislation that has passed recently, some of the pilot programs we are working on, we may get to a point where we will know better and we will not have people coming up to me at senior lunches saying, "You know, I paid into this program 30 years and I get $280 a month."

Here is a question for me and it also says Mr. Panelli. There you are. "If long-term care facilities are fewer but patients needing care multiply, there must be problems of no financial incentives for private investment in such facilities and/or are regulations unrealistic?" This is from Wanda Blohm.

I think, Mr. Cashdollar, maybe you do not need Mr. Panelli to answer this. If there is such a demand for these services, why isn't the private sector stepping in and building more facilities?

Mr. CASHDOLLAR. The private sector—and Mr. Panelli can speak to this as well. The private sector is building long-term care facilities. There is a brand new facility nearby that is coming on line and admitting residents and several more are planned.

The question is, will the new construction of long-term care facilities keep pace with the overwhelming growth of Nevada's elderly population.

Senator REID. So in short, there is money to be made in the private sector if they run an operation properly?

Mr. CASHDOLLAR. Long-term care facilities have been marginally profitable in Nevada and elsewhere, but I would take advantage of the question to say that policy-makers in Nevada and the United States do need to be careful about the regulations and policies that they pursue and reimbursement policies that they pursue.

You and I have spoken about the Boren Amendment. So up until recently——

Senator REID. Would you explain to them the Boren Amendment?

Mr. CASHDOLLAR. I will certainly try. The Boren Amendment, it is actually not that complicated even though it is a Federal law. The Boren Amendment was a Federal law that required states to pay nursing facilities and hospitals that are treating Medicaid beneficiaries rates that are reasonable and adequate. That Boren Amendment was repealed by the Congress——

Senator REID. Even though I voted against it.

Mr. CASHDOLLAR. Yes. I was certainly getting to that, sir. [Laughter.]

The Boren Amendment, which sounds like something everyone in the room could agree with, was repealed. So when I am asked today whether nursing facilities are fine and they are making plenty of money, I would say, "Well, let's see, because Nevada and other States no longer have this Boren Amendment that is a Federal requirement for adequate payment."

Now, Nevada's payment has been relatively good, but I do not want Nevada to be tempted by the repeal of the Boren Amendment to ransack the long-term care budget in this state. That would be a mistake. So I would encourage the Congress and the Aging Committee to keep an eye on state practices on reimbursement.

Senator REID. I would just interject here, the reason for that, the reason we want to make sure that the profit motive is protected with these institutions is otherwise, the Federal Government and the State Government winds up with all the problems. True?

Mr. CASHDOLLAR. In other words, we need to pursue reimbursement of regulatory policies that will allow long-term care capacity growth in Nevada, in the nation, and it is not just the beds, sir. We need people to provide the care that goes with those beds and that, I think, has to be maybe the number one priority of Nevada and the United States.

You have spoken to some parts of the caregiver work force, but there are nurses and nursing aide positions that we will need in great abundance in the years to come and that is something that we need to focus on.

Senator REID. Next question is, "What is the major difficulty in establishing a national health care registry?" There were a number of questions in this pile that deal with that same subject.

A number of states like the State of Nevada, which recently passed a law saying that people who are going to work in rest homes have to be fingerprinted. So there is some standard out there. It is also, every state requires doctors to go through some licensing procedure.

So establishing the registry for convalescence care workers is really not that difficult and I think we can do that with relative ease with the computerization we have in our society today. It will take a few dollars to set it up, but with the huge amounts of money we are spending in the health care field, it would be a de minimis amount of money. So I do not think it is going to be that difficult.

In that Senator Grassley is a sponsor of this legislation, he is the Chairman of the committee, also he is a member of the Finance Committee, as is Senator Breaux, the ranking member of the committee, I feel very comfortable that we can move this legislation.

We have a question for Dr. Takamura. We will hold that one. Another one for me from Ted Mendals. "Why put ailing people in facilities where they are given constantly synthetic drugs that cause risky side effects and are toxic when natural remedies, vitamins, minerals, et cetera, are available to help heal these people?"

I would say that there certainly is a lot of attention being focused now on alternative medicine. In fact, we allow certain payments under the Federal system where we did not before in alternative medicine. There has been, within the past three months, on the front page of Newsweek Magazine, featuring a doctor who is a Harvard Medical School graduate who believes in alternative medicine.

There have been a number of major programs on television dealing with this subject. So I would think that I would say to Mr. Mendals that there is a lot of work being done in this. Progress is being made. As you mentioned in your statement just a few short years ago, it was hard to find somebody who would come out for some of these alternative forms of medicine.

We are all even doing a program with the National Institutes of Health on alternative medicine. So this is moving right along.

Another question for you, Carla. For me, "The answer in long-term care coverage, what about partnership program already being used in California and other states?" I say to Kathleen Bauer that we have already talked about this. Mr. Cashdollar talked about this. I think this is really a step in the right direction and I would ask the Nevada legislature to take a close look at this and maybe we in the Federal level can give some type of incentives for states that go along with programs like they have in New York and California.

I am going to ask one of the staff to talk a little bit about this, medical savings accounts. We have Doris Morris who asks, "What qualifies to use MSAs?" Would you talk about that a little bit, Ken? Ken Cohen.

Mr. COHEN. Yes, Senator. Medical savings accounts are basically savings accounts to be used for medical expenses. Until recently, Medicare beneficiaries did not have access to medical savings accounts. As a result of the Budget Act last year, Medicare beneficiaries in a limited number will have access. They will have the opportunity to choose medical savings accounts as their choice.

Beneficiaries will learn more about this and other options when they receive mailings from the Health Care Financing Administration later this year discussing the new options allowed under the Budget Act.

Senator REID. Thank you very much. A question to me. "Is anything being done to change the lax requirements for long-term care?" Well, we have talked about that at some length today and we have done about the best we can.

I would also acknowledge, if we had people—and I am not going to ask to raise your hands at how many people have insurance to protect themselves for long-term care. There would only be a couple hands come up. After what we have said today about those insurance policies, I think some might be embarrassed as to really know how good they are, but it is a problem.

Ms. McConnell, here is a question for you. "What facility or facilities are you now associated with?" This comes from Len Grisdal of Las Vegas.

Ms. MCCONNELL. In terms of a facility, I am the administrator right now of Charleston Retirement and Assisted Living, and I also serve as the chair person for Governor Miller's Board of Examiners for Long-Term Care Administrators.

Senator REID. "Dr. Phillips, your organization, HMO, receives $530 per month per person, but does not always give quality care. How do you propose to provide the money to pay for long-term care?" This is from Cynthia Kraft.

Dr. PHILLIPS. Well, you are referring to Sierra Health Service and the $530, for those who do not quite understand how Medicare reimburses HMOs, it is based upon the average expenditure by the Federal Government for a Medicare-eligible recipient in a specific county or region. That is how that number is arrived at.

The 530, whether it is 530 or whether it is 500 or 600, is probably irrelevant to the question. The important point about the quality is, under Sierra Health and through the SHMO demonstration, we have developed a process to enhance reporting of services being provided with the intent that with a better reporting system we will be able to track our outcomes of someone who needs long-term care, whether that is home health, hospice, or nursing facilities.

We still have a ways to go, but I think from the standpoint of other HMOs in not only the State of Nevada but around the country, we have one of the most progressive quality programs in place right now.

We are hopeful that as we identify things that work well with long-term care, we will enhance those services. Things that are not working, as an organization, we are prepared to make changes. I think that is the same thing one could say whether it is an HMO or other health care provider.

Senator REID. Thank you very much. I am trying to get the questions that are not duplicates and some that I cannot read. "Much discussion this morning has focused on health professions education. I would like to remind the Senator and the committee that the Nevada Geriatric Education Center is poised to address this issue. Thank you very much." This is from Rose Yuhos.

A question from Margaret Laspeach. She is concerned about who is doing something about the regulation of home health care, long-term care insurance, and I think we have answered that adequately today. I will have the staff take another look at it and if it is necessary to elaborate on that, you can do that for her.

Some of these questions were written out before the testimony took place and some of them have been answered during these deliberations. Each of these questions, however, we will make sure that you get an answer even if it is duplicative of something we have already answered.

"Twenty-two years ago I joined the faculty of a school of social work on a grant to teach social work students gerontology and to stimulate their interest in working with the elderly. Continuing this focus would be very helpful in providing services that are appropriate to the needs of patients." We would all agree to that, that social workers trained properly can do a lot to help people in these extended care facilities.

Another question to me. "Currently Medicare does not assist family members in paying for adult day care. Current adult day care is not covered well." Is there anyone here that could talk to that? I know you, Carla, talked about what is available out there for adult day care. Would you come up here, please, and help us with this? I have got a couple of other questions for you while you are here.

Ms. SLOAN. I am thinking perhaps that the question concerns insurance payment for adult day care. Currently adult day care services are provided with some support from the Older Americans Act and that is true here in the State of Nevada. We fund a program in Henderson and in Las Vegas and in other areas.

While the cost of adult day care is much less costly than an institutional placement, it can still be a burden for a family and it is not an expense that is covered under Medicare. Medicaid contracts will provide for adult day care if it is under a waiver program, because most of the programs are non-medical in nature.

That is something that would be of great benefit if it were a covered expense under Medicare.

Senator REID. The situation, the example I gave you about my friends, there is no program for them. They take care of—she takes care of her mother and she is there day in and day out. Are there any programs that could give her a little help?

Ms. SLOAN. Yes, there are.

Senator REID. OK.

Ms. SLOAN. Yes, there are.

Senator REID. Let's talk about those. That is what this question is about.

Ms. SLOAN. One of the programs that is an excellent model for that type of respite care is through our Lend-a-Hand program in Boulder City and has now been replicated in Henderson and North Las Vegas is working on that. That is a volunteer program that matches folks.

So in the circumstance for your friends, if they wish to go to a movie, there would be a volunteer that was matched with that family that would go to the home and stay with mom or dad so that the family could go out for socialization or maybe a medical appointment or even a long weekend.

There are also facilities such as our adult day care sites that are working toward 24-hour care where they, too, can provide overnight respite. But it is available and we will help to try to locate what is appropriate for the family.

Senator REID. Another question for you. "Who is the community ombudsman advocate for the Las Vegas area?" This is from Alice Hobson.

Ms. SLOAN. Yes. We have a community ombudsman that is located in the Las Vegas office. Her name is Beverly Manor.

Senator REID. Just like the institution.

Ms. SLOAN. Yes. We also have a community ombudsman in Elko and Reno.

Senator REID. "What is Nevada's policy on recovery of assets from the estate or family of a deceased Medicaid beneficiary?" Does anybody know that?

Ms. SLOAN. A state recovery is something that we work under so that if a client is receiving Medicaid services, either under a waiver program or through other Medicaid services, that individual is advised at the time they enroll for those services that the estate recovery laws apply.

Senator REID. We have another question here that I think has been answered, but simply, "The fraud unit needs more contact with law enforcement. They need greater powers." That is what Frankie Sue talked about on a number of occasions today.

Here is a question that is one that I am sorry to say we have heard a number of times today. It is to Ms. Mason. I do not think you even need to answer it because you already have, but I think in fairness to Mary Ann Royer that we should read this.

"I'm disappointed and angry that my mother's home health care has been discontinued. She does not qualify for long-term care, nursing home. My needs are assisted living which is not within our financial means. So until legislation is passed, what would you suggest that I do to see that my mother's needs are met?"

Ms. MASON. First of all, I would call several different agencies because some agencies, for instance, I operate a hospital-based agency and am the only provider in a large part of the area and we take everybody. It does not matter whether they can pay or not. So I would suggest that you call a number of agencies.

Another thing you might look into in your community is if you have a senior services program. Many communities in Nevada have a senior center that can hook you up with some community resources, can help you with looking into those kinds of things. I would recommend that you call your community ombudsman to see what is available through that office.

But generally, it takes a little shopping until you can find an agency that is willing to give you a hand. Unfortunately, right now there is going to be a gap because there are agencies that are for-profit and this is America, it is free enterprise and they have every right to operate out there, but they are also able to say whether or not they want to take a client or not. Whereas, some not-for-profit agencies do not have that choice. So look around and see. There might be another agency that could provide this service.

Senator REID. A question from Laurie Moore who is a clinical social worker. "A psychiatrist reported to me that there have been recent changes in Medicare funding of mental health services for seniors which would reduce access to this important type of care." Now, I believe with the amendment that was offered by me, Wellstone, and Senator Domenici that we have expanded health care, we have not limited it.

So I would think that with the beginning of this year, I think there is an expansion there. We have tried to put health care, mental health care on a parity with other type of care.

Here is a question from Carol Egan, who is a registered nurse and wanting to know, "How can higher education systems be more accessible for working adults who wish to pursue degrees in the health care field. Example, no Master's program for nurses who are employed full-time during daytime hours. All classes are geared to those who can attend during the day and week days" I think this is something that we should take back to the university system.

Dr. Phillips, the business you are in, all the questions are not good ones, but I think in fairness, we should ask this question. "Your organization, Sierra Health Services, provide health care to my spouse and I since January 1992. We've experienced problems in the area of care from physicians, prescriptions, and waiting for appointments. What should we do about this? She's been unable to communicate with the officers of the corporation."

Dr. PHILLIPS. Well, I think that one advantage, that an HMO provides compared to non-HMO for Medicare recipients is if you have problems with access, if you have problems with your medications, you have an appeal process that is really protection for yourself as consumers.

That appeal process starts at the level of the health plan. So, for example, with Sierra, you contact member services of Sierra Health. You may already have done this. But the initial determination is provided by the HMO. If you do not like that decision, you have 60 days to appeal that initial determination.

That automatically takes it to a place in New York and it is outside of Rochester, NY. It is called the Network Design Group that is hired through HCFA, through Medicare——

Senator REID. But people do not have to go back there.

Dr. PHILLIPS. No, you do not go back, but you appeal and it is to a law judge. You have six levels of appeal. Having been a medical director of two separate Medicare Risk HMOs, I can assure you that if something is not right, the Federal decision through Network Design Group is in favor of the HMO member. You do really have more rights under an HMO than you do under traditional Medicare right now.

Senator REID. Dr. Phillips, this is one of the things we talked about in a number of the panels today and Dr. Weiss talked about. Consumers need to know what their rights are, and I think one of the problems of a lot of consumers, they simply do not understand what their alternatives are and thanks for explaining that.

Here is a question for Ms. Sloan. We have tended here today to focus on seniors, but assisted living, extended care also deals with other types of people who are there. This question is from Ilene Ardine. "Do you realize how many young spinal cord injured quads and paraplegics are living in unbearable conditions in homes and convalescent centers and what do you plan on doing for them?" Carla, this question was directed to you.

Ms. SLOAN. Well, our charge under the Older Americans Act for our long-term care ombudsman program is to serve persons aged 60 and older. When we are in facilities as in the role of an advocate and an ombudsman, we certainly are available to younger persons in the facility. As we put our new Silver Striper program together, that was of great concern to the administrator that is working with us on our pilot program, is that we address the needs of younger individuals in facilities as well.

We try to work closely with the advocates that are available through other resources. We work very closely with the Bureau of Vocational Rehabilitation and some of the groups for disabled services.

Senator REID. The final question is directed to Dr. Takamura. You need not come up here and answer this, but please hear the question. This is from one of the leading senior advocates in Nevada, Jean Maher. She is a member of the Silver-Haired Congress, which met in Washington and passed a number of resolutions.

One of the things that they did pass is a resolution dealing with elder abuse, which called for all licensed health care facilities to be subject to Medicare regulations and inspections. She would like to know if that is being followed up on. I would say to her that one of the things that you are doing is looking over all the resolutions that the Silver-Haired Congress came up with and hopefully assimilate some of those into policy changes.

I would like to excuse the panel and express my appreciation to this panel and all the witnesses today. As far as the Aging Committee is concerned, this was extremely helpful. I think we covered a wide array of issues, not only questions that were brought up here, but by the audience. We have a number of questions here that were duplicative; that is, they had already been answered. We also have some questions that could not be answered for a number of different reasons.

These will all be answered. There will be personal answers to each of you. You have your addresses on here and there is about maybe eight or nine that have not been answered. We will make sure we do that.

I have already thanked the witnesses. I want to thank the staff of the West Charleston Library for providing the logistical support, it has been tremendous. I want to extend my appreciation to Ted Totman, the majority staff director, for the support of the committee, and also to Ken Cohen, the minority staff director, for your attendance here today.

I listen to this testimony today and preside over the hearing, but the real work, if we are going to accomplish anything, has to be done by the staff of this committee. The staff of the committee, they are full-time working on issues relating to seniors. Senior issues are very important to me.

I am concerned about nuclear waste, the environment, crime, education. This is their full-time job. This is all they do and we are going to depend on them to come up with some answers for many of the things that were brought up here today.

I want to also thank the Sanford Center for Aging at the University of Nevada at Reno, the Division for Aging Services for their assistance. I think we made real progress in learning the right questions. We do not have a lot of the answers, but we have, I think, asked a lot of the right questions.

I appreciate the recommendations made by the panelists on what issues should be considered as we shape long-term care policy for the future. Nevada has much to offer in this dialogue. I am grateful that we were able to hold this hearing to hear from Nevadans and non-Nevadans who work in long-term care on a daily basis and learn their concerns.

We do have a public policy challenge on the horizon and today's hearing was both informative and educational and will do much to advance the issue. As many of you know, the Medicare Commission will soon begin meeting to chart the future for Medicare and how best to prepare the program for when baby boomers become eligible starting in the year 2011. Senator Breaux is a member of that commission.

I hope today's hearing sheds light on the topic for long-term care for their consideration. Exactly how our nation will address this long-term care challenge, and it is a challenge, remains to be seen. Whether we continue to rely on Medicare, Medicaid, private insurance, long-term care insurance, or establish a new social insurance approach remains to be seen.

I would hope that we will allow the private sector to take as large a role as possible in this. One thing, however, is certain. With the data suggesting at least two out of five of us will rely on long-term care in the future, it is imperative we all become conversant on the long-term care issue and ensure that our retirement planning includes a long-term care plan that is based on reality.

The long-term care challenge must be addressed at both the individual and the governmental level and must take into full consideration both public and private approaches.

Thank you all very much for your participation. This concludes this field hearing on the Senate Special Committee on Aging.

[Whereupon, at 11:45 a.m., the committee was adjourned.]

THE MANY FACES OF LONG-TERM CARE: TODAY'S BITTER PILL OR TOMORROW'S CURE?

TUESDAY, JANUARY 13, 1998.

U.S. SENATE,
SPECIAL COMMITTEE ON AGING,
Washington, DC.

The committee met, pursuant to notice, at 9 a.m., in the Mack Auditorium, Washoe Medical Center, 77 Pringle Way, Reno, NV, Hon. Harry Reid presiding.

Present: Senator Reid.

OPENING STATEMENT OF SENATOR HARRY REID

Senator REID. The Senate Special Committee on Aging is called to order. The first item of business, I want to extend my appreciation to all the many people who worked to make sure that we could have this remote hook-up with seven sites in rural Nevada. It was not easy because early this morning, one of the police officers at the University of Nevada, Reno, was murdered.

As a result of that, the campus has been blocked off, they have no classes today, and we have had to do this through, as I understand it, Las Vegas. But through the means of modern technology, everyone cooperated and we do and are able to have the remote sites brought into us.

We have a slight deviation from our schedule today. Congressman Jim Gibbons, who represents this area, has asked to testify at this hearing and I, of course, consented to that request. Congressman Gibbons has just arrived. Dr. Takamura and Dr. Bernick, just slide over. There is room for Congressman Gibbons there. There is a chair right behind you, Jim.

While Congressman Gibbons is getting ready to testify, let me just say a few words. This hearing has been worked on for about three months. This is the first of its kind. First of all, we are having a hearing outside Washington, DC. We are holding a hearing on convalescent care. We are holding a hearing simulcasting it to remote sites. There are a lot of firsts with this hearing.

This hearing is entitled, "The Many Faces of Long-Term Care: Today's Bitter Pill or Tomorrow's Cure." I welcome all of you here and especially our panel of distinguished witnesses. I want to first of all express my appreciation to the full committee chairman, Charles Grassley from Iowa, who has consented to this hearing being held here, along with the ranking member of the committee, John Breaux from Louisiana.

This is a bipartisan hearing we are holding this morning. I also very much appreciate Senators Breaux and Grassley graciously sending their staff directors Ted Totman and Ken Cohen, and helping to prepare for these hearings Ted Totman is the staff director for Senator Grassley. Ken Cohen is the staff director for Senator Breaux.

I became aware of two studies in the long-term care area that when viewed together really concern me. One study pointed out that 43 percent or two out of five, will, upon reaching the age of 65, require the assistance of long-term care facilities such as nursing homes and assisted living facilities.

Can you hear to the back of the room? Anyone that cannot hear? I have had this problem my whole life. I remember we had a judge and I used to try cases before him and he was getting a little hard of hearing. He used to get so mad at me because I would talk and only the jury could hear me. I, frankly, did it on purpose. The jury kind of felt sorry for me, this old man yelling at me. [Laughter.]

Anyway, I have always had a problem. I do not have a real loud voice.

One study pointed out that 43 percent or two out of five of us will, upon reaching the age of 65 require some type of long-term care. A second survey published—and this is the one that was striking to me, this was published in the Journal of American Geriatrics—suggested that a third of those polled said they would rather die than live in a nursing home.

It does not take a very smart person to see that a significant portion of the public has lost faith in the potential of our long-term care facilities. It is important to examine these concerns and do what it takes to restore confidence in such a large segment of the overall health care delivery system for older Americans.

I have served for 11 years on the Senate Aging Committee, and prior to that, four years on the House Aging Committee. In the House, I had the pleasure and distinction and I cannot think of enough words of praise to serve with the great Claude Pepper. What a great mentor he was. He traveled to Nevada for me, as he was very gracious to do for anyone that asked.

He was a good person and I certainly learned the vision that I think Claude Pepper had. While serving on these committees, I also learned about the many dimensions of long-term care. One thing I have learned is the importance of Federal standards for nursing homes.

I was a supporter of the Federal nursing home standards enacted in 1987 and remain a supporter of these standards today. While most facilities deliver compassionate and professional health care to residents, a system of well-defined standards with annual review is vital if we are going to ensure the maintenance of quality.

Today there are almost 40 million older Americans representing almost 13 percent of the United States population. By 2030, there will be approximately 70 million older persons, more than twice our population today. This group will make up 20 percent of the population, or said another way, one in five Americans will be over the age of 65 by the year 2030.

The need for long-term care will grow right along with population and it is not an option for us to bury our head in the sand and think we do not have a problem. Along with changing demographics, the face of long-term care is also changing. Today long-term care is no longer just care provided in nursing homes. Home health care—we had great testimony yesterday about home health care—assisted living, hospice care in addition to institutional care have become popular alternatives to nursing homes.

Although these industries are booming, our public policy has not kept pace with the changes that they have brought about. We must begin to answer critical questions. What should be the Federal role, the state role, the local role, the role of families, the role of the private sector?

How do we ensure quality in programs and safety of residents? Should a patient's eligibility for assistance dictate the care to be received, or should the patient's condition be the determining factor? In short, should money or illness be the guiding factor in care? It is obvious that it should be the health of the patient, but that is not the way it always is today.

I want to address the safety of residents issue. Senators Grassley, Kohl, and I have introduced legislation, S. 1122, The Patient Abuse and Prevention Act, to require the establishment of a national registry for confirmed abusers of seniors in long-term care facilities and require that staff undergo thorough background checks before working in these facilities. This is the least we could do to ease the mind of people who must place their loved ones in these facilities.

I am hopeful that Chairman Grassley, who determines what hearings will be held by this committee—who, by the way, as I have already mentioned, is a sponsor of this legislation—will hold a hearing. I am confident that he will in the near future allow us to move forward with this legislation.

Back to today's hearing. I want to tell you why I wanted to hold this hearing in Nevada. We have a lot of firsts here in Nevada. We lead the nation in senior suicide. We lead the nation in suicide generally. Nevada is in a unique position because we have the most rapidly growing senior population in Nevada and we need to build a future for those that require long-term care.

In 1996, there were about 210,000 seniors in Nevada, people over the age of 65. By the year 2020, that is a little more than 20 years from now, this group will grow to 335,000. The over-85 group in the Silver State numbered about 10,000 in 1993. By the year 2020, it will be about 35,000. It is this group for whom long-term care options become very crucial.

In spite of the growth, as recently as a month ago, it was reported that the state's growing senior population is putting a strain on the long-term care system. While the occupancy of available nursing home beds is 90 percent, it is expected the demand will far exceed availability as the baby boomers retire.

Vice President Humphrey once said, "The true moral test of government is how it treats those in the dawn of life, the children; those in the twilight of life, the aged; and those who are in the shadow of life, the sick, the needy, and the disabled." I believe that to be the case and that should be our guiding factor in this hearing and the work we do.

We must do all we can to ensure quality, safety, affordability, and accessibility in our nation's long-term care facilities. This must be done in partnership between Federal, State, and local government and the long-term care industry and the families who are involved.

Our first panel will address the Federal and State perspective as it relates to long-term care. We will also, of course, as I mentioned, hear from Congressman Gibbons. We will also hear about the prevalence of Alzheimer's and other dementia among older Americans and the impact that these diseases have on our long-term care needs.

Our second panel will tell the story from the patient's perspective, as well as the perspective of those who are charged with overseeing the quality and safety of the care provided.

On the third and final panel, we will hear from various witnesses, some of whom who will speak from the perspective of those who provide long-term care in nursing homes, assisted living facilities, home and community care settings. We will also hear about the type of long-term care delivery systems that should be in place to prepare for the future.

We will begin the hearing now. Witnesses have been instructed to keep to five minutes. We would appreciate your doing it. We have a long line of witnesses. We have brought from Washington, this is a Washington issue, these little lights up here. Green means you are okay, yellow means you had better start wrapping it up, and red means you are all through. So if you could do that, keep within the time constraints that will allow us to ask the questions that are necessary.

Also, the audience has been given question cards. Anyone who wants to ask a question, either here or in our remote sites, will be allowed to do so. Those that are in remote sites will fax the questions to us. We will do our very best to answer all these questions. We are going to answer all the questions. The question is whether we answer them all here, according to how the time goes, or whether you will have to receive a written response.

Having said that, Congressman Jim Gibbons.

STATEMENT OF HON. JAMES A. GIBBONS, A REPRESENTATIVE IN CONGRESS FROM THE STATE OF NEVADA

Mr. GIBBONS. Thank you very much, Senator. For the record, I am Jim Gibbons, U.S. Representative for the 2nd District of Nevada, which includes this area.

As I look out this morning at this audience, I believe that what we see here today is a reflection of not just the growing trend in Nevada, but a growing trend in America. When you have a room as large as this auditorium is and have only standing room only left for those people that want to hear the issues and the subjects that are going to be talked about today, it is very important for those of us that make decisions about these issues in Washington, DC. to pay particular attention to the ideas, the concerns, and the comments of the citizens in this audience.

Let me begin today by thanking Senator Reid for bringing this important hearing to Nevada so that all of us in Nevada have an opportunity not only to listen, but to contribute. With the formation of the U.S. Senate Special Committee on Aging, Nevadans are assured a voice on many critical issues that will be facing seniors in the future.

It is an honor and a privilege to extend a very special thanks to Senator Reid and all those who have dedicated their time, their energies, and the resources to making this hearing possible.

The people in the audience did not come here today to listen to a bunch of political speeches full of propaganda, and as your congressman, I came here, like you, to listen, to learn from the members of the committee, from the representatives in the health care industry, and from you, the citizens of Nevada.

I was especially pleased to learn about our fellow Nevadans in our rural communities around the state who will be able to join in this hearing through a satellite feed. The importance of providing quality health care to our rural hospitals should certainly be on our list of priorities.

For Nevadans, today marks the beginning of a renewed push for increased attention to America's system of health care. I speak for my colleagues when I say we do, we do understand that the current health care system is flawed. But it is up to all of us in this room to take responsibility and commit ourselves to making those necessary changes through improved delivery and the quality of health care, especially for our senior population.

Each of us has already taken the first step just by coming here today. Hearings that focus on the needs of our seniors, just like this one, are critical to the understanding, the challenges that face our aging population. Americans are making a difference. Nevadans are making a difference. Let's continue this cooperative working relationship to achieve our goals of positive reform in health care.

Senators, thank you very much for having this hearing and I look forward to today's proceedings, and I noticed the lights did not come on, so I must be okay.

[The prepared statement of Mr. Gibbons follows:]

U.S. Senate Special Committee on Aging
Hearing in Reno, NV
Tuesday, January 13, 1998

Let me begin by extending my appreciation to Senator Harry Reid for bringing this important hearing to Nevada. With the formation of the U.S. Senate Special Committee on Aging, Nevadans are assured a voice on many critical issues facing seniors. It is an honor and privilege to extend a very special thanks to Senator Reid and all those who have dedicated their time, energies and resources to making this hearing possible.

The people in the audience didn't come here today to listen to a bunch of political speeches full of propaganda. As your Congressman, I came here to listen and learn from the members of the committee...from the representatives in the health care industry...and from you, the citizens of Nevada.

I was especially pleased to learn that our fellow Nevadans in rural communities will be able to join in this hearing through satellite feed. The importance of providing quality health care to our rural hospitals should certainly be on our list of priorities.

For Nevadans, today marks the beginning of a renewed push for increased attention to America's system of health care. I speak for my colleagues when I say that we DO understand that the current health care system is flawed. But it's up to all of us in this room to take responsibility and commit ourselves to making the necessary changes. Each of us has already taken the first step...just by coming here today.

Hearings that focus on the needs of our seniors, just like this one, are critical to understanding the challenges that face our aging population. Americans are making a difference. Nevadans are making a difference. Let's continue this cooperative working relationship to achieve our goals of positive reform in health care. Thank you.

Senator REID. Thank you very much, Jim. You are welcome to participate as you see fit today. I would mention, before we start with our other two witnesses, this hearing, as I have indicated, we are very fortunate that we are able to simulcast this. As I did indicate, we had a very unfortunate incident on the University of Reno campus today where one of the police officers was killed, murdered, and there is an investigation going on.

But we were able to get the simulcast hooked up, as I have indicated. This is now being simulcast to the Great Basin College site in Battle Mountain; the Great Basin College site in Elko, NV; William Bee Ririe Hospital in Ely, NV; Mount Grant General Hospital in Hawthorne, NV; Pershing General Hospital in Lovelock, NV; Humboldt General Hospital in Winnemucca, NV; and Western Nevada Community College site in Yeringron, NV.

Scores of people are at these various sites. We appreciate very much their participation in these hearings. These hearings, as indicated in the testimony yesterday, are also concerned about rural America and rural Nevada.

It is my pleasure now to introduce Dr. Jeanette Takamura. We are lucky today to have the Secretary of Aging for this administration here in Reno. Dr. Takamura, this is basically her first trip outside Washington, DC. since her assignment. Prior to taking her job as Secretary for Aging, she served as Director of Hawaii Office of Aging.

She has worked in aging programs for many years. She has not only qualified by her experience, but also her academic background. She has a degree from the University of Hawaii, a Master's degree in social work from the same institution, and a Ph.D. in social policy from Brandeis University. We are very fortunate to have her with us today.

We also have with us Dr. Charles Bernick, who is one of the prizes that we have at the University of Nevada Medical School. He is associate professor of neurology, Chief of the Division of Neurology, University of Nevada School of Medicine. He is the founder and director of the University of Nevada Alzheimer's Disease Diagnostic and Treatment Centers. He is a member of the Alzheimer's Disease National Education Initiative and serves on the Advisory Board of the Nevada Geriatric Education Association.

Also, I wanted to just give you a flavor of the academic qualifications of this fine man. He is a graduate of Rice University, Phi Beta Kappa; University of Texas, where he also graduated with honors as a doctor. He has had an internship with San Francisco Alliance Hospital. He has had a residency in neurology at the University of Miami School of Medicine.

He has had a fellowship in neurology and neuromuscular disorders, University of Arizona, and on and on. We are very fortunate to have these two fine witnesses with us to help us understand more about aging in Nevada and in this country. Dr. Takamura.

47-539 98 - 7

STATEMENT OF JEANETTE C. TAKAMURA, ASSISTANT SECRETARY FOR AGING

Ms. TAKAMURA. Thank you, Chairman Reid, gentlemen. I appreciate the opportunity to be here to focus on an issue which is definitely uppermost in the minds of older Americans and their family members. I am especially pleased to participate this morning because you have been a true friend and a dedicated, effective advocate and leader on behalf of older Americans in our country.

Chairman Reid, I have submitted a written statement for the record. For the audience, you may wish to get a copy of it later. I will be extracting from that written statement.

Despite the evidence of improvements in the health status of older Americans, what we know is that we will continue to see increases in the need for long-term care partly because we anticipate the emergence of the baby boomer population as they begin to age. Thus, our concerns are not just only for our current elders, but also for our future elders and for their family members who we know are carrying the load as caregivers.

We know what the everyday reality of caregiving is like. In many instances, it is heart-breaking. Let me briefly highlight some of the more important federally-funded programs which serve older Americans and their family members.

As you know, the Administration on Aging, the agency which I head, grants and authorizes Older Americans Act monies to states and local communities for the development of aging and long-term care service delivery systems, and for the provision of gap-filling services among which are the more popularly known nutrition and transportation services.

Here in the State of Nevada, you have, and you are very fortunate indeed to have, some of my professional colleagues, Carla Sloan and her staff, who are very committed to serving you well. Under the Older Americans Act, they are your advocates, and they are, as I said earlier, committed to being sure that older Nevadans are well taken care of.

The Health Care Financing Administration within the U.S. Department of Health and Human Services, administers the Medicaid program, the largest source of public financing for long-term care services for both older adults and persons with disabilities. They also administer the Medicare program, which covers primarily acute care, but also offers some chronic and post-acute care benefits.

Of course, there is other Federal support and I will not be going through the litany of Federal programs. Support is available through a number of other agencies, including the Social Security Administration. I think many of you know that Supplemental Security Income is administered by Social Security and that income is used often by the aged, blind, and disabled to help cover their out-of-pocket costs for long-term care services.

Current resources for long-term care services are really not adequate to meet the growing needs of our older adults and their family members. In fact, we know that our family members are largely shouldering the burden of long-term care. In particular, I would note that women today are spending more time caring for older persons than they are in actually providing child care.

Among the long-term care issues facing national, state, and local officials are policy concerns around, first of all, the cost and financing of long-term care. Of note, the administration supported the 1996 Health Insurance Portability and Accountability Act, which clarifies the tax treatment of private long-term care insurance.

Moreover, the 1997 Balanced Budget Act offers provisions for the development of a prospective payment system for home care and for skilled nursing home facilities under Medicare. The Balanced Budget Act also provides for the repeal of the Boren Amendment under Medicaid.

Second, I would note, as an interest area for policymakers, the integration of acute and long-term care services through such mechanisms as managed care, and let me say particularly for those who are dually eligible.

However, and we must be realists, managed care organizations generally do not have an established track record in providing long-term care services. Those of us in the aging network are very much concerned about this and are truly very, very excited to be part of the discussion.

Third, assisted living facilities are sprouting up all across the country. As they grow in number, we remain concerned about the quality, their cost, and the market segments which they may or may not address.

Fourth, there is clear evidence of waste, fraud, and abuse in the Medicare and Medicaid programs, and the Administration, I would like to assure you, has taken some very bold steps by introducing Operation Restore Trust, which is a resounding success. As a result of this program, which has been able to identify specific instances of waste, fraud, and abuse, we are now moving forward and launching this effort nationwide.

The needs of most frail, older Americans and their family members are very simple. They simply wish to be cared for in their homes, to be able to afford such care, and to be assured that they will retain their dignity and ability to exercise choice in the process. These are some of the basic concerns which we must together strive to address.

As America's wonderful, and I underscore wonderful, gift of longevity touches more and more families and individuals, we must do everything that we can to ensure access, affordability, coordination, integration, and the appropriateness of services which will be needed, once again, by our current elders and also by our baby boomers.

Within this context, vigorous experimentation and the testing of new service delivery models and options, public/private partnerships and consumer education and protection, must be of the highest import.

Chairman Reid, I want to thank you again for this opportunity to focus upon long-term care issues. They are uppermost in the minds of older Americans and their family members. I look forward to working with you and I certainly am very happy to entertain any questions you might have. Thank you very much.

[The prepared statement of Ms. Takamura follows:]

DEPARTMENT OF HEALTH & HUMAN SERVICES

Washington, D.C. 20201

STATEMENT OF

JEANETTE C. TAKAMURA

ASSISTANT SECRETARY FOR AGING

DEPARTMENT OF HEALTH AND HUMAN SERVICES

BEFORE THE

SENATE SPECIAL COMMITTEE ON AGING

FIELD HEARING

JANUARY 12, 1998 - LAS VEGAS, NEVADA

JANUARY 13, 1998 - RENO, NEVADA

Mr. Chairman and Members of the Subcommittee:

It is a great privilege to be here with you today on behalf of Secretary Donna Shalala. I am indeed honored as the Assistant Secretary for Aging to be participating in this important forum with a true friend and advocate within the U.S. Senate for older Americans — the Honorable Harry Reid.

I have been asked today to provide insights into the current and future state of long-term care (LTC) at the national level. This is indeed an ambitious task, because LTC as a policy and program area is extraordinarily complex. I will attempt to provide a framework of federal LTC programs; indicate some of the key LTC issues facing policy makers at all levels; note HHS initiatives; and suggest possible future directions for LTC. I will also include a brief description of the LTC needs of older persons and their families and the importance of advocacy to ensure the emergence of a consumer-oriented, cost-effective LTC system. As I do this, I would ask you to keep in mind a number of trends. That is: 1) The older population will continue to grow. By the year 2020, there will be more than 70 million older persons in this country or more than twice the number today. The older population also is getting frailer. Despite recent evidence of declines in disability rates related to longevity, the need for LTC services will continue to expand. 2) Women, the family members who most often serve as the primary caregivers, are spending a significant amount of time providing eldercare. Indeed, some experts have indicated that women spend more years providing eldercare than child care. Concomitantly, women tend to be the primary consumers of LTC services because they generally survive their spouses, fathers, and brothers. 3) The older population is rapidly becoming more diverse as minorities live longer. For example, in 1990, 13 percent of persons 65 years and older were minorities. This percentage is projected to rise to 25 percent by 2030, almost doubling in 35 years. 4) Baby boomers, many of whom are now beginning to grapple in growing numbers with LTC concerns related to their parents, will join the ranks of our older Americans starting in 2011. By that time their own potential LTC needs will have taken on a measure of reality.

Let me briefly highlight some of the important federally funded programs which serve older Americans who require LTC beginning with those in the Department of Health and Human Services (DHHS). The Administration on Aging (AoA), the agency which I head, grants and authorizes the expenditure of funds under the Older Americans Act (OAA) to states and local communities for infrastructure development and the building of comprehensive and coordinated service delivery systems. These systems directly lend support to LTC needs through efforts to improve the coordination of other programs and funding streams. For example,

OAA funds provide gap-filling services such as transportation and nutrition services and are used for advocacy, coordination and other activities which help meet the needs and protect the rights of older adults. Here in Nevada, the Division on Aging Services under the leadership of my colleague, Carla Sloan, fulfills these responsibilities. Currently, Nevada receives $1.6 million for supportive services, including $50,000 for protective elder rights services such as the LTC Ombudsman and elder abuse activities; $2 million for congregate meals; $600,000 for home delivered meals; $87,000 for disease prevention, health promotion activities; and $52,000 for the provision of in-home services for the frail elderly. I have attached for the record a summary of some other programs administered by DHHS that address LTC.

With regard to federal funding of LTC, the Health Care Financing Administration (HCFA) administers the Medicaid program -- the largest source of public financing for LTC services for older adults. In FY 1996, approximately $16.7 billion in federal funds were expended for care in nursing facilities for the elderly. This included approximately $28.2 million for nursing home care for the elderly in Nevada. Approximately an additional $2 billion in federal funds was spent nationally for home and community-based alternative care for the elderly, including home health, personal care, and home and community-based waivers. Nevada received approximately $2.2 million of these funds. HCFA also administers Medicare, a program which mainly covers acute care benefits. However, the Medicare home health benefits cover some chronic care as well as post-acute care. In FY 1996, more than $16.7 billion was spent for home health benefits to meet chronic and post-acute care needs. A share of these funds has gone to serve the needs of older persons in this state.

Among the important agencies involved in LTC services outside DHHS are the Department of Housing and Urban Development (HUD) and the Social Security Administration (SSA). HUD, for example, administers the Supportive Housing Program for the Elderly (Section 202). In FY 1997, $645 million was appropriated to support this program nationally. SSA administers a variety of income security programs including the Supplemental Security Income (SSI) program to provide cash assistance to aged, blind, and disabled individuals and their dependent family members. Many older persons use their SSA benefits, including SSI, to pay out-of-pocket LTC expenses, including board and care.

At the federal level we are also emphasizing quality through a number of means. Last Spring, the President appointed a Commission on Consumer Protection and Quality in the Health Care Industry for which Secretary Shalala serves as a co-chair. This Fall, the Commission approved a Consumer Bill of Rights which was endorsed by the President. Additional Commission recommendations are expected later this Winter addressing requirements for protecting consumers in managed care and fee-for-service plans.

These recommendations and their implementation will have important implications for consumers of LTC.

The OAA authorizes state LTC ombudsman programs. In all 57 states and territories and 550 localities, LTC ombudsmen investigate and resolve complaints related to the care of nursing home and board and care residents. In a number of states, ombudsmen also monitor the quality of home care. This program provides a community presence in long-term care facilities by monitoring private and publicly-subsidized care.

The LTC issues which face national, state and local officials are complex. To offer a sense of this, let me just list a few major LTC policy issues.

Assisted living facilities are one of the fastest growing residential care options for older persons. Many states are wrestling with how much regulation is necessary to protect residents and ensure quality of care while assuring sufficient flexibility to sustain a home-like environment, accommodate individual residents' preferences, and avoid discouraging developers.

Industry-driven Medicare home health benefits are being utilized increasingly to meet the LTC needs of older adults. However, the Office of the Inspector General (OIG) and the General Accounting

Office have found this benefit to be very susceptible to abuse. The OIG evaluated a sample of 3,745 services in 250 home health claims in four states and estimated that 40 percent of the services did not meet Medicare reimbursement requirements.

Over at least the last two decades, Medicaid spending on nursing homes has risen. States are making efforts to control costs and increase the provision of home and community-based services. The rates of increase for nursing home expenditures have been declining and nursing home utilization rates are beginning to come down. However, estimates of nursing home expenditures continue to increase at rates beyond the overall inflation rate, e.g., 7.8 percent in FY 1995. Nursing home spending continues to be a significant part of total Medicaid expenditures for older persons, e.g., almost 64 percent in FY 1995, with an additional 8 percent spent on home care.

Out of an interest in creating a more seamless, cost-effective system of care, federal and state officials alike are giving increased attention to strategies for integrating acute and LTC through mechanisms such as managed care, especially for those older persons who are dually eligible for Medicare and Medicaid. Managed care organizations, primarily concerned with primary and acute care in the past, generally do not have an established track record in LTC and many advocates are concerned about this lack of experience. For these reasons, we need to monitor closely provider performance.

From the beginning of his administration, the President has maintained a strong and continuing commitment to health care reform. This commitment has been reflected in LTC efforts by DHHS and other federal agencies. At the 1995 White House Conference on Aging, President Clinton unveiled Operation Restore Trust (ORT) to combat fraud and abuse in the Medicare and Medicaid programs, targeting in particular nursing homes and home health agencies with questionable fiscal and care practices. Within DHHS, the Office of the Inspector General, HCFA, and AoA, partnered, along with the Department of Justice, to carry out ORT demonstrations in five states. The ORT demonstration has proved so successful that a full-scale national effort is now underway.

The Administration supported the 1996 Health Insurance Portability and Accountability Act (HIPAA) authored by Senators Kassebaum and Kennedy. The HIPAA clarifies tax treatment of private LTC insurance and directs the Department of Treasury to prepare regulations for the implementation of these provisions in consultation with DHHS.

Through the 1997 Balanced Budget Act (BBA), the President took important steps toward improving and expanding health care access and quality. The BBA includes provisions for developing a prospective payment system for home care and skilled nursing home facilities under Medicare and the repeal of the Boren Amendment under Medicaid, all of which are expected to reduce nursing home and home health costs. The BBA also provides for an expansion of the PACE program, which represents one model for integrating LTC and acute care using Medicare, Medicaid, and other dollars.

The AoA has been engaged for the last three decades in partnership with State and Area Agencies on Aging in the development of a LTC infrastructure. More than half of all State Units on Aging nationwide are administering Medicaid waiver programs, two-thirds are administering the widely-appreciated Health Insurance Counseling and Assistance Program, and one half are administering programs for adults with disabilities. Many area agencies have taken on similar responsibilities at the local level.

While the scope and operation of LTC systems are complex and the issues pertaining to the system of services, costs and quality of care are challenging, the needs of most frail older Americans and their families are relatively simple. The majority of older Americans live at home or in small community residential settings. As survey after survey has shown, older adults and their families — the payers of the major portion of LTC costs, prefer to have services provided in their homes and communities rather than in institutions. Long-term care, particularly when it is delivered in the community, does not generally involve expensive medical care. For the most part, it entails basic assistance with dressing, eating, using the bathroom, and other activities of daily living. Personal care, meal preparation, or chore services — whether provided by one of the millions of volunteer caregivers, family members, neighbors, friends, or by a paid service provider — can help older persons remain in their homes as long as possible. As simple as the needs of a frail older person may be, some basic infrastructure must be in place and accessible to them. For instance, an ideal home and community-based care system would include the following services, as appropriate: personal care, homemaker, and chore services; congregate and home-delivered meals; adult day care; rehabilitative care; assisted transportation; home health care; supportive services for caregivers; and assisted living. Because older Americans often have multiple and changing health and social service needs, effective HCB service programs also require administrative arrangements that facilitate the coordination of and access to HCB and institutional services, including discharge planning, case management, pre-admission screening, and linkages to medical providers.

In light of the gift of longevity with which a growing majority of Americans are now blessed, we must engage as a nation in ensuring that we have an architecture for longevity in place; i.e., a design for the future which acknowledges long life as a reality, is sensitive to the needs of current elders, and is informed by the likely requirements and contributions of the largest cohort of older adults this world has yet to see — the baby boomers. Let me thus suggest four areas where more attention must be focused at the federal level if we are to empower all Americans as well as develop a LTC system which resonates with the broadest spectrum of our population.

- **We must ready America for longevity.** That is, those of us in federal positions of responsibility must be sure that all Americans are aware of and prepared for the challenges and opportunities which lie ahead for our communities, families, and ourselves as the gift of longevity begins to manifest itself in even more pronounced ways. To the extent that life expectancy is increasing and disability rates among the elderly are declining, we need to foster a climate of "active aging", where society can continue to draw on the talents of its older citizens. At the same time, frail elders with disabilities need access to appropriate long-term care services in their communities.

- **We must give greater emphasis to consumer education and protection.** Although increased choices are leading to healthy market competition and in most cases improved potential consumer options, the number and magnitude of these choices is bewildering to many older persons. As you know, HCFA is launching a number of consumer education efforts around the new preventive benefits and managed care options under the BBA. We support these and are working closely with them. In addition, last year we transmitted to the aging network our managed care principles which suggested broad roles in advocacy, information and assistance, benefits counseling, quality assurance, care management, and consumer protection, including adopting the ombudsman function in managed care. Because the aging network is so concerned about the relationship of managed care to LTC, it is important that we encourage them to establish a clear understanding of what approaches they will adopt in relation to managed care organizations, particularly in regard to advocacy and consumer protection.

- **We must encourage public-private partnerships as well as partnerships among federal agencies which can generate more resources, new creative approaches, and which recognize and address the diverse needs of a longevous population.** There is hardly enough that we can do in this regard, particularly if we are committed to fostering the development of more coordinated and effective services. The AoA and I take the coordination and advocacy responsibilities seriously. We are already beginning to plan how these might be carried out through partnerships with others.

- **We need vigorous experimentation and testing to determine what is working and at what cost.** The HCB waiver program has expanded dramatically and supports reforms that can make HCB services a more attractive alternative to institutional care. I submit that the Title IV research and demonstration program under the OAA is another important vehicle for doing the type of demonstrations that are needed in LTC, particularly for non-nursing home eligible older persons. As most people in the field recognize, Title IV has been the testing ground for many important developments in LTC, e.g., On Lok (the predecessor of PACE), case management (particularly under the channeling projects), the LTC Ombudsman Program, and national LTC resource centers and state planning grants.

This concludes my assessment of the current state of LTC at the national level and some of the future possibilities for improving services for older persons. Obviously there is much we all must do at every level of government to institute needed changes in the way LTC is organized, financed and delivered. The AoA is just one of many agencies that has an important role to play in this endeavor. Nonetheless, it is an important role. The OAA authorizes the AoA to be an "effective and visible advocate for older persons" within DHHS and other departments and agencies, and to coordinate federal, state local and private programs to "establish a nationwide network of comprehensive and coordinated services" for older persons. As the new Assistant Secretary for Aging, I am anxious to begin initiating discussions with others with the goal of promoting the development of more effective LTC systems for older persons and all those needing LTC.

Finally, I would like to thank you, Senator Reid, for providing me with this opportunity to be here with you in Nevada and to present testimony before the Senate Special Committee on Aging on this important topic. I look forward to the rest of this morning's hearing, and working with you as we move forward toward improving LTC services. I will be happy to answer any questions you might have.

ATTACHMENT 1

SUMMARY OF OTHER DHHS PROGRAMS RELATED TO LTC

The Administration for Children and Families (ACF) administers the Social Services Block Grants which are awarded to states and may be used to provide a broad array of supportive, social, and personal care and assistance services to persons in need of home and community-based assistance, including the elderly. In FY 1997, $13.9 million was allocated to Nevada.

The Substance Abuse and Mental Health Services Administration (SAMSHA) administers, among other programs, the Community Mental Health Block Grants which are formula grants to each state to carry out comprehensive community mental health services for all populations regardless of age. In FY 1997, Nevada received $1.4 million under this program.

The Health Resources and Services Administration (HRSA) has administered since 1992 a State Alzheimer's Disease Demonstration Program which is designed to demonstrate new approaches to providing home and community-based services to Alzheimer's victims and their families. Currently, $6 million is allocated to 15 states. While Nevada is not one of these states, the new approaches under development will be of use in planning community-based approaches to addressing the issues of Alzheimer's disease.

The <u>Office of the Assistant Secretary for Planning and Evaluation (ASPE)</u> funds a large number of national policy research studies relative to disability, aging and LTC. Currently, two of their most significant ones are the evaluation of the Cash and Counseling demonstrations funded by the Robert Wood Johnson Foundation and a national study of assisted living. The cash and counseling demonstrations are designed to test new methods of providing consumer-directed services for the elderly and the disabled. The assisted living study is examining the state-of-the-art of the emerging area of assisted living and how it fits into the development of LTC systems around the country. Both of these studies have important policy implications for Nevada and other states.

Senator REID. Dr. Bernick.

STATEMENT OF CHARLES BERNICK, M.D., DEPARTMENT OF INTERNAL MEDICINE DIVISION OF NEUROLOGY, UNIVERSITY OF NEVADA SCHOOL OF MEDICINE

Dr. BERNICK. Senator Reid and members of the field committee, I very much appreciate this opportunity to address the committee regarding the unique demands that patients with Alzheimer's disease are going to place on long-term care systems in the future.

The fact that Alzheimer's disease is a major public health problem, I think, is widely recognized. The numbers speak for themselves. Close to 10 percent of individuals over the age of 65 and probably 40 percent of people over the age of 85 have Alzheimer's disease.

With the over 85 years of age group being the fastest growing segment of our population in Nevada and the nation, it has been estimated that the number of people afflicted by this disease by the year 2050 will rise from its current level of 4 million to 14 million Americans.

The effect of Alzheimer's disease, though, goes beyond those numbers. I think it really relates to the nature of the disease itself, which is one that robs people of their memory and other mental and cognitive abilities to the point that we know that every one of those 14 million will need, at some point in their course, 24-hour supervision and care and many of them will require institutionalization.

The needs of these people, though, do change as the disease progresses. Early on, they may just need modest supervision with finances and medications, but as the disease progresses, more troublesome behaviors could occur for caregivers to deal with. It could be aggressiveness, agitation, wandering, getting lost, help in daily activities such as toileting and bathing.

It is really not surprising that 50 percent of people that are caregivers are themselves depressed. Unfortunately, the services to shore up this fragile part of our system is pretty sparse. I think most caregivers have to either depend on family members, adult day care, or paid home health aides or companions to get the respite time that they need.

For many people, these services either are not available or are not affordable. For example, because of the geographic separation of families these days, there may not be any family members around. Or if you do live in a rural area, you may not have adult day care available. If these services are available, you may not be able to afford them because day care and home health aides are not a benefit of Medicare. So many people have to pay out of pocket.

Because of this, eventually most or many people with Alzheimer's disease do have to be placed. The caregivers cannot handle it. I think that placement is a very difficult decision because of many concerns by the family. One is the concern of the quality and appropriateness of the care that they are going to get in residential care. There are many concerns about it.

Are the staff trained to deal with Alzheimer's patients? Do they have activities and programs that are appropriate for them? Are these people going to be over-medicated just to keep their behaviors under control or isolated?

And besides that, I think there is a tremendous burden financially on patients. Individuals will have to pay out of pocket for assisted living or group care, or they have the option of spending down, that is depleting all their savings, so that they can qualify for Medicaid. And even then, their only choice really is in a skilled nursing facility.

I think the potential exists for private insurance to cover long-term care, as you mentioned yesterday, but at the moment, many policies are very restrictive and are too expensive for most elderly individuals.

So in sum, I think in the coming years, Alzheimer's disease will place an increasing burden on our long-term care system. I think there are going to be several issues that I know we are going to hear more and more over and over again today on what we need to address.

One is developing programs and expanding services to assist families and caregivers so that people can stay at home longer. We know that is cost-effective. It costs $12,000 to keep someone at home compared to $40,000 if you are going into a nursing home.

We need to reduce the gap between the care that is needed and the services that are provided by residential care facilities, and this may mean designing new forms of residential care in holding these facilities accountable for the quality of their care.

We need to find alternative ways to finance this care, which you have discussed yesterday. I think there is going to need to be some combination of public and private sources. I think we need to continue funding research into this disease because that ultimately will be the only way to shore up this flood of cases we are going to be seeing in the future. I thank you.

[The prepared statement of Dr. Bernick follows:]

UNIVERSITY OF NEVADA
SCHOOL OF MEDICINE

Dept. of Internal Medicine
Division of Neurology
901 S. Rancho Lane
Suite 105
Las Vegas, Nevada 89106
(702) 474-0532
Fax # (702) 477-0033

THE MANY FACES OF LONG TERM CARE: TODAYS BITTER PILL OR TOMMORROWS CURE?

Testimony before the

Senate Special Committee on Aging Field Hearing

January 12, 1998
West Charleston Library
Las Vegas, Nevada

January 13, 1998
Washoe Medical Center Auditorium
Reno, Nevada

Presented by
Charles Bernick, M.D.

Senator Reid and members of the field hearing committee. My name is Charles Bernick and I am the director of the University of Nevada Alzheimer's Disease Diagnostic and Treatment Centers for the state of Nevada. I very much appreciate this opportunity to address the committee regarding the unique demands placed by patients afflicted with Alzheimer's Disease and related dementias on long term care systems.

That Alzheimer's Disease is a major public health problem is widely acknowledged. Close to 10% of individuals over the age of 65, and 40% of those over 85 years of age, suffer from Alzheimer's Disease and other forms of dementia (which I will subsequently lump together with Alzheimer's Disease in this testimony).With the 85 and older age group being the fastest growing segment of the population in Nevada and the nation, it is estimated that the number of patients with Alzheimer's Disease (AD) will rise from the 4 million currently affected to 14 million by the year 2050.

More than just the numbers, AD has a significant impact on long term care due to the nature of the condition. Alzheimer's Disease relentlessly and progressively impairs memory and other cognitive function; every individual with AD will at some point in their disease require 24 hour care and supervision, with many eventually needing institutionalization.

The type of care needed by AD patients changes with disease progression. Though it is often recognized that 50% of nursing home patients have AD, what is less known is that unpaid family caregivers represent a critical and hidden part of long term care in the United States. Approximately 80% of AD patients are cared for at home by family. Initially, caregivers may only have to supply moderate supervision such as managing finances and medication, in addition to dealing with the repetitiveness and frustration that may come with memory decline. As the disease advances, caregivers may need to cope with more troublesome behaviors such as wandering, paranoia, agitation, physical abusiveness, sleep impairment and need for assistance with self care tasks (eg bathing, dressing and feeding). Some family member leave or reduce paid employment to assume the caregiving role. It is not surprising that studies show 50% of caregivers are themselves depressed and suffer from impaired health.

Services to shore up this fragile part of the long term care spectrum are sparse. Most caregivers must either depend on other family members, adult day care services or paid home health aides or companions for badly needed respite time. Unfortunately, these resources may not be available or financially feasible for all caregivers. For example, adult day care or sitter services are not covered by Medicare and only on a limited basis by Medicaid programs. Furthermore, in rural areas that are far from a major city, as we have in Nevada, there may not be any respite services short of family and friends.

When family caregivers are no longer able to provide care at home, the AD patient is placed into some type of residential care, either a group home or nursing home. Placement decisions are extremely difficult for caregivers due to both emotional and economic concerns.

One recurring worry of caregivers is the quality and appropriateness of care provided by these facilities, and for good reason. These is frequently a gap between the services available and the care an AD patient needs. In the case of group homes, there is a concern regarding the type of training staff members receive in handling dementia patients, along with the social activities provided. Some of the same issues apply to nursing homes, which traditionally have emphasized care of residents with physical illness in need of skilled nursing facilities. Nursing homes have in the past been accused of "warehousing" AD patients, using strategies such as isolation and employment of physical and pharmacological restraint in response to disruptive behaviors.

The past ten years has seen a proliferation of Special Care Units (SCU) in nursing homes. These units purport to offer programs more tailored to dementia patients. The efficacy of SCUs has not yet been systematically demonstrated. More disturbing, studies indicate that not all SCUs offer the same degree of specialized care, with some units only differing from the rest of the facility by being locked.

The cost of residential care becomes another tremendous burden for families. Group home care must be payed out of pocket. Because Medicaid will fund nursing home care, families are often forced to spend down their assets to qualify for welfare. This is indeed a "bitter pill to swallow" for many who have worked their entire life, yet accumulated limited savings. The potential exists for private insurance policies to cover long term care. However, many policies offer only restricted coverages or are too expensive for most elderly persons.

In summary, in the coming years, AD will place an increasing burden on long term care. Several issues deserve further consideration:
1) Because institutionalization of AD patients is often determined by the interplay between disease progression and caregiver vulnerability, programs and services aimed at assisting families with caregiving are needed. More recognition should be directed at family caregivers, as this unpaid force is a dam against the flood of AD cases that are anticipated.
2) Strategies to reduce the gap between the care required by a dementia patient and services provided by residential facilities need further development. These strategies might include alternative forms of residential care, programs to increase social activities and new design principles in refurbishing or building new facilities.
3) Alternative ways to finance the care of AD patients should be evaluated. Some of the reforms that have been proposed include increasing the availability of long term care insurance, extending the health maintenance organization model of prepaid financing to cover long term care services, allowing AD patients to cash in life insurance policies early, allowing more flexibility in funds from Medicaid to cover group home and home health services, and providing tax credits or other forms of relief for family caregivers.
4) Research into treatments for AD needs to be continually supported. A treatment that would simply delay the onset of the disease for 5 years would reduce in half the number of individuals afflicted with AD.

Thank you for your consideration.

Senator REID. Doctor, would you be kind enough to tell everyone assembled, what is Alzheimer's disease? How would you describe the disease? We know how disabled people become, but talk about the disease and what we are doing to find out what we can do to delay the onset of the disease and hopefully some day to cure the disease.

Dr. BERNICK. Well, Senator, to be very brief about it, Alzheimer's disease is a degenerative disease of the brain. That is, nerve cells are dying in certain areas of the brain which manifests itself by the loss of memory and other mental abilities. Fortunately, there is a lot of research going on and we know that if we can find a treatment that will just delay the onset of the disease for five years, not cure it, just delay the onset, we will reduce in half the number of people with this disease.

I think that is a realistic expectation. There are many studies going on now, even traditional drugs such as anti-inflammatories, and estrogen replacement in women to try to delay the onset of the disease. There are two drugs on the market already to improve symptoms of the disease. I think there is truly optimism in finding ways to manage this disease, slow its progression, and prevent its onset, which we should be able to see in the near future.

Senator REID. What is the medical research community doing about this as far as Federal monies to help, state grants? What is being done? Private institutions helping? What is happening?

Dr. BERNICK. Well, I think all of those sources contribute to the research that is going on. Certainly Federal monies are very important in large-scale research efforts. Interestingly, industry is also involved. As you might imagine, the pharmaceutical industry has a vested interest in developing treatments that may be effective to this huge population.

So there is a lot of activity going on. Of course, there always can be more and I think from the Alzheimer's Association standpoint, the request for further Federal funding is always going to be there until we find a cure for the disease.

Senator REID. It is interesting to note that with all the tremendous cutbacks in the past five years in almost every program, the two programs where there has not been a cutback is in Immigration and Naturalization Service and the National Institutes of Health. Last year alone, the National Institutes of Health had a 7 percent increase, which I think speaks well of this country's desire to attack some of these diseases.

I would say and ask, Dr. Bernick, if you and Dr. Takamura would agree that spending money for research now has the potential for saving us lots of money in the out-years. That is clearly true, isn't it?

Ms. TAKAMURA. I think that is true. I also would like to mention that there is a wonderful partnership between HRSA, the Health Resources and Services Administration, and the Administration on Aging to provide demonstration programs to actually support caregivers who are providing services to family members with Alzheimer's.

I think anything we can do to find a cure, find a way to retard the progression of the disease, and to support caregivers is certainly money well spent.

Senator REID. It did not go over my head and I am sure it did not go over anyone's head here, that the average cost of keeping someone who is ill with Alzheimer's or Parkinson's at home is about $12,000 a year or $1,000 a month. But to put them in institutional care is $40,000 a year or $3,500 a month, or something like that. So there is clearly the case we need to do more.

I would like to hear, Dr. Takamura, you talked a little bit about this Operation Restore Trust. You passed over that quickly. Tell those within the sound of our voices what this is all about.

Ms. TAKAMURA. Thank you for giving me the opportunity to briefly talk about Operation Restore Trust. It is a wonderful initiative that represents a partnership between the Office of the Inspector General, the Administration on Aging, the Department of Justice, and other branches of the Federal government to really pursue welfare—excuse me, not welfare—Medicare and Medicaid waste, fraud, and abuse.

We are finding ourselves highly successful. We have found many billing systems, for example, have not been as efficient as we would like. We have found over-billing in some instances. We have been very successful in recovering money and we think that this is an essential effort.

Senator REID. I think the figures are that for every dollar we spend in going after fraud, waste, and abuse, we bring back over ten dollars to the Federal coffers.

Ms. TAKAMURA. That is right.

Senator REID. So it is an area also where we have to be generous in the beginning because in the long run we wind up saving a lot of money. Congressman Gibbons, we are going to wind this panel down. I want to make sure you have an opportunity to ask them any questions or make a statement if you care to.

Mr. GIBBONS. Thank you, Senator. I think one of the more important things we can do here is what can we do as policymakers in terms of assisting in helping reduce the cost. I was very taken by the fact that caring for an Alzheimer's patient in the home is $12,000 a year versus $40,000.

I think one of the policy things that we can do is to improve not just the quality of life of the patient who is involved, but the quality of life of those who care for those individuals in the private sector. It is important for us to make sure that we do enact policies that help reduce the cost, reduce the burden on those individuals that help us care for our loved ones.

One of the issues that I always am very taken by is the cost of prescription drugs in our medical society. It is an important issue in terms of a growing senior population who becomes less and less capable of spending higher and higher dollar amounts on more and more expensive drugs.

I think a policy of this nation ought to be to help ensure a reduction in the cost of those drugs, either through some program to help in the research, as we talked about earlier, and development of less expensive medicines and to help also seniors be able to include the cost of prescriptions in some of their insurance, whether it is in Medicare or through another insurance program.

I think there are some ideas and policies that we as policymakers in Congress can work on.

Senator REID. Your point is well-taken, Congressman, because Dr. Bernick said one of the ways we are going to delay the onset, it appears at this stage, is through medication, which is not covered with the traditional Medicare program. So you certainly bring out a very important point.

Also, the point that you mentioned was mentioned both by Dr. Takamura and Dr. Bernick in passing and that is, we really have to be concerned about the caregivers. We believe, as Dr. Bernick said, that 50 percent or more of the caregivers of patients with Alzheimer's are depressed themselves, not because of any reason other than the tremendous burden they have to take care of these problems.

I have to say that it helps, of course, for people to have money to care for their mother, father, whoever it is, but even with people with money, the burden of caregiving is extremely difficult. We keep mentioning in this hearing today about yesterday. We had a hearing yesterday where we covered many of these same areas and that is why we keep referring to them.

One of the things we talked about yesterday is respite care. People who take care of those who are sick for long periods of time, they need a break, whether it is to go out to dinner, go to a movie, take a drive, but some of them are simply unable to do it because of the restrictions at home.

I think what we found, there are a few programs, but most of them are voluntary in nature. Most of the programs where you get respite care are those where people, good-hearted people in this state, have agreed to come in and spend a little time to relieve someone. The problem we have with that, of course, is the problem we have with a number of areas in this area of health care.

We had a woman yesterday who came in and talked about some problems she was having with her mother. Her mother is 79, has very serious arthritis. She has sold everything that she owns except her job to take care of her mother, and she is on her last legs and now she is trying to get her mother in a rest home. Her mother was there with her yesterday.

But she went through some of the horror stories of advertising in the newspaper for people to come in and take care of her mother. One stole all their jewelry. One went out a window in the middle of the night with some of her possessions. Another had a nervous breakdown on the job. I mean, she could have written a short story on her problems dealing with her mom.

So these are all serious problems that we have not found answers to yet. As I said yesterday when we finished this panel and I think I will probably say the same thing after the next two panels, we do not have all the answers, but at least we are now asking some of the questions, which has not been done before.

Here at the table with me are the people who are going to go back to Washington and carry forward with the work. Congressman Gibbons and I are going to go out when this hearing is over and worry about nuclear waste and worry about grazing fees and what is happening up at Lake Tahoe and the railroad going through Reno.

We have a lot of things we are working on. These staff directors at this table are concerned only about aging problems and this hearing is something that they will take back to Washington, share with the chairman and the ranking member of the committee, and hopefully move forward with policy for the entire Senate.

I did not introduce my staff director, Jerry Reed, no relative, no relation, there is no nepotism here. He spells his name R-E-E-D, although he does such a good job I would like to claim him as a relative.

So anyway, panel, thank you very much for your time and efforts.

Mr. GIBBONS. Thank you, Senator. [Applause.]

Senator REID. We are now going to change the order of people testifying. We are going to begin Panel 2. Panel 1, as you know, was entitled the present, in effect, and we hope provided some insights into the current and future state of long-term care at the national level, discussions of the strengths and weaknesses of long-term care, and future initiatives for improvement of the programs.

Today's second panel will articulate concerns over patient safety, law enforcement, financial issues, quality of care issues, and options for care. The panelists will share personal experiences with long-term care within the context of their relevant personal and professional roles. Ombudsman programs, patient advocates, the 1987 OBRA Act, licensing requirements, and other facets of facility regulation and oversight will be addressed.

Let me say again how much we all appreciate the diligent work of the University of Nevada and Washoe Med for allowing us to work with our friends in rural Nevada. Seven sites. We could not have done it without Washoe Med and the University of Nevada.

We are first going to hear from Carol Hunter. We had today scheduled that her mom would be able to come with her, but her mother is a nursing home resident and she simply was not capable of coming here today. We are very fortunate to have Carol Hunter with us. Please proceed.

STATEMENT OF CAROL HUNTER, MOTHER OF JANET HUNTER, A NURSING HOME RESIDENT

Ms. HUNTER. Thank you, Senator Reid. Good morning and again, thank you for the opportunity to participate in this panel. My mother, Janet Hunter, is currently residing at a skilled nursing facility in Reno. The goal of my testimony today is to provide information to you, other caregivers, and managers of skilled nursing facilities on what nursing home placement represents to those involved in the process.

Truly, the most difficult task I ever fulfilled was to assist my mother with her placement into a nursing home. Many years before, my mother had to facilitate a similar placement for her mother and I know the anxiety she experienced with that placement.

While my mother always declared she would never put her daughter through this type of process, we both knew the decision to transfer to a skilled facility was the best and only option. My apprehension was based on many years of experience as an advocate for elder rights. I am all too aware of the transgressions associated with nursing home placement, even in the best of facilities.

While it remained mostly unspoken, my mother's reaction was a combination of fear and defeat. Fear based on the transgressions suffered by her own mother as well as friends and colleagues placed in nursing homes, and defeat based on the absolute knowledge that her long-held independence was in critical jeopardy.

Sadly, many of her fears were realized. Her entry into the facility can be described as planned chaos. Several staff members arrived to take a variety of tests, administer instructions, and acknowledge her entry. Yet, no single person in a position of authority came to welcome her, explain routines, inquire about her anxieties and expectations. Suddenly she was one of many.

Subsequent to admission, our anxiety was heightened. A fall due to improper supervision, loss of many dearly-held personal rights, and a persistent reduction in what she had known as the quality of care. Overnight, she was dependent on an ever-changing array of strangers for the most personal of needs. The timeliness of the care depended on her workload or the interest of the staff on duty at the time.

Her daily routine of many years no longer existed. Her dignity was challenged and her spirit noticeably diminished. I must note that my mother enjoys the advantage of having a personal caregiver who assists her through companionship, attendance to personal needs such as showers and laundry. Her caregiver has earned our implicit trust and consistently excels in her assumption of the role as friend, companion, and advocate.

Unfortunately, having a caregiver created a new set of concerns. Her caregiver gradually assumed duties that were clearly the responsibility of the facility staff, linen changes, assistance with personal hygiene. She frequently assumed these duties because staff could not, due to an overwhelming workload, 12-hour shifts, persistent overtime, or staff who would not due to lack of personal initiative.

Be assured that my comments are not intended as an indictment of the long-term care industry. Rather, I feel my mother's care is overall better than expected. Where the industry does fail is in the recognition of what nursing home placement represents.

I encourage intensive, hands-on training for all staff, including administration, on the aging process. Experience what it is like to no longer see clearly, hear clearly, move without assistance, fulfill the most personal of tasks, recognize and experience the radical transition from independence to dependence, acknowledge the fear and isolation that comes with placement, acknowledge the resident's rights and needs.

I care and fear the most for those residents that have no family, friends, or colleagues who will advocate for their rights. The long-term care ombudsman program is a critical resource for these residents. Ms. Gilda Johnstone and the local Aging Services Office has been an invaluable resource as well as a tenacious advocate for the rights of residents.

Further, appreciate the predicament of the families suddenly confronted with an unintelligible maze of bills, medical jargon, and responsibilities complicated by the guilt, fear, and frustration that is inherent with the placement of a loved one into the care of strangers. Truly my mother is an exception in the process. She is blessed with financial resources as well as a combination of strong will, family, lifetime friends, influential colleagues, as well as an exceptional medical and professional team.

Most importantly, recognize that the system has serious gaps in the consistency of care. Work diligently to close these gaps, focus on client and staff needs, and be driven by a commitment to a quality of care that you would want for yourself.

Senator REID. Thank you very much. We are going to have questions for you, so be patient.

[The prepared statement of Ms. Hunter follows:]

1. TESTIMONY: U.S. SENATE SPECIAL COMMITTEE ON AGING

" The Many Faces of Long-Term Care: Today's Bitter Pill or Tomorrow's Cure?"

Conducted January 13, 1997, Reno, Nevada at Washoe Medical Center Auditorium

Carol F. Hunter, Las Vegas, Nevada

Janet Hunter, Reno, Nevada. Currently residing at Skilled Nursing Facility in Reno, Nevada

▲▲▲▲▲▲▲▲▲▲▲▲ ▲▲▲▲▲▲▲▲▲▲▲

Senator Reid and Committee Members:

I am Carol Hunter, daughter of Janet Hunter. My mother is currently residing at a Skilled Nursing Facility, located in Reno, Nevada. A goal of my testimony today is to provide information to you, other caregivers and managers of skilled nursing facilities on what nursing home placement represents to those involved in the process.

Truly the most difficult task I ever fulfilled was to assist my mother with her placement in a nursing home during August, 1997. Many years before, my mother had to facilitate a similar placement for her parent, Mrs. Francis Holcomb. I knew the agony my mother experienced with this placement, including the mixed reactions of all other family members and friends. The pressure to "do the right thing" was intense; nursing home placement, in spite of monumental misgivings, was the best answer.

While my mother always declared she would never "put her daughter through the same process", we both knew when the decision to transfer to skilled care was the best, and only, option. Yet, the decision was not made without tremendous misgivings. My apprehension was based on many years of experience as an advocate for Elder Rights; I am all too aware of the hurdles, pains and personal violations associated with nursing home placement - even in the best of facilities.

While it remained mostly unspoken, my mother's reaction was a combination of fear and defeat. Fear, based on the transgressions suffered by her own mother as well as friends and colleagues placed into nursing homes, and defeat, based on the absolute knowledge that her long held independence was in critical jeopardy.

Sadly, many of her fears were realized. Her entry into the facility can be described as planned chaos. Several staff members arrived to take a variety of tests, administer instructions and acknowledge her entry. Yet, no single person in a position of authority came to welcome her, explain routines, inquire about her anxieties or expections. Suddenly, she was "one of many". Subsequent to admission, our anxiety was heightened: a fall due to improper supervision, loss of many dearly held personal rights and a persistent reduction in what she had known as quality of life. Overnight she was dependent on an ever changing array of strangers for the most personal of needs - the timeliness of this care dependent on the workload or interest of the staff on duty at the time. Her daily routine, of many years, no longer existed. Her dignity was challenged at every turn and her spirit noticeably diminished to frightening levels.

I must note that my mother enjoys the advantage of having a personal caregiver who assists her through companionship, attendance to personal needs such as showers, laundry and other related duties. Her caregiver has earned our implicit trust and consistently excels in her assumption of the role as friend, companion and advocate. Unfortunately having a caregiver creates a new set of concerns; her caregiver gradually assumed duties that were clearly the responsibility of the facility staff, e.g. linen changes, assistance with personal hygiene, advocacy to assure the preservation of her personal rights. She frequently assumed these duties because staff did not, due to overwhelming workloads, twelve (12) hour shifts and frequent overtime: or staff who would not, due to lack of personal initiative.

Be assured that my comments are not intended as an indictment of the long term care industry. Rather, I feel my mother's care is overall better than expected. Where the industry does fail is in the recognition of what nursing home placement represents. I encourage intensive, hands-on training for all staff, including administration, on the aging process. Experience what it is like to no longer see clearly, hear clearly, move without assistance and fulfill the most personal of tasks. Recognize and experience the radical transition from independence to dependence; acknowledge the fear and isolation that comes with placement.

Acknowledge the resident's needs and rights - under all circumstances. I care and fear the most for those residents that have no family, friends or colleagues who will advocate for their rights. The Long Term Care Ombudsman program, a component of Nevada's Division for Aging Services, is a critical resource for these residents. I can assure the quality of this resource through personal experience. Ms. Gilda Johnstone, an Ombudsman in the Reno Aging Services office, has been an invaluable resource - as well as a tenacious advocate for the rights of resident's.

Further, appreciate the predicament of the families: suddenly confronted with an unintelligible maze of bills, medical jargons and responsibilities - complicated by the guilt, fear and frustration that is inherent with the placement of a loved one into the care of strangers.

47-539 98 - 8

Truly, my mother is an exception in this process. She is blessed with financial resources as well as a combination of strong personal will, family, life-time friends, influential colleagues as well as an exceptional medical and professional team. Yet, note that her experience, even with this team of advocates, has included violations of her personal needs and rights.

Most importantly, recognize that the system has serious gaps in the consistency of care. Work diligently to close these gaps, focus on client and staff needs and be driven by a commitment to a quality of care you would want for yourself.

47 539 664

Senator REID. We will now hear from our Attorney General, Frankie Sue Del Papa.

STATEMENT OF FRANKIE SUE DEL PAPA, ATTORNEY GENERAL, STATE OF NEVADA

Ms. DEL PAPA. Senator Reid and members of the committee, in Nevada, the Medicaid Fraud Control Unit of the Attorney General's Office has primary jurisdiction to investigate and prosecute patient abuses in long-term care facilities, and that would be fiscal abuse and also physical abuse.

Our Medicaid Fraud Control Unit has received almost a 50 percent increase in the number of complaints and referrals of patient abuse and neglect in the last year. Over the last two years, the Medicaid Fraud Control Unit has reviewed over 130 complaints and referrals and opened over 20 criminal investigations.

These numbers may reflect the need to address the serious problem of patient abuse and neglect in our state, but these numbers may also reflect the increased reporting of abuse cases thanks to ongoing public education and awareness efforts.

In the fall of 1995, the Attorney General's Office, in conjunction with the Department of Human Resources and county social services agencies, formed a long-term care task force to help meet the needs of a rapidly growing senior population in our state. This task force produced the report, "Choices for Seniors," which addressed the following.

The need to develop choices among a range of service options which are responsive to seniors' needs, the responsibility to assure the availability of these choices in settings where quality of care can be assured, and the commitment to educate all factions of the community regarding elder abuse, neglect, and exploitation.

To help with this commitment, the Attorney General's Office published a practical guide to long-term care, a pamphlet containing tips on how to choose a long-term care facility, information on the rights of residents, and information on alternatives to nursing home care.

In order to better meet the needs of growing long-term care needs of senior Nevadans who require varying degrees of assistance and medical attention, the State and Federal governments need to explore the possibility of extending Medicaid and Medicare funds to assist seniors who could live in less-restrictive settings than skilled nursing facilities.

Additionally, it is critical that the jurisdiction of the Medicaid Fraud Control Units be similarly expanded. In fact, the National Association of Attorneys General has asked for flexibility or some relaxation of the rules in order to better coordinate with other law enforcement agencies.

As more and more seniors make Nevada their home, it is important to provide strong systems for their safety and well-being, whether or not they reside in long-term care facilities. In the fall of 1996, my office joined forces with Betsy Kolkoski, the elders rights attorney for the Division for Aging Services, to come up with a more comprehensive plan to address the growing problem of elder abuse, neglect, and exploitation.

We met with, among others, senior advocates from both private and public sectors and used their input to publish an action plan to better protect Nevada's elderly. The passage of legislation proposed in the action plan at this past legislative session included A.B. 242, which made Nevada one of the first states to recognize the intentional and unjustified isolation of the elderly as a serious crime.

S.B. 80, which doubled the damages and authorized recovery of attorney's fees in civil litigation involving elder abuse, neglect, exploitation, and isolation. A.B. 9, Assemblyman Mark Manendo's bill to increase the minimum penalty for criminal elder abuse was amended to add funeral home employees as mandatory elder abuse reporters and to authorize an elder abuse reporting hotline.

A.B. 155, which was proposed by Assemblywoman Vivian Freeman and Assemblyman Jack Close, was strongly supported by participants in the action plan. This bill requires the fingerprinting and mandatory criminal background checks for long-term care employees.

In addition to the legislation that I have just mentioned, implementation of the goals of the action plan has led to the publication of this guide for mandated reporters. Actually there are thousands of copies that have been distributed with reference to that.

We have also developed protocols to help law enforcement and protective services agencies better coordinate and communicate with reference to their response to the investigations of elder abuse. We have distributed statewide a video entitled, "RX for Abuse," which was produced by the Division for Aging Services to provide health care professionals with information on how to detect and report cases of elder abuse.

We have done public service announcements. We have done a guardianship survey. We have obtained funding for additional elder abuse videos and materials to provide education to law enforcement officers. And we are in the process of creating the elder abuse reporting hotline in northern Nevada.

In conclusion, I would like to applaud Senators Reid, Kohl, and Grassley for co-sponsoring the Patient Abuse Prevention Act, and encourage Congress to pursue the establishment of a national registry identifying persons who have been convicted of patient abuse, neglect, and other related crimes.

Finally, we must support every local, state, and national effort to educate the public about long-term care alternatives, how and where to report abuse, neglect, and what resources already exist for relatives and friends and family and other loved ones who will be or who are already receiving long-term care.

[The prepared statement of Ms. Del Papa follows:]

STATE OF NEVADA
OFFICE OF THE ATTORNEY GENERAL
100 N. Carson Street
Carson City, Nevada 89701-4717
Telephone (702) 687-4170
Fax (702) 687-5798

FRANKIE SUE DEL PAPA
Attorney General

BROOKE A. NIELSEN
Assistant Attorney General

TESTIMONY OF ATTORNEY GENERAL FRANKIE SUE DEL PAPA BEFORE THE SENATE SPECIAL COMMITTEE ON AGING FIELD HEARINGS HELD JANUARY 12 AND 13, 1998.

Thank you for the opportunity to address this important issue, one that is critical to Nevada. Our state was originally nicknamed "The Silver State" because of the valuable silver ore buried deep beneath the Nevada soil. Today, with the fastest growing population of persons 65 years of age and over, Nevada is still the "The Silver State" because of the valuable silver haired citizens who live here and who, in significant numbers, are continuing to choose to move here and make Nevada their home their home and to live through their twilight years by enjoying the multiple forms of recreation and relaxation our state offers.

In Nevada, the Medicaid Fraud Control Unit of the Attorney General's Office has primary jurisdiction to investigate and prosecute patient abuse cases in long term care facilities. Our MFCU has received almost a 50% increase in the number of complaints/referrals of patient abuse and neglect in the last year. Over the last two years, the MFCU has reviewed over 130 complaints/referrals and opened over twenty criminal investigations. On the one hand, these numbers may reflect the need to address the serious problem of patient abuse and neglect in our state. But on the other hand, these numbers may also reflect increased reporting of abuse cases thanks to ongoing public education and awareness efforts.

In the fall of 1995, the Attorney General's Office in conjunction with the Department of Human Resources and County Social Services Agencies formed a Long Term Care Task Force to help meet the needs of a rapidly growing senior population. That task force produced the report "Choices for Seniors," a copy of which has been provided to you. This report addressed the following:

- The need to develop choices among a range of service options which are responsive to senior's needs.
- The responsibility to assure the availability of these choices in settings where quality of care can be assured.
- The commitment to educate all factions of the community regarding elder abuse, neglect and exploitation.

To help in this commitment, the Attorney General's Office published "A Practical Guide to Long Term Care," a pamphlet containing tips on how to choose a Long Term Care Facility, information on the rights of residents and information on Alternatives to Nursing Home care.

In order to better meet the growing long term care needs of senior Nevadans who require varying degrees of assistance and medical attention, the state and federal governments need to explore the possibility of extending Medicaid/Medicare funds to assist seniors who could live in less restrictive settings than skilled nursing facilities. Additionally, it is critical that the jurisdiction of the Medicaid Fraud Control Units be similarly expanded. In fact, the National Association of Attorneys General has asked for flexibility, or some relaxation of the rules, in order to better coordinate with other law enforcement agencies.

As more and more seniors make Nevada their home, it is important to provide strong systems for their safety and well being whether or not they reside in a long term care facility. In the fall of 1996, my office joined forces with Betsy Kolkoski, the Elder Rights Attorney from the Division for Aging Services to come up with a more comprehensive plan to address the growing problem of elder abuse, neglect and exploitation. We met with, among others, senior advocates from both private and public sectors, and used their input to publish "An Action Plan to Better Protect Nevada's Elderly." A copy of that plan has also been provided to you. Committees were formed to implement the goals of the Action Plan which was made public in March of 1997. Since then, much has been accomplished on behalf of our state's elderly population:

- Passage of legislation proposed in the Action Plan including:

AB 242 which made Nevada one of the first states to recognize the intentional and unjustified isolation of the elderly as a serious crime;

SB 80 which created double damages and authorized recovery of attorneys fees in civil litigation involving elder abuse, neglect, exploitation and isolation.

AB 9, Assemblyman Mark Manendo's bill to increase the minimum penalty for criminal elder abuse was amended to add funeral home employees as mandatory elder abuse reporters and to authorize an elder abuse reporting hotline.

AB 155, which was proposed by Assemblywoman Vivian Freeman and Assemblyman Jack Close was strongly supported by participants in the Action Plan. This bill requires the fingerprinting and mandatory criminal background checks for long term care employees.

In addition to the legislation I have just mention, implementation of the goals of the Action Plan has led to:

- The publication of the "Guide for Mandated Reporters of Elder Abuse." This guide is a resource for all persons concerned about the elderly and explains the role and responsibility of state and local agencies who respond to reports of elder abuse, neglect and intimidation. You have all been provided with a copy of the guide which should also help you better understand the roles of various state and local agencies involving cases of Elder Abuse.

- Development of Protocols to help law enforcement and protective services agencies better coordinate and communicate their response to, and investigation of, reports of Elder Abuse. Last week, these Protocols were signed by representatives from eleven different state and local agencies with varying responsibilities to respond to reports of Elder Abuse. A copy of those Protocols has been provided to you.

- Statewide distribution of the video "Rx for Abuse," which was produced by the Division For Aging Services to provide health care professionals with information on how to detect and report cases of elder abuse. The video stars Shirley Jones and Marty Ingles.

- Public Service Announcements to encourage better reporting of Elder Abuse which aired both in the north and the south.

- Guardianship survey, in which providers and advocates statewide were surveyed regarding the need for guardianship.

- Obtained funding for additional Elder Abuse videos and materials to provide education to law enforcement officers throughout the state.

- Creation of an Elder Abuse reporting Hotline in Northern Nevada.

In conclusion, I would like to applaud Senators Reid, Kohl and Grassley who are co-sponsoring the Patient Abuse Prevention Act and encourage Congress to pursue the establishment of a national registry identifying persons who have been convicted of patient abuse, neglect and other related crimes.

Finally, we must support every local, state and national effort to educate the public about long term care alternatives, how and where to report abuse and neglect and what resources already exist for relatives and friends of family and other loved ones who will be or who are already receiving long term care. Thank you.

Senator REID. Thank you. Frankie Sue, before you finish, would you hold up, so the people in the rural sites can see, those publications? Turn it around the other way. You all help her here. Turn it around, hold it up.

Ms. DEL PAPA. Great. This is the elder abuse action plan. You can see this is a fairly comprehensive document which includes recommendations on how to address elder abuse and a timeline included therein.

I should mention, Senator Reid, that there was a meeting last week. Your staff has been very supportive, obviously, in this regard. We are proceeding to amplify even what is included in this plan.

Senator REID. These are available free of charge?

Ms. DEL PAPA. These are available free of charge through our office; also through the Department of Human Resources. We have partnered a great deal with the Department of Human Resources. Obviously they are involved in everything we do in this regard. This document is on long-term care. This is the task force on long-term care.

Senator REID. Turn it just a little bit. There we go.

Ms. DEL PAPA. The smaller documents which are available—and I should say that Betsy Kolkoski will be doing a 15-county rural tour shortly. These are just the very inexpensive documents to produce, but they are handy to have. One is on long-term care. One is on elder abuse and a lot of comments with reference to it.

Finally, there is this document which is the guide for mandated reporters. Frankly, every document we do, we encourage people to plagiarize and widely distribute it as far and wide as they can. This document is in such—I mean, literally, there are thousands and thousands of copies that have already been produced and are in the process of being produced as well.

Senator REID. Thank you. All these documents are in the packets that were available at the door, too.

We will now hear from Carla Sloan, the Administrator for the Division of Aging Services for the State of Nevada.

STATEMENT OF CARLA SLOAN, ADMINISTRATOR, DIVISION FOR AGING SERVICES, DEPARTMENT OF HUMAN RESOURCE

Ms. SLOAN. Thank you, Senator Reid. I am honored to participate on this panel to present Nevada's long-term care ombudsman program for patient advocacy. The position of ombudsman was originally created by the Swedish government in 1809. This government official was given independence, power, and prestige for the impartial hearing and resolution of citizen complaints.

It was not until after World War II that the idea of an ombudsman position spread throughout the rest of the world. This was tied to the growing popular feeling that there was an increasing distance between government and citizens.

Media attention in the 1960s about accounts of abuse in nursing homes brought attention to the need for advocates for institutionalized seniors in the United States. In 1978, amendments to the Older Americans Act required each state to establish an ombudsman program. Long-term care ombudsmen take on a variety of roles at different levels.

Under the direction of the resident, ombudsmen act on their concerns and violations of their rights. In addition to resolving individual problems, the work of the ombudsmen lay the foundation for systemic change within the long-term care system. Aggressive enforcement of government regulation of the industry is essential for the protection of residents.

We applaud the commitment and commend the work that the Nevada Health Division does on a daily basis to ensure regulatory compliance of the long-term care industry. Aging Services collaborates with the Health Division and provides feedback on a regular basis to the survey process. The divisions frequently conduct joint investigations.

During the last three years, we have seen a 3 percent increase in the number of complaints in nursing homes. Seventy-three percent of the complaints come from facility staff. As the number of nursing facilities has not increased, this high level of self-reporting shows a cooperative effort by the industry to coordinate complaint investigation and resolution.

Residential facilities for groups are rapidly growing in Nevada to meet the ever-increasing demand for long-term care alternatives. Inappropriate level of care complaints have increased by 22 percent in the last three years. Since this segment of the industry is relatively new, self-reporting of incidents and complaints has not reached the same level as in nursing homes. There is much education to be done with this part of the continuum of care.

Fifty-five percent of the complaints investigated by Nevada ombudsmen were substantiated during the past year. The major complaint categories were care plan and assessment; staff supervision; accidents and improper handling; abuse, neglect, and exploitation; dignity, respect, and staff attitudes.

Our program is one of the few nationally that investigates complaints of abuse, neglect, and exploitation. In a 1995 survey of ombudsmen programs by the Administration on Aging, Nevada was responsible for investigating 13 percent of abuse and neglect complaints reported nationally.

The ombudsman program's focus on expanding community presence into nursing homes and other residential care settings has become the most effective vehicle for combating the abuse and neglect of residents, and promoting quality of care and quality of life. The program is unlike any other. Its sole purpose is supporting and protecting the resident.

The State of Nevada, through Governor Bob Miller and the legislature, have been very supportive of this critical program. A Federal Older Americans Act grant funds 38 percent of our program. State funding of 62 percent of the program expense allows the division to provide professional service to the most vulnerable of our elderly population.

Nevada's sincere commitment to elders and long-term care is evident by its continual support of our ombudsman program. Nevada is also committed to volunteerism. Governor Miller and the 1997 legislature approved a new state annual appropriation of nearly $250,000 for senior volunteer programs.

The retired senior volunteer programs in both southern and northern Nevada have agreed to provide the volunteer management for a pilot program called the Silver Stripers. The Silver Striper program seeks to enhance the quality of life for residents in long-term care facilities by providing them with an opportunity to experience friendship and support from trained older volunteers.

While volunteer initiatives such as the Silver Striper program are essential to enriching the lives of elders, as the patient advocacy demands of the senior population increase, we will see continued and increased support from the Administration on Aging, the Congress, the state legislature, and from local community partners to preserve and expand ombudsmen services.

Thank you for this opportunity to speak on behalf of the elders served by the Division for Aging. As the state with the fastest growing 65 and older population, we are pleased to offer our experience to the Senate Special Committee on Aging in your efforts to identify the strengths and weaknesses of national policy on long-term care.

[The prepared statement of Ms. Sloan follows:]

UNITED STATES SENATE
SPECIAL COMMITTEE ON AGING
FIELD HEARINGS
JANUARY 12 AND 13, 1998

"THE MANY FACES OF LONG-TERM CARE:
TODAY'S BITTER PILL OR TOMORROW'S CURE?"

PANEL 2
TODAY'S PERSPECTIVE
NEVADA'S LONG TERM CARE OMBUDSMAN PROGRAM
FOR PATIENT ADVOCACY

PRESENTED BY:
CARLA SLOAN, ADMINISTRATOR
NEVADA DIVISION FOR AGING SERVICES
340 N. 11TH STREET, SUITE 203
LAS VEGAS, NEVADA 89101
PHONE (702) 486-3545
FAX (702) 486-3572

The Many Faces of Long Term Care: Today's Bitter Pill or Tomorrow's Cure?

Panel 2 - Today's Perspective
Nevada's Long Term Care Ombudsman Program for Patient Advocacy

Carla Sloan, Administrator
Nevada Division for Aging Services
Department of Human Resources

Introduction

The position of ombudsman was originally created by the Swedish government in 1809. This government official was given independence, power, and prestige for the impartial hearing and resolution of complaints by citizens. The classical definition of an ombudsman is described as a neutral third party who investigates and makes reports regarding grievances.

A broad conceptualization of an ombudsman is a "citizen defender" who advocates between citizens and the authority, with the power to personalize bureaucratic red tape, to increase government responsiveness, to implement a complaint resolution system, and to recognize appropriate services for citizens.

It was not until after World War II that the idea of an ombudsman position spread throughout the rest of the world. This has been tied to the growing popular feeling that there was an increasing distance between government administration and citizens and their needs.

Media attention in the 1960s about accounts of abuse in nursing homes brought attention to the need for advocates for institutionalized seniors in the United States.

The Office of the Long-Term Care Ombudsman was federally mandated in 1971. President Nixon proposed initiatives in 1975 creating ombudsman units whose focus would be on individual residents, thus compensating for the limitations of quality assurance and regulation. In 1978, amendments to the Older Americans Act required each state to establish an ombudsman program. In 1981, decisions by Congress added board and care facilities to the ombudsman federal mandate. Although this legislation did not change the qualities of the ombudsman program, it greatly increased the population that required ombudsman services.

The scope of the ombudsman program's responsibilities and authority are described in Title VII, Chapter 2 of the Older Americans Act. The programs are directed at responding to needs of institutionalized seniors by:

1) Investigating and resolving complaints made by or on behalf of residents of long term care facilities;

2) Establishing procedures for ombudsman access to facilities and patients' records;

3) Creating a statewide reporting system to collect and analyze data relating to complaints;

4) Mandating procedures to assure client confidentiality;

5) Providing information to public agencies regarding the problems of long term care facilities' residents; and

6) Other responsibilities include educating the public, training staff and volunteers, and helping to develop resident and family councils in facilities.

Ombudsmen take on a variety of roles at different levels. Two levels of advocacy include resident-level and systems-level. On a systems-level, ombudsmen attempt to solve broader or underlying causes of problems by advocating for policy change. This is done by evaluating laws and regulations, educating public and facility staff, analyzing program data, and promoting resident and family councils. On a resident-level, the ombudsmen's responsibilities include working cooperatively with outside agencies and providing assistance and training to facility staff. It is important that ombudsmen ensure residents have timely access to the ombudsman program and resolution to complaints.

In pursuit of these activities, the ombudsman must maintain relationships involving tension between the individual and the system. On the one hand, the ombudsman must be critical of the facilities and other agencies they review, and then be able to work cooperatively with the same agencies to ensure that residents receive proper services and protection of rights. This can be difficult considering that ombudsmen have the ability to affect administrators and staff and to induce change within the long term care system.

Whatever power the ombudsman has, whether real or perceived, adds to the tension of the ombudsman relationship. The long term care ombudsman's powers range from conciliatory to coercive action, including education, coordination with other agencies, win/win negotiations, pursuing the involvement of regulatory agencies, administrative and civil, or criminal, legal actions, or public disclosure activities such as using the media.

Impact of 1987 OBRA

The Division for Aging Services supports a strong survey and enforcement process that assures that each resident receives the care and services that he or she needs to achieve the highest attainable level of well-being. Because of the Nevada Division of Health's survey process, we feel the long term care industry in Nevada has improved and continues to provide a commitment to quality of care and quality of life.

We applaud the commitment and commend the work that the Health Division does on a daily basis to ensure that residents of long term care facilities receive quality of care and quality of life. The Division for Aging Services collaborates with the Health Division and has given feedback on a regular basis to the survey process. The Health Division has been responsive to all Aging Services referrals, and on many occasions the divisions have conducted joint investigations.

Ombudsman Program Data

During the last three years in Nevada, we have seen a 3% increase in the number of complaints in long term care facilities. 73% of the complaints received come from facility staff and administration. Based on the fact that the number of nursing facilities has not increased in the past three years, this high level of self-reporting shows a cooperative effort by the industry to coordinate complaint investigation and resolution.

Residential facilities for groups are rapidly growing in Nevada to meet the ever increasing demand for long term care alternatives. Inappropriate level of care complaints have increased by 22% in the last three years. Since this segment of the industry is relatively new, the self-reporting of incidents and complaints has not reached the same level as in nursing homes. There is much education to be done with this part of the continuum of care.

55% percent of the complaints investigated by the ombudsman were substantiated during the past year. The major complaint categories during this past year were:

1) care plan and assessment,
2) staff supervision,
3) accidents and improper handling,
4) abuse, neglect, and exploitation, and
5) dignity and respect, staff attitudes.

The ombudsman program in Nevada Is one of the few nationally that does investigate complaints of abuse, neglect and exploitation. In a 1995 survey of ombudsmen programs by the Administration on Aging, Nevada was responsible for investigating 13% of abuse, neglect complaints reported nationally to ombudsman programs.

Recommendations for the Future of Quality Care

The Long Term Care Ombudsman Program's focus on expanding community presence into nursing homes and other residential care settings has become the most effective vehicle for combating the abuse and neglect of residents and promoting quality of care and quality of life. The program is unlike any other - its sole purpose is supporting and protecting the resident.

Ombudsmen provide a regular presence in long term care facilities. In doing so, they become familiar with the facility, the management, employees, residents, visitors and families. By regularly speaking with residents throughout the year, the Ombudsmen form a strong rapport with them, enabling the residents to develop skills that will allow them to have their viewpoint heard and respected and their needs met in a constructive and proactive manner.

Under the direction of the resident, Ombudsmen act on their concerns and any violations of the their rights. In addition to resolving individual problems, the work of the ombudsmen lays the foundation for systemic change within the long term care system.

The State of Nevada through Governor Bob Miller and the Legislature have been very supportive of the Ombudsman program. Title VI of the Federal Older Americans Act grant funds 38% of Nevada's Long Term Care Ombudsman Program. State funding of 62% of the Ombudsman Program expense allows the Division for Aging Services to provide professional service to the most vulnerable of our elderly population. Nevada's sincere commitment to patient safety, quality of care, and quality of life for elders in long term care residence is evident by its continual support of the Long Term Care Ombudsman Program.

As the patient advocacy demands of the senior population increase, the Division for Aging Services will seek continued and increased support from the U.S. Administration on Aging, the U.S. Congress, the State Legislature, and local community partners to preserve and expand ombudsman services.

Thank you for this opportunity to speak on behalf of the elders served by the Nevada Department of Human Resources Division for Aging Services. As the state with the fastest growing 65 and older population, we are pleased to offer our experience to the Senate Special Committee on Aging's effort to identify the strengths and weaknesses of national policy on long-term care. We pledge our continued partnership in seeking solutions and recommendations for future improvements.

Presented to the
United States Senate
Special Committee on Aging
Nevada Field Hearings
January 12 and 13, 1998

Senator REID. We will now hear from Rick Panelli, who is the Chief, the Bureau of Licensure and Certification, Nevada State Health Division.

STATEMENT OF RICK PANELLI, CHIEF, BUREAU OF LICENSURE AND CERTIFICATION, NEVADA STATE HEALTH DIVISION

Mr. PANELLI. Senator Reid, thank you very much for the opportunity to be here and be part of this activity. The Bureau of Licensure and Certification is the regulatory agency in the State of Nevada which does the inspection and certification for state licensure in Medicare and Medicaid certification.

The agency currently licenses in excess of 700 facilities which provide health care and care for the dependent. This does not include home health and hospice care which are also a portion of the long-term care provisions for individuals.

The annual survey and certification process for each facility focuses on quality of life, quality of care, resident behavior, and facility practices. The Health Division would encourage facilities or it does encourage facilities come into compliance by requesting or requiring a plan of correction to all deficiencies noted.

We feel that this process needs to be a partnering process between the state and the facilities in order to come up with resolutions that will best provide the actual quality of care and quality of life that is necessary for our aging population.

For facilities or for providers that fail to come into compliance, there are remedies and sanctions that can be imposed. They stem all the way from directed plans of correction, monetary sanctions or civil monetary penalties, and probably the most effective that we have found is a ban on all admissions to a facility. If the facility is having problems providing care based on staffing ratios or other issues, we do a ban on admissions, do not allow the facility to take on more people than they can care for, and hold them at that level until they do provide adequate care.

There are two categories of compliance or non-compliance which we cite facilities for and facilities actually are kind of labelled by these two areas. One is substantial compliance with regulations. The other one is a facility that provides substandard quality of care. In the United States, 75 percent of all of the long-term care facilities, these skilled nursing facilities have been found to be not in substantial compliance with the Federal regulations on their first survey process.

In Nevada, we have had numbers as high as no facility on their first survey was found to be in substantial compliance. We will talk a little bit later about what that might mean.

But the real true indicator, I think the best indicator of a facility's ability to provide adequate quality of care is in the designator of providing substandard quality of care because this looks at actual outcome and it looks at what actually is happening with the patients. This is the most important piece that we can be looking at in a facility.

There are several negatives that could come out of this labelling that goes on. One of those is that it produces a negative reaction to the long-term care industry, and as a whole, if you see everybody as not in substantial compliance with regulations, you think that every facility is providing poor quality of care and that is not necessarily true.

I think that one of the things that it does do, and we have seen this in Nevada, is that it keeps people out of the catch-and-fix situation, which is one where they are out of compliance of regulations, we go in and we sort of catch them, they fix their problems. The next time we are back, they are out of compliance with those regulations.

I think that the reports and the numbers would indicate that Nevada facilities are no longer—or most of the Nevada's facilities are no longer in this situation. They are catching their problems themselves, they are fixing their problems, and they are moving on. We are not having to go back and have these repeat-type deficiencies.

One of the largest and most rapidly growing areas of long-term care is in the residential facilities for groups. These are facilities that are similar to assisted living in some other States. We have increased that particular number. In 1991, we had about 188. We are now up to about 600 facilities in this State. These facilities provide a very home-like atmosphere.

The key issue, I think, for us in the future is to look at new regulations, partnering with the industry to develop these types of regulations that will allow for a continuum of care. People need to be able to stay in place. They need to be able to age in place and not be moved into the highest levels of care which are most expensive. Take advantage of the home health that can be provided in an individual's home.

Finally, we have about 359 currently registered homes in this State, what we call registered homes. Those are the homes that provide care to two and under non-related individuals. We would be glad to answer any questions that anyone would have and I hope that people contact our agency for help in locating homes.

[The prepared statement of Mr. Panelli follows:]

UNITED STATES SENATE
SENATE SPECIAL COMMITTEE ON AGING
Field Hearings – January 12-13, 1998

Richard J. Panelli, Chief
Bureau of Licensure and Certification
Health Division
Department of Human Resources
State of Nevada

Bureau of Licensure and Certification (BLC) is responsible for statewide inspection surveys of Medical and Dependent Care Facilities for compliance with Federal certification regulations for Medicare and Medicaid and Nevada state licensure regulations

Code of Federal Regulations (42 CFR)
Nevada Revised Statutes Chapters (NRS 449)

1997	700 facilities	321	Homes for Individual Residential Care
		265	Residential Facilities for Groups
		45	Skilled Nursing Facilities/Nursing Facilities (SNF/NF)
1991	222 facilities	0	Homes for Individual Residential Care
		188	Residential Facilities for Groups
		34	SNF/NF
1997	pending facilities	29	Residential Facilities for Groups
		6	SNF/NF

BLC conducts annual on-site surveys of all health and care facilities to determine compliance with regulations

Annual on-site surveys focus on:

- Quality of Care
- Quality of Life
- Residential Behavior/Facility Practices

- Health Division encourages facility compliance through requiring a Plan of Correction (POC) for each deficiency found

Sanctions and Remedies:

- Directed POC
- Directed In-Service Training

- State Monitoring
- Monetary Fines (CMPs)
- Ban on Admissions
- Seriousness, frequency, pervasive nature
- Revoke, deny, suspend license, terminate Medicare/Medicaid reimbursement

The regulatory system not only establishes minimum standards for provision of Health Care it also:

- Educates providers
- Protects recipients - who are among our most vulnerable citizens.

43 SNFs / 2 NFs

Survey Activity July 1995 through October 1997

- No facility in substantial compliance on annual survey (75% the National Average).
- 13 facilities providing Substandard Quality of Care (5 in FY97).

"Substantial Compliance" - is not a good indicator of:

- Quality of Care
- Quality of Life
- Resident Behavior/Facility Practices

WHY?

- "Potential" for poor outcome
- 1 resident / pattern is not necessary

"Substandard Quality of Care" - is a good indicator of:

- Quality of Care
- Quality of Life
- Resident Behavior/Facility Practices

WHY?

- Actual harm or poor outcome has occurs
- Pattern/wide spread
- Major system failures

Negative Issues:

- Produces negative reaction to Long Term Care (LTC) industry as a whole
- Makes it more difficult for consumers to differentiate based on survey findings
- Increases costs – Follow-up survey process

Positive Issues:

- Helps to eliminate "catch and fix" compliance (only 2 repeat Substandard Quality of Care)
- Scope and Severity
- Remedies/Sanctions – CMP / Ban on Admissions

291 Residential Facilities for Groups
39 Residential Facilities for Alzheimer's and related Dementia

- 3 beds to 125+ beds
- 1 care level step above retirement/independent living
- Similar to "Assisted Living":

    Provide very "home-like" living conditions – many 6-bed facilities

    Limited Supervision

- New regulations:

    Allow for continuum of care where individuals remain in the same facility until they require daily skilled nursing

    Home Health may be utilized to meet care needs

    Less costly than a SNF/NF

359 Homes for Individual Residential Care:

2 or fewer residents

Complaint investigations is the only state oversight

Changes Resulting from the Regulation

- ☐ Eliminates the distinction between Level A and Level B participation requirements.
- ☐ Makes available to HCFA the full range of OBRA enforcement remedies. *§488.406*
- ☐ Codifies informal dispute resolution process (with no delay in enforcement) *§488.331*
- ☐ Offers one hearing — under either Federal or State procedures. *§488.330(e)*
- ☐ Classifies seriousness of deficiencies for the purpose of imposing a remedy through the use of scope and severity. *§488.408*
- ☐ Establishes and defines "substantial compliance" *§488.301*
- ☐ Defines "substandard quality of care" *§488.301*
- ☐ Establishes two civil money penalty ranges *§488.438*
- ☐ Explains "repeat deficiencies" for purposes of increasing a civil money penalty when deficiencies are found on a subsequent standard survey. *§488.438(d)*
- ☐ Establishes "tie breaker" rules which apply when there are disagreements between HCFA and the State about compliance, choice of remedies or timing of remedies. *§488.452*

Unchanged from Current Practice (Already Implemented)

- ☐ Survey frequency - no greater than 15 months between standard surveys and States cannot exceed a Statewide 12 month average. *§488.308*
- ☐ Unannounced surveys *§488.307*
- ☐ Mandatory imposition of Denial of Payment for New Admissions after three months of noncompliance. *§488.417(b)*

Background

- ☐ The Survey, Certification and Enforcement of SNFs and NFs was published as a Notice of Proposed Rulemaking (NPRM) in August 1992.
- ☐ HCFA received nearly 28,000 public comments in response to the NPRM.
- ☐ The final rule was published on November 10, 1994.
- ☐ This regulation becomes effective on July 1, 1995.

Health Care Financing Administration
Health Standards and Quality Bureau
Office of Survey & Certification
Division of Program Operations

6325 Security Boulevard, ME 2-D-2
Baltimore, Maryland 21207

A94-2355 f

SURVEY, CERTIFICATION AND ENFORCEMENT OF SKILLED NURSING FACILITIES AND NURSING FACILITIES

(HSQ-156-F)

POCKET REFERENCE GUIDE

Available Remedies

- Temporary Management *§488.415*
- Civil Money Penalties (CMPs) *§488.430 - 488.444*
- Denial of Payment for New Admissions *§488.417*
- Secretarial authority to deny all payments *§488.418*
- State Monitoring *§488.422*
- Directed Plan of Correction *§488.424*
- Directed In-service Training *§488.425*
- Closure of a facility or transfer of residents, or both *§488.426*
- Termination of Provider Agreement *§488.4[illegible]*

Notice/Disclosure Requirements

Disclosure:

- Survey information may be disclosed to the public 14 calendar days after such information is made available to the facility. *§488.325 (.)*
- The State MUST disclose certain information to the State's long-term care ombudsman. *§488.325(f)*
- Substandard quality of care - The State must notify the State board for licensing nursing home administrators and the attending physician of residents. *§488.325(h)*

Notice:

- 15 days — non-immediate jeopardy for all remedies, except CMPs. *§488.402(f)*
- 2 days — immediate jeopardy for all remedies, except CMPs. *§488.402(f)*

	Isolated	Pattern	Widespread
Immediate Jeopardy to Resident Health or Safety	PoC Required: Cat. 3 Optional: Cat. 1 Optional: Cat. 2	PoC Required: Cat. 3 Optional: Cat. 1 Optional: Cat. 2	PoC Required: Cat. 3 Optional: Cat. 2 Optional: Cat. 1
Actual Harm that is not Immediate Jeopardy	PoC Required* Cat. 2 Optional: Cat. 1	PoC Required* Cat. 2 Optional: Cat. 1	PoC Required* Cat. 2 Optional: Cat. 1 Optional: Temporary Mgmt.
No Actual Harm with Potential for More than Minimal Harm that is not Immediate Jeopardy	PoC Required* Cat. 1 Optional: Cat. 2	PoC Required* Cat. 1 Optional: Cat. 2	PoC Required* Cat. 2 Optional: Cat. 1
No Actual Harm with Potential for Minimal Harm	No Remedies Commitment to Correct Not on HCFA-2567	PoC	PoC

Substandard quality of care: any deficiency in §483.13 Resident Behavior and Facility Practices, §483.15 Quality of Life, or in §483.25, Quality of Care that constitutes: immediate jeopardy to resident health or safety; or, a pattern of or widespread actual harm that is not immediate jeopardy; or, a widespread potential for more than minimal harm that is not immediate jeopardy, with no actual harm.

Substantial compliance

Remedy Categories

Category 1 (Cat. 1)	Category 2 (Cat. 2)	Category 3 (Cat. 3)
Directed Plan of Correction State Monitor; and/or Directed In-service Training	Denial of Payment for New Admissions; Denial of Payment for All Individuals, Imposed by HCFA; and/or Civil Money Penalties: $50 - $3,000 per day	Temporary Management Termination Optional: Civil Money Penalties: $3,050 - $10,000 per day

DENIAL OF PAYMENT FOR NEW ADMISSIONS must be imposed when a facility is not in substantial compliance within three months after being found out of compliance.

DENIAL OF PAYMENT AND STATE MONITORING must be imposed when a facility has been found to have provided substandard quality of care on three consecutive standard surveys.

Note: Termination may be imposed by the State or HCFA at any time when appropriate.

**** Required only when decision is made to impose alternate remedies instead of or in addition to termination.***

Senator REID. Mr. Panelli, both you and Ms. Sloan mentioned the different complaints received in different ways. You do a more active—I mean, you go out and inspect and the administrator spends a lot of their time responding to complaints that people make. Do you think that the number is going up as to the number of deficiencies? Is it because we report better than we used to?

Mr. PANELLI. I think there are several things. One of them is that we report better than we did in the past. The system now has us looking more at actual—we are getting away from recordkeeping. We are looking at the residents. Another thing is that the public is becoming more aware. People are becoming more educated and that also generates and drives more complaints for us to look at.

Senator REID. It sure would be nice if we could do that with Medicare and Medicaid, be more concerned about quality rather than the paperwork.

Mr. PANELLI. Yes. I think that that is a key issue that has to be looked at. We have to get away from paper compliance. This does not give us what the total outcome is.

Senator REID. I think one of the things that Dr. Takamura is interested in, in her efforts to make sure that we eliminate fraud, waste, and abuse, is to make sure that people who are cheating the system get taken out of the system. But people who are trying to work their way through some of these complicated programs are not penalized in some way.

It is a fine line, but we have to make it because we have to simplify the recordkeeping in all areas of health care delivery in this country.

Mr. PANELLI. It is a very difficult thing. Sometimes it is very difficult to see if care is being provided, especially like in a home health agency without some of those recordkeeping issues, but they need to be minimized.

Senator REID. Now, one of the things that I am interested in, in Ms. Hunter's testimony, as I was with a woman by the name of Rose George yesterday, is how you make a decision in placing your loved one in a facility. It is difficult to go get the information, is it not?

Ms. HUNTER. It is extremely difficult. Fortunately, in my background, I have 15 years of experience including working with the Aging Services Division, and even at that, I did not have all the background. When we knew the placement was coming, there was a plethora of this is what you have to do, this is what you are going to do, and the next thing you knew, you had placement.

Senator REID. The lady that testified yesterday, somebody came up to me afterwards and said, "Are you going to help get her in a rest home?" I said, "Yeah, but that is not the problem. The problem is the thousands of other people who do not have her ability to come before thousands of people and plead her case."

We need to make sure that there is more protection, there are more advocates for people getting in these facilities. I was impressed with your written statement, and you covered part of this in your oral statement, and that is, people caring, good people, but if they are not qualified, not trained to handle this difficult transition from bringing somebody from your home into one of these facilities.

Think of the trauma of one of us being placed in a brand new home and then have people—and then not, as you have indicated clearly in your statement, not being able to hear quite as well or see quite as well or walk quite as well, and people who do not understand how difficult the transition is.

We really need a better job of training people for taking care of all the problems connected with growing older.

Ms. HUNTER. And I would sincerely agree. I think that is the biggest weakness in what I have seen. My mother is in a very good facility, but the training has to be constant and it has to go all the way up to the administrative level. They all need to understand what is experienced not only by the client and by the patient, but by the family.

Senator REID. This is not just in rest homes. It is with physicians themselves. I was stunned to learn we have a very, very big shortage of physicians trained to take care of seniors. People trained in geriatrics simply are very few and far between. Medical schools, all medical schools require courses in pediatrics, but only a handful of the 120-plus medical schools require courses in geriatrics.

As Carla Sloan mentioned, I think it was her or maybe it was Dr. Bernick, that people spend more time taking care of elders than they do their children. So we really need to do better and that is why there are a number of us pushing legislation that would give incentives for people to go into geriatrics and to give incentives to medical schools to require those courses.

Attorney General Del Papa, if we accomplish nothing else in these hearings, and I think we will accomplish a great deal, but if we accomplish nothing else in these hearings other than you coming forward and stating yesterday and today that we need to increase flexibility of state fraud units, you have convinced me.

I am headed to Washington. I am going to work on that legislation. It is very important, and please explain to our viewers what we are talking about here in making this improvement. Move that microphone.

Ms. DEL PAPA. Well, currently the Medicaid fraud control units, which in our state happens to be located in the Attorney General's Office, do not have the flexibility under the Federal law to go outside those facilities that—you have to have a Medicaid connection. It has to be a Medicaid facility.

What the National Association of Attorneys General is asking for is to relax that restriction so that you in particular could do greater investigations with reference to Medicare. Right now, our hands are tied. Although we do work with other facilities, and certainly Nevada is a small enough state, we have got a very receptive, for instance, U.S. Attorney here.

We do consumer efforts together. We do these types of things together, but I just think on a national basis and certainly within our own state, to have that relaxation. Again, when you look at the percentage——

Senator REID. Attorney General, would you tell us what difference it makes though. Let's say that you have the ability to have more flexibility than you now have. What mechanically could you do that you cannot do now?

Ms. DEL PAPA. Well, Senator, the problem is, as you know being trained in the law, if it is not within your jurisdiction, and particularly if there are Federal restrictions on exactly how you can and cannot spend your time, it restricts your ability to do these types of cases.

We became—and, of course, there are great incentives at the national level, there were great incentives to implement these Medicaid fraud control units. Nevada, we were the 40th state to take advantage of that. I mean, when I first became Attorney General seven years ago, I was astounded that we did not have a fraud control unit because, number one, your Medicaid fraud control units act as a deterrent on the front end.

That is really good when you look at the Federal dollars and when you look at state dollars that are being expended for these health care programs and you look at—and all the national statistics show you that anywhere from 5 to 15 percent of your health care dollar may have some fraud element in it, an overcharge, and we all know that.

The trick is how do you systematically attack it, and in our state what we have done, through the Medicaid Fraud Unit, is to go after providers and, as I said, also go after patient abuse, both fiscal and physical abuse.

By way of an example, just in a provider case, the first case that we had was a young psychiatrist from Las Vegas who was cheating the Medicaid system. He cheated us out of $30,000. He would see patients for five minutes and charge for two-hour increments. He was charging for more hours than there were in a day. When our investigators caught him, what he said was, "Well, five minutes with me is the equivalent of two hours with someone else."

Of course, we did not buy that. But it is complicated and the paperwork, Lord knows, anyone who has been through any kind of medical treatment, it is difficult to read these medical documents. And so, you have to have these fraud control units. We have auditors, we have investigators. I am really into computer forensics. I just think because we live in the age of the Internet, we are trying to be on the cutting edge of attacking it.

The flexibility, Senator, believe me, would go a long way towards helping not only this state but the entire country.

Senator REID. So what you are saying is if you are doing investigation on a Medicaid fraud case and you see that the same person or institution is also cheating or deceiving in Medicare, you can go forward with your investigation?

Ms. DEL PAPA. It would be better, right. If at the Federal level they would relax those rules, there would be a greater ease of doing these cases, and I think that we would all be better off in doing it. I mean, we try to cooperate now, but I am just saying it is not systematic. Again, when you do not have jurisdiction, as you know, when you do not have jurisdiction to go forward, it sometimes get complicated in trying to bring these cases.

Senator REID. When you have an investigation going forward, you are already doing the work, you have interviewed witnesses, now under the present law, you have to call the United States Attorney saying, "Look what I found," and she has got bank robbers and drug cases and all this other stuff and you have to get her to start investigating.

Ms. DEL PAPA. Right. And we already have the system. See, the wonderful thing is you have got these—every state now has a Medicaid fraud control unit and you want to have dedicated bodies who do that type of work and do not do anything else because it is just like locally with your local district attorneys now.

They are so inundated with bank robberies and murder that it is hard for them to branch out and do the other types of consumer cases, et cetera. That is why you have got to have it centralized in an office such as the Attorney General's Office or in the Medicaid fraud control unit.

Senator REID. Ms. Sloan, in your testimony, you mentioned the ombudsman program in Nevada is one of the few nationally that does investigate complaints of abuse, neglect, and exploitation. What do you mean by that statement?

Ms. SLOAN. Abuse, neglect, and exploitation in facilities? Our protocols—and we have worked very hard with our partners in the last several years and in cooperation with our Attorney General and others. We just signed a document last week in which law enforcement, many of the social service agencies have agreed to how investigations will take place.

In nursing facilities, our ombudsmen are charged with the investigation of abuse, neglect, and exploitation. That is quite unique to the ombudsman program nationally. It would be more typical that if an ombudsman had an indication that such a crime was taking place, they would then call in the adult protective services unit or perhaps they would call in the law enforcement. In Nevada, our ombudsmen investigate those.

Senator REID. Panel, thank you very much. All of your written statements will be made part of the record. I appreciate all of you summarizing your statements. As I have indicated, the full statement the court reporter has will be taken down and be made a part of this complete record that will be disseminated in the U.S. Senate. Thank you very much. [Applause.]

We are now going to hear from Panel 3 entitled, "Tomorrow's Cure." This panel is to ensure available, affordable, quality care for the future and this will be the focus of the final panel. Long-term care, in all of its diverse forms which includes nursing homes, community care, home care, hospice, has had a changing role in the spectrum of health care options in recent years.

The role will continue to change as the older population grows. Specific issues such as financing options; health insurance coverage; the SHMO, which you will hear something about; and other new long-term care concepts all play a role in the formulation of national policy. These will all be addressed by the third and our final panel today before we take questions from the audience and address questions to this final panel.

Those of you who want to submit questions, make sure that you fill out the paper, and if you have a question, hold it up and staff will pick up those questions and start bringing them to us. We will find, as we proceed with the questions, there will be a lot of people—I should not say a lot, but several people will ask the same questions. Therefore, the staff and I will sort through the questions to take only one of the same subject. We will try to get to all of them, as I indicated earlier.

We are first going to hear from Dr. Lawrence Weiss, Director of the Sanford Center for Aging, University of Nevada at Reno. I want to say publicly, Dr. Weiss, that in these hearings, you have been so involved in them. The Sanford Center has been helpful with resources, planning. I cannot express my appreciation enough for the great work that you have done. Please proceed.

STATEMENT OF LAWRENCE J. WEISS, PH.D., DIRECTOR, SANFORD CENTER FOR AGING, UNIVERSITY OF NEVADA, RENO

Mr. WEISS. Thank you. Thank you, Senator, for allowing me to present testimony at this hearing today. I am representing the Sanford Center for Aging at the University of Nevada, Reno. Our center is dedicated to programs that benefit all older persons through a commitment to education, research, and community service.

Our faculty, staff, and volunteers explore innovative ideas and aggressively seek new opportunities that enhance successful aging in the 21st century. The issue being addressed today is long-term care and its impacts each and every one of us, if not today, it will tomorrow. We must assure that our nation can add quality to our remaining years even after chronic illness befalls us.

On our panel, the third, we have the task to talk about tomorrow's cure. In order to deal with this tremendous imperative that is haunting our personal health care system today, we have to establish affordable, accessible, quality care systems that maximize health, choice, and independence. I propose to address these imperatives by proposing the establishment of an integrated delivery system.

Today there are over 100 million people who have chronic conditions. It accounts for over 70 percent of the personal health care dollars. That translates into 425 to 659 billion. A person who has more than one chronic condition uses six times the health care resources. To me, this is a mandate to look to establish more integration in our care delivery.

How do we go about doing that? Integrated delivery services is the first step. We must provide a full array of comprehensive services not just hospital or physician care, not just nursing home care. We have to expand the definition of what long-term care is. Beyond the institution, it has to come back to the home.

It has to span the continuum of care, incorporating all the different services, over time, cross-discipline. We have to think about pooling our resources. We have to develop integrated financing mechanisms. We cannot continue in this same path today where we have Medicare, we have Medicaid, we have the Older Americans Act all operating independently. We have to pool that financing, find ways of doing that.

There are some examples through managed care organizations, but they are only scratching the surface, the Social HMO which you will hear about later from Dr. Phillips. The program for all-inclusive care for the elderly is another model that we can emulate.

We have to empower the consumer, educate, and make decisions jointly, collaboratively with professionals and consumers.

Coordination of care occurs through inter-disciplinary action, through teams that work together across settings. And we have to utilize information technology. It is a powerful tool for data and coordination. And we have to do this through a variety of educational and research mechanisms.

In summary, I request that the U.S. Senate Special Committee on Aging propose a national policy on long-term care that will prepare our country for the 21st century. We cannot continue down the current path. Certainly the baby boom generation will not tolerate it. The current non-system is too costly in terms of dollars and lacks a quality of life.

We must develop integrated delivery systems that are affordable, comprehensive, person-centered, empower the consumer, employ market forces, and incorporate integration techniques in a continuum of care concept. We can work together as academics, researchers, government officials, and providers to experiment through various research demonstrations to accomplish this. Thank you.

[The prepared statement of Mr. Weiss follows:]

TESTIMONY Presented to the U.S. Senate Special Committee on Aging Field Hearing, Reno and Las Vegas, Nevada, January 12 and 13, 1998

The Many Faces of Long-Term Care: Today's Bitter Pill or Tomorrow's Cure?

LAWRENCE J. WEISS, Ph.D.
Director, Sanford Center for Aging
University of Nevada, Reno
Reno, Nevada 89557-0133

Thank you Senator(s) for allowing me to present testimony at this hearing today. I am representing the Sanford Center for Aging at the University of Nevada, Reno. Our center is dedicated to programs that benefit all older persons through a commitment to education, research, and community outreach. Our faculty, staff, and volunteers explore innovative ideas and aggressively seek new opportunities that enhance successful aging in the 21st century.

The issue being addressed today is long-term care (LTC) and that its impact effects each and every one of us. If it does not effect us today, it will tomorrow. I will briefly convey to you what the problems are, their impact on tomorrow's seniors, and make some suggestions on what we must do to assure that we as a nation can add quality of life to our remaining years, even after chronic illness befalls us.

Establish an Integrated Delivery System: Tomorrow's Cure

In order to deal with the tremendous imperatives that are haunting our personal health care, we as a nation must establish an affordable, accessible, quality care system that maximizes health, choice, and independence. I propose to address these imperatives by discussing four major issues in the establishment of an integrated delivery system:

1) Expand the definition of LTC, incorporate the concept of the "continuum of care" which treats the person across settings and over time;
2) Enhance the role of the consumer and market forces to develop a new model of care;
3) Employ service integration techniques, especially focused on acute and chronic care;
4) Establish quality care outcomes through research.

47-539 98 - 9

First, let me define what LTC is or should be. LTC is not just nursing home care. LTC is any service, formal or informal, that addresses a person's level of functioning due to chronic disabling illnesses. Traditionally, our health care system only reimburses for "acute" care issues. Medicare only pays for care while the person is improving, not for on-going LTC services. Although in recent times, through the home health Part B benefit, some have argued that the tremendous increase in utilization has resulted in a more lenient view of Medicare Part B home care benefits to cover LTC services. The federal program has left the coverage of LTC services to the states through the Medicaid program. States only provide benefits for nursing home care for the Medicaid eligible persons. The eligibility requirements are very limiting, especially financially, resulting in the need to become impoverished before qualifying.

In addition, most states also provide very limited coverage under some Medicaid waivers to persons with moderate functional limitations of daily living activities through a home and community-based program. In Nevada that program is called CHIPS. Statistically only a small number of persons are served by these state programs. In

Nevada, only 1152 persons are served. The need is much greater. In short, for all practical purposes only the nursing home is an option for people in need of LTC. This limited definition of viable options for covered LTC services needs to change.

Our nation's health care system needs to define its service system along a continuum, not as isolated incidents that occur at a single point in time. The care system needs to be person-centered, across service settings, involve treatment of different conditions, different disciplines, and adjust to individuals changing needs over time. Lip service is paid to establishing the continuity of care. Only after preventive, primary, rehabilitation, and other long-term care services are a covered benefit will a continuum of care be effective. Form follows financing, so a system needs to pool its financial resources, extend the service options, and focus on the enhancement of individual functioning within a continuum of care.

Second, I support the enhancement of the consumer's role and market forces in developing a new model of care. We all value controlling our own destiny, having independence and autonomy, privacy, and some decision-making capability. The health care system is currently built on the medical model, which is not adequate to deal with the complexity of chronic illnesses and the lack of a "cure". Generally, the consumer or "patient" does not participate in his or her own health care decision-making process. Government is afraid to empower consumers, concerned that they will over-use services and therefore cost more. Some research activities that have studied the impact of the role of consumers do not display overuse and increased expenditures. When given a role in the decision process, consumers generally use less service. Increased participation by the consumer and their family should then increase the effectiveness of the care system by spreading of available resources and personal involvement. This collaborative model of care needs to be incorporated into LTC, acute care, and the continuum of care.

Most consumers and their families who have the resources to pay for services want to make decisions about which providers to use and most do. Unfortunately, those consumers who do not have their own resources do not make decisions. When it comes to LTC, we assume that the consumer can not make decisions, either about service type, provider, or day-to-day services. Therefore, public agencies go to great lengths to establish rules and regulations to try and ward off abuse, neglect, and try to assure some quality. Unfortunately, public agencies can not monitor care closely enough and the abuse continues. If caught in an infraction, public agencies do not have the clout or willingness to enforce the rules. When you have a service, such as nursing homes, in which one-third of the public would rather die before using, you have a problem. I maintain that if the consumer and their family were empowered, had the service options available, and the resources to make decisions, the quality of care across the industry would improve. Let market forces play a role, as they do in other industries.

Third, the whole array of services needs to be integrated into an easily accessible and appropriate system of care that centers on the person. Currently, a person gets lost in entitlements, eligibility requirements, and lack of communication between the many providers and service systems. Developing a truly seamless integrated delivery system is a critical feature in the establishment of effectiveness, efficiency, and quality in health care. Integrating LTC with acute care is especially needed given the incidence and cost of chronic conditions conveyed earlier.

One simple example of integrating acute and chronic care came out of a model program, Evercare, created by the United Health Care program in Minneapolis. This program provided a geriatric team, especially a geriatric nurse practitioner, to nursing home residents in order to provide primary care. Their results have shown a dramatic decrease in acute hospital admissions. Even though this model is limited in providing primary care only to the LTC nursing home residents, the benefits are obvious.

Other model demonstration programs that begin to develop integrated delivery systems are the Social Health Maintenance Organization and the Program for All-inclusive Care for the Elderly (PACE). Both of these models incorporate some of the integration techniques but are limited in scope or size.

Clearly, we as a nation need to learn from these models, develop variations on the theme, and employ service integration within our delivery of health and LTC care. In order to accomplish this, we need to utilize integration techniques. One important integration technique is the use of automated technology that provides a person-centered health data and communication system. Such a system can track all health related issues, communicate that information to all providers, and aid in the coordination of services, while simultaneously comparing the care with standards or benchmarks. Other integration techniques that need to be considered in designing a system of care include:

- Pooled financing or a single payor method;
- Individually tailored plans of care;
- Interdisciplinary clinical care coordination; and
- The full array of services (including low cost housing, assisted living, transportation, social, mental health, personal care, home and community-based services, and other services that provide functional enhancement, prevention or primary care).

The fourth and final imperative in developing the future integrated delivery system is the need to establish quality care outcomes through research. We certainly have reached a level of sophistication in our health service research that we can employ scientific techniques in trying to determine what works and what does not work.

Experimentation with different techniques in the provision of care is essential in determining what is most effective and efficient. The allocation of limited health care resources depends on determining what works from an economic perspective and what works from a quality of life perspective. Research demonstrations are essential in that quest for the ideal model of care.

The Case for a Long-Term Care System

Why should I make the above recommendations and why should we be concerned about LTC? There are many reasons why we should focus on LTC and shape a national policy, which currently does not exist. First, the major cause of illness, disability, and death are chronic conditions. The number of chronic health conditions has increased dramatically since the turn of the century. Those persons who have a chronic condition live longer today, especially with cancer and cardiovascular diseases, and are most likely to require LTC services. This is especially true for those 65+. Today, there are 100 million persons who have a chronic condition. By the year 2040, the number will increase to 160 million. Of those who are disabled, 20% need help with basic daily activities and 60% of those are 65+ years. Please note that most of the figures reported are taken from a very excellent publication, Chronic Care in America: A 21st Century Challenge, produced by the Robert Wood Johnson Foundation and authored by Dr.'s Catherine Hoffman and Dorothy Rice.

Second, we are living longer. Since 1900, life expectancy has increased about 30 years, to where people now routinely live into their 70's and 80's. Today, there are 33 million persons 65+ or about 13% of the total population. The net increase in growth of 65+ persons, is one per minute, according to the 1993 census. By the year 2040, there will be 87 million persons 65+ or 21% of the population. Nevada's 65+ population is growing in faster due to the in-migration of retirees. But more devastating to LTC services is the tremendous growth in 85+ persons. Currently, we have about 3-4 million persons 85+ or 1% of the 65+ population. By the year 2040, the 85+ population will grow to 4% or greater of the 65+ population, totaling 12-23 million people. This is the fastest growing age group of any in the population. Life expectancy demographic research predicts that by the year 2040, males will reach 75-86 years and females will reach 83-92 years of age.

Third, the incidence of disability and chronic conditions increase with age. It is well known to seniors and service providers alike that with increasing age, disability and chronic conditions increase. A study by the Scripps Gerontology Center, Miami University, found that both moderate and severe disability increase with age. Based on an Ohio sample of seniors that were representative of the nation, those that were 65-69 years of age had 10% incidence of disability, those 85-89 years of age were 44% moderately or severely disabled, and those 95+ had 74% incidence of disability. Admissions to nursing home level of care correspond to these figures. In addition, those persons with more than one chronic condition increase with age. In other words, two-thirds of those who have a chronic condition and are 65+ years, have more than one chronic condition.

Fourth, those who have chronic conditions account for 70% of the national expenditures on personal health care. The direct medical care costs for persons with a chronic condition account for $425 billion. If you add indirect costs for morbidity and mortality, the total becomes $659 billion annually. As expected, hospital care and physician services account for two-thirds of the total personal health care dollars, whereas 12% is spent on nursing home care. Medical care costs more for people with chronic conditions. In fact, having more than one chronic condition dramatically increases the total health care cost by six-fold over those with only acute care conditions. These figures are overpowering. We need to focus on these financial issues, change our methods and incentives of reimbursement, and develop integrated systems of care.

Fifth, chronic care is financed primarily by individual out of pocket expenses and public sources. If you exclude acute care expenses, the individual accounts for 33% or $23 billion of nursing home care expenses nationally, Medicaid accounts for 52% or $36 billion, Medicare accounts for 9% or $6 billion, and private insurance 2% or $2 billion annually. Long-term care costs for home health primarily come from Medicare, 39% or $8 billion, individual expenses account for 21% or $4 billion, Medicaid 16% or $3 billion, and private insurance accounts for 12% or $3 billion annually. None of these figures calculate the economic value of informal care. Informal care is estimated to be 75-80% of the total expenditures.

So if it is estimated that $100 billion was spent on formal services, then it could be estimated that $400-500 billion is spent on informal care of chronic conditions. The impact on individuals and their families as well as public sources, especially state governments, is enormous. The economics of LTC demand a national policy.

In summary, I request that the U.S. Senate Special Committee on Aging propose a national policy of LTC that will prepare our country for the 21st century. We can not continue down our current path, certainly the baby boom generation will not tolerate it. The current "non-system" is too costly in terms of dollars and lacks quality of life. We must develop integrated delivery systems that are affordable, comprehensive, person-centered, empower the consumer, employ market forces, and incorporate integration techniques and a continuum of care concept.

Senator REID. Our next witness is someone with a name as long as Frankie Sue's. We have Wendy Van Curen Simons, who is the Administrator, Park Place, Assisted Living Residential Neighborhood for Seniors. Please proceed.

STATEMENT OF WENDY VAN CUREN SIMONS, ADMINISTRATOR, PARK PLACE, ASSISTED LIVING RESIDENTIAL NEIGHBORHOOD FOR SENIORS

Ms. SIMONS. Thank you, Senator. In 1953, I had the honor of sitting in the lap of an elderly gentleman named William Cornwall who happened to be a senior engineer on the Oakland Bay Bridge in California. I was three years old at the time and he would tell me fabulous stories about creatures beyond the imagination.

I asked him one day—and bear in mind I was three and I had to really conceptualize what he said afterwards—"How did you build the bridge?" Far too simple a question. The response was powerful and stuck with me to this very day and even invoked the design concept that I came up with. His reply was, "Design to function in multi-dimensions." And I remember that. I was three. I had to really work to remember and that took a lot of work, but it stuck.

As our country is being challenged to think outside the norm with regard to long-term care options, this elderly man's statement came back to mind. It is a time for us to think beyond linear black and white we are so familiar with and move into more creative systems of long-term care. You are hearing this over and over again.

Nationwide we are seeing one creative approach, the trend of assisted living, explode. The residential style social model of care has been in existence since the 1940s known formally as residential care homes. The current mass development of assisted living is being dictated by consumers of health care who do not consider other options of the past acceptable.

The trend of assisted living is being generated and supported by private sector dollars. It is growing through market demand and with the creative designs of the individuals developing this housing alternative, combining independence with personal care in a warm, dignified community setting.

To date, assisted living is recognizing individuality and choice due to the fact that no significant reimbursement is available from the Federal level and no Federal regulations have been generated to cripple the creation of this option and the creativity of this option.

Nevada has been a leading state in piloting and pioneering regulatory guidelines. Regulations have been in place since 1955, two years past my conversation with Bill Cornwall, with multiple revisions and evolutions. During the past five years, dramatic changes have occurred.

Administrators must be licensed and certified. Caregivers must be fingerprinted and undergo continuing education criteria. Facilities must be bonded as well as licensed, and in 1998, new administrators in the State of Nevada will be required to take a national standardized exam to be licensed.

The most significant item to note is that the assisted living residential care industry in Nevada and the regulatory agency, Bureau of Health facility, which you heard Rick Panelli earlier, worked in a public/private sector relationship to write the regulations and the law governing this industry in Nevada.

This demonstrates the value of a state recognizing its own regulatory needs, consumer desires, and industry input to create a system of aging in place. It is important not to fall into the traps of the traditional past, but to forge a strong, proactive relationship with all the providers of service of our seniors, consumers of long-term care and governmental agencies.

It is further important to think beyond what we are familiar with and enter the multi-dimensional thought process for solutions for the future. We continue to hear that today. Had Steven Spielberg limited himself to traditional thinking, Jurassic Park would not have been created and been as wonderful for us to all experience.

We, too, must continue a course of thinking outside the lines to generate long-term care solutions for change and we must be willing to risk a bit as well. Items to consider. Regulations, I believe, should remain with the states. Each part of the country has its own particular demographic profiles. A Federal standard would repeat the mistakes of previous long-term entities. Consumer choice and quality business practices will dictate the success and failure.

Incentives for creating training programs and partnering with educational institutions, as we have explored already with Larry Weiss and the universities, should be considered. Given a national shortage of workers in long-term care settings, (just as we are considering educational incentives for our children's education), we should consider incentives for the late life worker reentering the work force and encourage them to become employed in the health care industry with the value of their lifelong experience.

A new commitment to training and education of future health care workers needs to come from the industry as well and partnering with the educational institutions, and community-based workshops will continue to educate our public and our caregivers.

Managed care and managed care organizations need to recognize assisted living as a partner in cost savings. Long-term care insurance policies are recognizing this. This should be encouraged. And assisted living as a component of the multi-dimensional care system must be encouraged.

With the increasing number of individuals entering the aging arena as well as the Alzheimer's demographics that we are now seeing today and as cited in JAMA, we are finding that individuals can function in an assisted living level providing that the guideline and criteria at that level are not so crippling and facility-based.

Thank you, Senator, for the opportunity to participate. It is impossible for me to speak in less than five minutes. That is why I submitted to you so much text. Those of you that know me well. [Applause.]

[The prepared statement of Ms. Simons follows:]

FIELD HEARING OF THE

U.S. SENATE SPECIAL COMMITTEE ON AGING

"The Many Faces of Long Term Care: Today's Bitter Pill or Tomorrow's Cure"

Las Vegas, NV – January 12, 1998
Presentation by:

Margaret McConnell, R.N., M.A.

Owner/Administrator
The Charleston Retirement and Assisted Living

Reno, NV – January 13, 1998
Presentation by:

Wendy V.C. Simons

Administrator/Partner
Park Place Assisted Living Residential Neighborhood for Seniors

The Charleston
Retirement & Assisted Living Center

BIOGRAPHY

Margaret McConnell

Margaret McConnell is a native Nevadan, born, raised and educated in Reno, Nevada.

Margaret is a Registered Nurse with a Bachelor's Degree in Nursing from the University of Nevada, Reno, and a Master's Degree in Marriage and Family Counseling from UNR.

She worked for 17 years as a psychiatric nurse and psychologist for the State of Nevada's Mental Health programs in both Northern and Southern Nevada.

About 13 years ago, Margaret and her husband entered the private industry through the purchase of The Charleston Retirement and Assisted Living facility. Margaret is the Administrator of The Charleston.

Margaret is Chairperson of Governor Miller's Board of Examiners for Long Term Care Administrators, Co-Chair of the National Board of Examiners Residential Care/Assisted Living Examination Committee. Margaret is also active in her professional work association and seniors abuse prevention work, is on the Nevada Geriatric Education Advisory Board, and is Vice President of the Nevada Tennis Association. Margaret is both an avid golf and tennis player.

2121 W. Charleston, Las Vegas, Nevada 89102 • Fax (702) 382-8407 • (702) 382-7746

The Charleston
Retirement & Assisted Living Center

BIOGRAPHY

Margaret McConnell

Margaret McConnell is a native Nevadan, born, raised and educated in Reno, Nevada.

Margaret is a Registered Nurse with a Bachelor's Degree in Nursing from the University of Nevada, Reno, and a Master's Degree in Marriage and Family Counseling from UNR.

She worked for 17 years as a psychiatric nurse and psychologist for the State of Nevada's Mental Health programs in both Northern and Southern Nevada.

About 13 years ago, Margaret and her husband entered the private industry through the purchase of The Charleston Retirement and Assisted Living facility. Margaret is the Administrator of The Charleston.

Margaret is Chairperson of Governor Miller's Board of Examiners for Long Term Care Administrators, Co-Chair of the National Board of Examiners Residential Care/Assisted Living Examination Committee. Margaret is also active in her professional work association and seniors abuse prevention work, is on the Nevada Geriatric Education Advisory Board, and is Vice President of the Nevada Tennis Association. Margaret is both an avid golf and tennis player.

2121 W. Charleston, Las Vegas, Nevada 89102 • Fax (702) 382-8407 • (702) 382-7746

FIELD HEARING OF THE U.S. SENATE SPECIAL COMMITTEE ON AGING

LAS VEGAS NV – JANUARY 12, 1998

The Many Faces of Long Term Care: Today's Bitter Pill or Tomorrow's Cure

BY

Margaret A. McConnell, R.N., M.A.
Owner/Administrator : The Charleston Retirement and Assisted Living

A VISION FOR THE FUTURE
OF
LONG TERM CARE

The statistics relating to the care of the elderly are reviewed daily and are absolutely staggering. As has already been discussed numerous times today, we must acknowledge our rapidly growing elderly population. In this decade alone, from 1990 to the year 2000, the elderly population is projected to grow by more than 40%. Along with this incredible increase comes the challenge of offering a quality lifestyle to our elderly, without overburdening taxpayers with the costs. To meet the demands of our elderly, we must work together nationwide to offer services that are creative and cost-effective, while meeting each individual's needs.

Turning to the future of long term care and its problems, I will discuss several steps that I believe must be taken to ensure quality of life for residents of long-term care facilities. In discussing this topic, I think it useful to refer to the Assisted Living Facilities Association of America's outline of future trends in long term care.

- **The general public and health care professionals must increasingly recognize and accept the assisted living residence as an appropriate and viable long-term care alternative.**

Once a senior is no longer able to function at home, we must make services available to deal with their changing lifestyle. Assisted living is the next step in the evolution of housing and health care as an option for those who cannot live alone, but do not need the twenty-four hour supervision of a nursing home.

At this time, there is no question that assisted living is the fastest growing segment of health care. Assisted living is a "special model" of care for our elderly, where the resident comes first. This philosophy of responding to the individual needs of each resident has resulted in a dramatic increase of assisted living facilities across the United States. Since the late 1970's, when professionally managed assisted living was first introduced, the industry has grown to over 30,000 licensed residences. These residences house an estimated one million individuals.

There are several characteristics which distinguish assisted living from other forms of long-term care and lend to its growing popularity. These characteristics include: independence, privacy, increased choices, and a nurturing spirit. As Americans live longer, more individuals and their families are seeking compassionate, low-cost care in non-institutional environments with a high quality of life. These people are increasingly turning to assisted living facilities as a solution to their housing problems.

- **Many nursing homes will convert into assisted living residences and states will begin to increase the regulation of assisted living residences as more companies enter into this market.**

In the past decade, there has been a gradual shift away from nursing homes, as people have increasingly recognized the limitations of this restricted, but most necessary level of care. Throughout the country, regulations have become increasingly stringent on nursing homes. Most significantly, this has included heightened demand on care takers for documentation and accountability. Unfortunately, in spite of these efforts, we continue to hear of quality of care problems in our nursing homes. Let us learn from the nursing home experience and not repeat the same mistakes in retirement and assisted living centers. Although legislation and regulation is essential to a smooth running, organized country, it is essential that we not over regulate retirement and assisted living facilities. Instead, we must allow individual states to oversee and regulate the assisted living industry. In most states there are significant differences in the needs of elderly. It is important to recognize these differences and allow flexibility at the state level to monitor assisted living facilities. In addition, we should encourage professional organizations in assisted living to support, educate, counsel, and nurture private care facility operators. This peer monitoring could provide checks and balances to assure quality care in the assisted living environment.

- **States should increase the use of public funds to support low-income persons in assisted living residences in lieu of nursing homes.**

As I said earlier, assisted living is the fastest growing segment of health care, allowing our seniors to reside in a less restrictive setting than a nursing home. However, most of the new construction currently being done is aimed at the senior who can afford $1,500.00 to $3,000.00 per month in rent. This leaves over 80% of our nation's population who are not able to afford this monthly fee. Since approximately 90% of assisted living costs are paid privately and since the costs of most assisted living residences are too high for most seniors to be able to afford, it is essential that alternatives be developed to enhance and expand payment mechanisms for assisted living.

One alternative for enhanced reimbursement is the Medicaid Waiver Program. As most of you are aware, Medicaid is the primary payment mechanism for nursing home residents. The reimbursement rate in a nursing home is approximately twice the monthly cost of assisted living, on a monthly basis. It has been estimated that as much as 50% of today's national nursing home population could be served in assisted living residences. The dollar cost savings could be astronomical if thousands of appropriate seniors were moved to assisted living residences from nursing homes with Medicaid Waiver reimbursement as the payment mechanism.

More than twenty states nationwide are now implementing the Medicaid Waiver Program as State officials realize that they can not only save money but also serve people more appropriately in assisted living residences. These officials state they were driven in this direction by the concepts behind assisted living—the privacy, the maximized independence, and the dignity for each resident. In Nevada, the Medicaid Waiver Program is relatively small at this time, due primarily to budget constraints, and has an extensive waiting list of several months.

Another manner in which states can increase the use of public funds to support assisted living is by augmenting the Supplemental Security Income (SSI) program. SSI financially supplements our nation's neediest seniors. The monetary reimbursement per month for retirement and assisted living centers needs to be increased as this would allow seniors more choices in quality care living arrangements. The current SSI reimbursement rate is so low, about $750.00 per month in Nevada, that most facilities are unable to offer services to the SSI recipient. The trend over the past few years has been that fewer and fewer assisted living operators can accommodate these seniors. I am unaware of any new facility coming on line in Nevada, that will be able accept SSI recipients. Since SSI recipients comprise a significant percentage of our consumers, we have a serious issue confronting us.

❖ **Partnerships will be developed to better offer services to residents as they age in place.** In Nevada, our Licensing Board for Long Term Care Administrators is actively working with the Sanford Center for Aging to offer continuing education to our long-term care administrators.

These efforts are aimed at insuring that administrators are up to date and working with Nevada's elderly population in the most innovative and practical ways. Caring for Nevada's frail elderly is a huge responsibility and it is imperative that this work be carried out by qualified, well-informed caregivers.

To further insure quality care for our seniors, programs, courses and curriculum could be added to our colleges and universities nationwide to prepare administrators, supervisors and caretakers to work with the frail elderly in the community, in assisted living, or in the nursing home setting. Curriculum should include subjects such as fiscal, organizational, and dietary management, along with resident care.

Long-term care industry workers must understand the whole person, not just the person's medical, dietary, or daily hygiene needs. These workers must embrace the importance of encouraging each resident to be as independent as possible.

In closing I'd like to commend the committee today for holding this special hearing. It is through fact gathering, planning, and openness to new ideas that we can together find an answer for the compelling issues of long term care today. In establishing a national policy on long term care, I encourage you to include consumers, families, long term care representatives, and educational and policy makers from throughout the United States.

Thank you,

Margaret McConnell
1-12-97

Wendy V.C. Simons
Consultant
1530 Pass Dr. • Reno, NV 89509
(702) 323-7706 • (702) 323-3102 Fax

December 30, 1997

Honorable Charles E. Grassley
Chairman
United States Senate
Special Committee on Aging
Dirksen Senate Office building
Room G-31
Washington, D.C. 20510

Dear Senator Grassley and Senate Committee Members:

Thank you for the opportunity to participate as a panelist in your Senate Special Committee on Aging field hearing on Tuesday, January 13, 1997 in Reno, Nevada. The topics to be discussed are of great importance and the course of future planning needs to be progressive and innovative.

Through my presentation I hope to cite the exceptional communication that has developed within our state and identify how this communication has allowed Nevada to step beyond the traditional patterns of thinking into a potential blending and multi-dimensional track of service to our seniors. We are just beginning to feel the great influx of the over 65 population and the many providers of services to them are identifying similar needs. The public and private sector must partner to develop flexible solutions to future challenges.

I am grateful to be considered for your panel and remain deeply committed to charting new pathways of service to this senior population whom I have spent my whole life with.

I remain,

Sincerely,

Wendy V.C. Simons

FIELD HEARING OF THE U.S. SENATE SPECIAL COMMITTEE ON AGING

In

RENO, NEVADA – JANUARY 13, 1998

"The Many Faces of Long Term Care: Today's Bitter Pill or Tomorrow's Cure"

Presentation by:

Wendy V.C. Simons
Park Place Assisted Living Residential Neighborhood for seniors

FIELD HEARING OF THE U.S. SENATE SPECIAL COMMITTEE ON AGING

Reno, Nevada – January 13, 1998

TESTIMONY OUTLINE

SECTION I

SECTION II

SECTION I

DESIGN TO FUNCTION: MULTI-DIMENTIONAL THINKING

In 1953 I had the honor and pleasure of sitting in the lap of an elderly gentleman, William Cornwall, who happened to be a senior engineer on the Oakland/Bay Bridge in California. I was 3 years old at the time and he would tell me fabulous stories about creatures beyond the imagination. I asked him one day, how he built the bridge. He replied, "Design to function in multi-dimensions."

As our country is being challenged to think outside of the norm with regard to long term care options, this elderly man's statements come back to mind. It is a time for us to think beyond the linear black and white we are so familiar with and move into more creative systems of long term care.

Nationwide, we are seeing one creative approach, the trend of "assisted living" explode. The residential style, social model of care has been in existence since the 1940's known formerly as residential care homes. The current mass development of assisted living is being dictated by the consumers of health care who do not consider skilled nursing facilities as an option of choice. The trend of assisted living is still being generated and supported by private sector dollars. It is growing through market demand and with the creative designs of the individuals developing this housing and health care alternative combining independence with personal care in a warm, dignified, community setting. To date, assisted living is recognizing individuality and choice and due to the fact that no significant reimbursement is available from the federal level and no federal regulations have been generated to cripple the creation of this option in the long term care continuum.

Nevada has been a leading state in pioneering regulatory guidelines. Regulations have been in place since 1955, with multiple revisions and evolutions. During the past 5 years, dramatic changes have occurred. Administrators must be licensed and certified, caregivers must be fingerprinted and undergo continuing education criteria, facilities must be bonded as well as licensed, and in 1998, new Administrator's will be required to pass a national standardized test. The most significant item to note is that the assisted living/residential care industry in Nevada and the regulatory agency, Bureau of Health Facilities, worked in a public/private sector relationship to write the regulations and laws governing the industry. This demonstrates the value of a state recognizing it's own regulatory needs, consumer desires and industry input to create a system of aging in place.

It is important not to fall into the traps of the traditional past, but to forge a strong pro-active relationship will all the providers of service to our seniors, consumers of long term care components and governmental entities. It is further important to think beyond what we are familiar with and enter the multi-dimensional thought process for solutions in the future.

Had Steven Spielberg limited himself to traditional thinking, Jurassic Park would not have been created to be the spectacular product it became. We too, must continue a course of thinking outside the lines to generate long term care solutions for change, and we must be willing to risk a bit as well.

Wendy Simons 1/98

(2)

ITEMS TO CONSIDER

- **REGULATIONS SHOULD REMAIN WITH THE STATES.**

Each part of the country has it's own particular demographics and profiles. A federal standard would repeat the mistakes of previous long term care entities. Consumer choice and quality business practices will dictate success and failure.

- **INCENTIVES FOR CREATING TRAINING PROGRAMS FOR EMPLOYEES OF LONG TERM CARE PROGRAMS SHOULD BE CONSIDERED.**

1. There is a national shortage of workers for long term care settings. Just as we are considering educational incentives for our children's education, we should consider incentives for the late life worker re-entering employment in the health care industry.
2. A new commitment to training and education of future health care workers needs to come from the industry as well. Partnering with educational institutions for program and curriculum development for caregivers and other allied fields must be a priority for all in the long term care industry.
3. Community based workshops offering educational opportunities for individuals to understand aging issues and preventative health must be encouraged.

- **A REVIEW OF THE EXPENDITURES OF FEDERAL DOLLARS FOR INDIGENT CARE IN SKILLED NURSING FACILITIES SHOULD BE CONDUCTED.**

1. While the private sector is choosing Assisted living or home based care as an alternative, State and Federal dollars continue to be spent in skilled nursing facilities for individuals who would be appropriate in an assisted living setting. Some attention has been given to this area, and by no means are the Medicaid clients a source of great revenue to the skilled facilities, however many individuals are forced to "spend down" to be eligible for Medicaid assistance in a skilled setting. If slightly supplemented in an assisted living setting, some individuals would have resources last longer resulting in savings to the Medicaid program.
2. Individuals who would choose to be in an assisted living facility and who are on the SSI/Medicaid program are unable to be supplemented above the base rate without penalty. Families should be allowed to contribute without fear of deduction from the Medicaid dollars. (Nevada has just initiated this program.)

Wendy Simons 1/98

(3)

- **LONG TERM CARE INSURANCE POLICIES ARE RECOGNIZING THE DOLLARS SAVED IN ASSISTED LIVING.**
  Many Long Term Care insurance policies are now reimbursing for Assisted Living as an alternative to skilled nursing facilities. This should be encouraged when appropriate.

- **MANAGED CARE AND MEDICARE MANAGED CARE NEED TO RECOGNIZE ASSISTED LIVING AS A COST SAVING.**
  1. Often times, an individual in an Assisted living facility undergoing a health crisis can be maintained for a brief period of time through supportive services coming to the facility. Currently, some managed care and Medicare managed care programs require hospitalization for services to continue. This is not a good use of dollars if the alternative is appropriate.
  2. Community based "house call" programs should be considered in assisted living facilities. This would reduce the cost of some medical offices and allow physicians and nurse practitioners to evaluate their patients in their own setting.

- **SAFETY NETS NEED TO BE ENCOURAGED, BUT INDIVIDUALS SHOULD NOT BE IN A COCOON.**
  1. Continued communication between all the components of the health care continuum needs to be encouraged. No one agency should have complete control, power or turf over another. When considering financial reimbursement for programs, "funding formulas" often slant service away from those most in need.
  2. Financial incentives should be considered for community based care programs that allow a multi-dimensional flow. Sometimes an individual needs a Band-Aid other times a meal or a hug, but rarely a "mummy wrap" of services.
  3. If all the funds are wrapped up in one agency there is a tendency for that agency to spend on it's own special interests. We need to consider a blending of services.

- **ASSISTED LIVING, AS A COMPONENT OF THE MULTI-DEMENSIONAL CARE SYSTEM MUST BE ENCOURAGED.**
  1. Creative designs must be allowed and no one facility should be required to be like another. (Just as we choose car types, home types and store types, consumers should be allowed to choose the type of assisted living design they find appropriate.)
  2. With the increasing numbers of aging individuals and the projected numbers of individuals with probable Alzheimer's dementia, flexibility in design and housing as well as personal care options will be critical to best save health care dollars. As was cited in JAMA, October 22/29, 1997- Vol 278, No.16, "Alzheimer disease costs (medical, Long term care, home care, and lost productivity for caregivers totals a direct and indirect dollar expenditure approaches $100 billion each year. This figure will increase in the future and truly challenge our creativity and resources.

- **ADDITIONAL RESEARCH DOLLARS NEED TO BE DIRECTED TO THE STUDY OF ALZHEIMERS DISEASE AND RELATED AGING ISSUES.**
  To effectively plan and implement care options, strategies must be based on anticipation of effective care systems in this, the greatest component need.

Wendy Simons 1 98

AN OVERVIEW OF ASSISTED LIVING/RESIDENTIAL CARE HOMES IN NEVADA

By
WENDY V.C. SIMONS

I. BRIEF HISTORY OF THE EVOLUTION OF RESIDENTIAL CARE

History in Nevada
Changes and National trends

II. CLARIFICATION AND TERMINOLOGY

Board and Care, Adult Group Care, Residential Care, Foster Care, Domicilliary Homes, Rest Homes, Assisted Living Facilities

III. WHERE DOES IT FIT IN THE OVERVIEW OF OPTIONS?

Retirement Communities, Home Based Care, Skilled Nursing Facilities Licensure Requirements, Inspecting Agencies, Etc.

IV. WHAT SERVICES ARE PROVIDED?
WHAT ARE THE REIMBURSEMENT RATES?

Room and board, assistance with personal hygiene, personal laundry, medication supervision, socialization, activities, heath care co-ordination, other activities of daily living assistance

V. FUTURE DIRECTIONS

New designs and interest in alternative living
In home support agencies
New levels of professionalism, yet home environment

Wendy V.C. Simons 1/98

RESIDENTIAL CARE HOMES / ASSISTED LIVING IN NEVADA

By Wendy V.C. Simons

BRIEF HISTORY

Residential Care Homes have been in Nevada since the 1940's. During the early years they were actually more boarding home type facilities, created in existing residences in local communities and usually by an individual who had some nursing background. In fact, Margaret Von Fluee (my mother) opened the first such facility in downtown Reno at 315 Hill Street in response to several agencies stating they had no place to locate "old folks" in a safe environment outside of a hospital setting.

The following years saw the creation of Skilled Nursing Facilities as we know them today, when reimbursement became available from Medicare/Medicaid programs. Yet during the expansion of long term health care options, residential care homes (board and care homes) maintained their existence and evolved as non-medical models of care; providing room, board and some personal care assistance. The majority of these early homes housed from 10-20 individuals and would expand through additions to accommodate more clients. In the ensuing years, a few larger complexes were built in the Reno and Las Vegas areas.

Initially, group care homes were licensed by the Nevada State Welfare division and the early regulations to govern them were created around 1955. In 1974 the Nevada State Health Division took over the responsibility of licensure and inspection of larger facilities. Stricter life safety codes were enacted and many facilities were retrofitted with sprinkler systems. There were about 11 such facilities in the state at this time. Nevada State welfare continued to license "Family Care Homes" caring for 3 or fewer residents.

The most significant transition occurred in 1986 when the Bureau of Health Facilities became responsible for regulations and licensure for the smaller care homes. Categories and regulations were created for facilities caring for "six or less" and "seven or more" individuals. The state licensure list jumped from (15) fifteen facilities to over three hundred (300) statewide.

It is interesting to note that during my affiliation as a Director with the National Association of Residential Care Facilities (NARCF) I discovered that Nevada's regulation of facilities was years ahead of many states, and that in 1990, only twenty-one (21) states had regulations in place for these facilities!

(2)

During the past three years, Nevada has undergone a dramatic change and evolution in the regulations of residential care/ assisted living. Through a significant joint venture effort among facility providers and the state regulatory agency, Bureau of Licensure and Certification, a complete revision of the standards and regulations governing residential care facilities was adopted in December 1997. The new regulations allow for more of an aging in place philosophy of care providing certain conditions and standards of care are established. The blending of a standard created by regulators and the provision for **consumer choice** in residential care options would have never occurred if not for the visionary thinking of the Chief of the Bureau of Licensure and Certification, Sharon Ezell, and the leaders of the residential care/ assisted living industry gathering together to discuss and create the current regulatory document.

Since 1955 Nevada has remained pro-active in charting the future course of residential care/assisted living. The newest regulations are evidence of that as well as the requirement in 1994 that administrators of facilities have certification and licensure in addition to the facility license. In 1998, Nevada's Board of Examiners for Long Term Care (BLECA) will adopt a new national exam for administrators thanks to the efforts of longtime Nevada provider, Margaret McConnell. The 1997 Legislature adopted the requirement for fingerprinting of caregivers and bonding of facilities. Nevada has remained in the forefront as a leader in collaborative efforts between agencies and providers in the residential care industry and has demonstrated that a State can direct its needs better than a federal entity. In this manner, Nevada can serve as a model for others to follow.

The massive growth in assisted living/residential care facilities has been created by a consumer interest and desire for increased options in long term care. This social model of care has evolved not by the availability of federal dollars creating physical plants, but by individuals seeking a less institutional standard of service.

The future of residential care and the newly developing assisted living care system should be dictated by individual states. Each section of the country has specific demographics and human profiles that are best controlled by the individual areas. It is predictable that most aging individuals and their families will choose the setting they are most comfortable with, both esthetically and financially. Ultimately, as we anticipate the future history of this type of care system, consumer choice and individual preferences will write the text.

Wendy Simons 1/98

(3)

CLARIFICATION OF TERMINOLOGY

In Federal studies this industry is termed "Board and Care Homes". Nevada refers to them as "Residential Care Facilities for Groups" or "Adult Group Care Homes". The V.A. system used the term "Domicillary Care homes". Some states call smaller homes "Foster Care Homes for the Elderly", and sometimes they are called "custodial care" and the newest term for recently designed facilities is "Assisted Living Facilities".

Ultimately, all these titles and names apply to a non-medical model of care, unlike skilled nursing facilities which fall into the category of medical models of care.

WHERE DO RESIDENTIAL CARE/ ASSISTED LIVING FACILITIES FIT

One must clearly understand the spectrum of elderly housing options to understand where Residential Care/Assisted Living homes fit in the continuum of care.

Ideally, everyone would prefer to age in place in his or her own home. However, when an individual no longer has sufficient physical or mental abilities to prepare meals, handle financial affairs, manage medications, attend to personal hygiene and daily living necessities then it is time to research and engage support systems and alternatives. These may include:

1. Home based support- usually the first choice, such as caregivers, home health services, etc.
2. Community living complexes- (Retirement communities) which provide shelter and meals for those not in need of supervision and assistance.
3. Residential Care/ Assisted Living facilities- which provide meals, lodging, activities of daily living (ADL's) assistance, and medication supervision.
4. Extended Care Facilities- which provide residence and skilled nursing services in a medical setting.

It is easy to see that Residential Care/ Assisted living is between home and nursing home.

It is also prudent to note that individuals may move in and out and between any of the above systems of service.

Wendy Simons 1/98

(4)

SERVICES PROVIDED IN RESIDENTAL CARE/ ASSISTED LIVING

Residential Care/ Assisted Living facilities provide twenty-four hour supervised living, meals, laundry, medication supervision and assistance, socialization, activities and health care co-ordination in a non-medical residential group living environment. The design and types of homes are unique to each operator.

Keep in mind these are not medical facilities, but residential style environments, many managed by the owner/operator in the case of the smaller homes. Some facilities operate with managers and other staff, depending on the size of the home and the number of clients. Eighty-five (85%) percent of the licensed facilities in Nevada are small facilities of 6 or fewer residents. The owners are usually individuals who have been involved in the health care field and have an entrepreneurial spirit. The reason for the success of these homes is due to the fact that many families prefer a home-style setting for their aging relative and want to avoid the nursing home setting.

Currently we are seeing a dramatic increase in the number of newer Assisted Living Complexes. Their focus remains the same as the smaller setting, a non-medical, social model of care allowing consumer choice of services and care needs.

WHAT TYPE OF CLIENT IS APPROPRIATE

The residents of these facilities must be ambulatory, or if in a wheelchair, able to transfer independently. Residents must be mentally and physically able to evacuate the facility with or without assistance in case of an emergency. Residents must be free of communicable disease. Residents must be able to self-medicate with supervision and should have some capacity for self care. If a resident is accepted with one of the new "allowable conditions" as stated in regulations, provisions must be made to provide supervision by an appropriately skilled medical person for the allowed conditions. Incontinence is allowed and is managed according to each facilities philosophy.

The typical resident is an individual who living alone would not eat properly or care for himself/herself properly. The individual may or may not need assistance with one or more activity of daily living (ADL). The usual assisted living individual is a widow about 85 years of age who was in a subtle state of decline in an independent living setting. It is not uncommon for couples to move in to an assisted living setting due to the care needs of one of the individuals. Residents in assisted living may come as a result of caregiver burnout, lack of community resources and/or relocation by a family member living in the area.

Wendy Simons 1/98

(5)

Most recently we have seen the increase of facilities who are willing to take what might have been considered and ICF I or II (Intermediate care) level client that would been normally place in a skilled nursing facility. Curiously enough, many of these clients do well in a small residential setting and it is not uncommon for an individual who needed a wheel chair in a larger building to be walking in a residential home setting. Individuals that might seem quite confused in large living environments often do better in a home-like setting as well. Behavioral issues often disappear in a more residential setting.

CHARGES AND REIMBURSEMENT SOURCES

At this writing, the cost of placement in residential care/ assisted living facility in Nevada ranges between $ 748.66 (for the state assisted/ SSI client) and $3000.00 per month. Private pay facilities usually scale their rates based on the services needed by the resident. Unfortunately there is a decline in the number of available placements for the state assisted client and no new facilities have been built in the last ten (10) years that accommodate the SSI client. The newly built assisted living facilities accept only private pay individuals. Some low income individuals have qualified for the Medicaid waiver program while placed in residential care settings which increases the rate of reimbursement to the $900.00 range. However, this is still not an incentive to accommodate the SSI subsidized client when the private pay market is strong.

FUTURE DIRECTIONS

The growing **consumer interest** with regard to long term care options will impact this industry greatly in the future. Already we are seeing larger corporations such as Mariott, Kennsington, Sunrise, Manor Care, Standish, Alternative Living Services, ARV and numerous others developing "assisted living" facilities across the nation. Many of these corporations have recognized the **consumer demand** for non-medical care options for their loved ones. The "assisted living" trend is being dictated by the **interest of the public** in this alternative level of care. It is evident that our country and our state must pay attention to this **expressed choice of individuals** and break away from the limited options of the past and allow for a multi-dimensional care system.

Our challenge is to think much as Steven Spielberg did when he created "Jurassic Park". We must evolve beyond lateral flat-screened thinking in care options and allow for the development of new creatures. Computer technology and the willing to risk allowed Spielberg to develop what could not exist before.

Creative thinking in health care options must allow us to develop what has not existed before. This is what we are seeing in the development of "assisted living" as an entity to itself. It is an industry with multiple designs and multiple personalities. Assisted living remains aware of the need for "high touch" service and not just high tech documentation.

The creative challenge continues. To individuals, to states and to future economic decisions of the government.

Wendy Simons 1/98

(6)

BOB MILLER
Governor

STATE OF NEVADA

CHARLOTTE CRAWFORD
Director

MYLA C. FLORENCE
Administrator

DEPARTMENT OF HUMAN RESOURCES
WELFARE DIVISION
2527 N. Carson Street
Carson City, Nevada 89706-0113
(702) 687-4770

November 20, 1997

WENETTE VAN CUREN-SIMONS
PARK PLACE
2305 IVES CT
RENO NV 89503

This letter informs all Adult Group Care Facilities (AGCFs) of the upcoming increase in Supplemental Security Income (SSI) payments.

Beginning January 1, 1998, the federal SSI payment will increase 2.1 percent. In addition, the state supplement for aged and blind individuals will increase 6 percent effective January 1, 1998 from $311 to $329.66. Due to systems requirements, this increase will be delayed approximately six weeks. Retroactive payments for January and February 1998 will be sent by the Social Security Administration around the second week of February. The new schedule of payments for aged and blind individuals will be as follows:

Federal Payment	State Payment	Total Payment
$494.00	$329.66	$823.66

A disabled individual's federal payment is $494 with no state supplement.

Welfare Division policy requires each client in an AGCF receive a personal needs allowance. For 1998, the personal needs allowance is increased to $75 per month. The balance of the combined federal/state SSI payment is available for room and board costs.

Should you have any questions, please contact Jeanette Hills, Chief, Eligibility and Payments, at (702) 687-4386.

Sincerely,

Myla C. Florence

Myla C. Florence
Administrator

MCF:CR/saL1.11

pc: Division for Aging Services
Mental Health/Mental Retardation
Washoe County Social Services
Clark County Social Service

Working for the Welfare of ALL Nevadans

WENDY V.C. SIMONS

INTRODUCTORY SUMMARY

Wendy is a native Nevadan, born and raised in the "old folks" home, as her mother opened the first senior care home in the state in the late 1940's. She has been considered a senior advocate for many years through numerous affiliations and dedications to senior care issues. She is the creator of a unique design in assisted living called Park Place, and has gained the reputation of being proactive in legislative and regulatory issues in Nevada.

WENETTE (WENDY) V.C. SIMONS
1530 Pass Drive
Reno, Nevada 89509
(702) 323-7706 (H) * (702) 323-3102 (FAX)
(702) 746-1188 (W) * (702) 746-1189 (FAX)

BIOGRAPHICAL SKETCH

- Second generation care provider –Margaret Von Fluee (mother) developed the first residential care home in the state of Nevada in 1948. Born and raised in the "old folks home", have been active participant since childhood; eventually taking over as administrator in 1992 upon graduating from University of Nevada at Reno.
- Developed and operate Park Place Assisted Living Facility in Reno, a 60 resident assisted living neighborhood: a unique design concept still unduplicated.
- Professional reputation for being "the person to contact" with regard to care choices and counsels families on the multitude of options available in the state of Nevada.
- Have presented in numerous provider workshops and seminars for Washoe Medical Center and Saint Mary's Hospital personnel, created a joint venture seminar with the Bureau of Licensure and Certification on the new state regulations adopted in 1997 with a emphasis on admission assessment and regulatory compliance.
- Made presentations nationally for the Assisted Living Federation of America Institute and the American Association for Homebuilders as well as the National Association of Residential Care Facilities. (1984 in Minnesota, 1989 in Boston, 1990 in Tulsa, 1990 Washington, D.C., 1996 in Nevada ALFA Institute)
- Presenter in the V.A./ U.N.R. Conference in 1992 on Alternatives to Long Term Care.
- Subject of cover story on Residential Care in 1991 October issue of Senior Spectrum.
- Expert witness, 7th Judicial Court, State of Nevada, in client assessment for alternative placement from a long term care facility.
- Presenter before numerous State legislative committees since 1976.
- Co-producer and Host of the "Senior Scope" television show for KOLO Channel 8 for 10 years. Topics of the program have included: Care options for families; Senior abuse, neglect, exploitation; Medications and the elderly; Health and cost containment issues; Managed care; Late life romances; Sanford Center for Aging; etc.
- Member of the NAAB "Pass Point" Committee for the National Exam for Residential Care Administrators, 1997

CURRENT PROFESSIONAL AFFILIATIONS

- Member of the Founders Council of the Assisted Living Federation of America
- Member and past Vice Chairman of the Sanford Center for Aging Studies, Community Advisory Board at University of Nevada, Reno.
- Member of the Nevada Adult Care Association and past President.
- Past President and member of the Executives Association of Reno
- Member of the Sierra Continuity of Care Association
- Member of the Senior Coalition of Northern Nevada

OTHER ORGANIZATIONS AND AFFILIATIONS AND HIGHLIGHTS

- Member of the Executive Committee of the Assisted Living Federation of America 1991-1993
- Past member of the Washoe Zephyrs Toastmasters and Evaluator of the Year 1991
- Past Chairman for Nevada ALFAA Council of States
- Past President of the Older American's Advisory Council of Northern Nevada by Governor appointment for 1990-1992
- Selected one of Reno's "10 Most Watchable Women" 1992
- Past member of the Nevada Junior Livestock Show Board by Governor Appointment, 1987-1991
- Past President of the Swope Middle School Parent's Group.
- Past Secretary of the Reno High School AAA Parent's Group
- Coordinator and Commentator of the Governor's Conference on Aging Fashion show 1990
- Lecturer at UNR Animal Science Department 1976-1982
- Miss Reno Rodeo 1970
- Judge of Horse Shows, Drill Team Competitions and Parades for over 30 years.

EDUCATION

- **B.S. in Education from the University of Nevada, Reno**
- **Licensed Residential Care Facility Administrator, RCFA 5611**

Senator REID. One thing I did not mention is that Wendy's mother opened the first senior care home in the State of Nevada in the late 1940s.

Ms. SIMONS. That is correct. Rather than observing this industry, I have lived it and I love it.

Senator REID. We will now hear from our next witness, Winthrop Cashdollar, who is the Executive Director of the Nevada Health Care Association.

STATEMENT OF WINTHROP CASHDOLLAR, EXECUTIVE DIRECTOR OF THE NEVADA HEALTH CARE ASSOCIATION

Mr. CASHDOLLAR. Senator Reid, representatives of the Senate Special Committee on Aging, and members of the audience, my name is Winthrop Cashdollar. I am the Executive Director of the Nevada Health Care Association, an association of Nevada's long-term care providers. The Nevada Health Care Association is affiliated with the American Health Care Association, which is the nation's largest association of long-term caregivers.

Senator, I want to thank you again for holding these hearings and for the opportunity to sit on this panel, particularly, looking for "tomorrow's cure." There is an awful lot of work that we will need to do to be ready for the demographic tidal wave of America's elderly in the future and the sooner we start, the better. I commend you for rolling up your sleeves and getting down to work on what can be a daunting issue.

I also sincerely appreciate what you and Dr. Bernick had to say about long-term caregivers. Whether these caregivers are in the home or in nursing facilities, they deal with disability, disease, and death day in and day out. It is a very difficult job and we need to consider the work that they do every day and give them respect and recognition. We must also pursue public policies that will make sure that we have enough qualified caregivers now and in the future. It should be a priority of our long-term care policy.

I would like to speak briefly today about three components of tomorrow's cure for long-term care, access, quality, and financing. Regarding access, the current governmental division of responsibility for acute health care and long-term care for the nation's senior citizens is confusing, places beneficiaries more according to program rigidities than clinical needs, and causes too many of our frail elderly to fall between the cracks of the system.

In order to rationalize the full continuum of acute care and long-term care services, it is time that we better integrate acute care and long-term care. A number of speakers have already spoken to the need for a seamless health care system for the elderly, an integrated system of service delivery.

I would go further and would suggest that what we need is a single program for acute care and long-term care for America's elderly, a single program that includes the entire continuum and which can be partnered with private sector coverage that will fit together like a puzzle.

I am going to be submitting for the record, with your permission, Senator, this brief brochure entitled, "SecureCare," and I believe the audience was given an opportunity to pick up a package that includes this brochure and I commend this to the audience and to the Senate Special Committee on Aging.

Senator REID. That will be the order. That will be made part of the record.

[The information of Mr. Cashdollar follows:]

SECURECARE

Secure Care

MEETING

THE NEEDS

OF AN

AGING NATION

Secure Care

FACT: The average Ancient Greek lived until age 18. The median life span of a Puritan was 33 years. In 1991, the average American life expectancy was about 72 years for men, 79 years for women. ■ FACT: In 1994, about one in eight Americans was age 65 or older. By 2030, one in five Americans will be a senior citizen. ■ FACT: In 1994, 7.3 million Americans needed long term care services. By 2000, this number will rise to 9 million, and by 2060 it will skyrocket to about 24 million.

Society Is Changing And So Must Our Long Term Care System

Americans are living longer and healthier lives, thanks to better diet, better medical care, and safer living and working environments. But no one is immune from the effects of aging that far too often result in chronic illness and reduced physical or mental ability. *Consider one more fact: two out of every five Americans will require nursing home care at some point in their lives.*

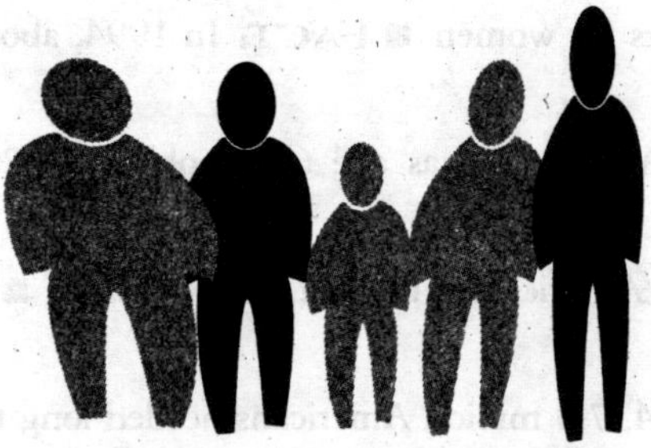

Two out of five Americans will be cared for in a nursing home at some point in their lives.

SOURCE: *New England Journal of Medicine*

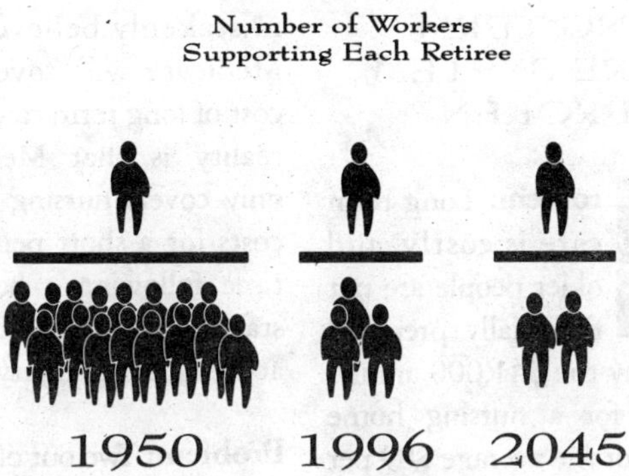

Ratio of Retirees to Workers

In 1950, there were 16 workers to every retiree. Today there are three. By 2045, there will only be two workers to support each retiree.

SOURCE: *New York Times*

Our population and our lifestyles are changing in ways that significantly affect how we provide for those in need of long term care.

Change is everywhere:

In the workplace—The number of workers to support each retiree is declining.

In our families—Our mobile society means that sons and daughters live farther from their parents than ever before.

In our homes—The number of single-parent and two-working-parent households continues to grow.

All these changes mean a greater burden for our families and our society in providing and paying for the long term care that a growing number of our citizens will require.

THE CURRENT LONG TERM CARE SYSTEM IS BROKEN

Problem: Long term care is costly, and older people are not financially prepared to pay the $41,000 annual cost for a nursing home stay or the average $89 per visit fee by a home care registered nurse.

Problem: Most people mistakenly believe that Medicare will cover the cost of long term care. The reality is that Medicare only covers nursing home costs for a short period of time following a hospital stay to recuperate from an acute illness or injury.

Problem: Two out of three nursing home residents are forced onto Medicaid to

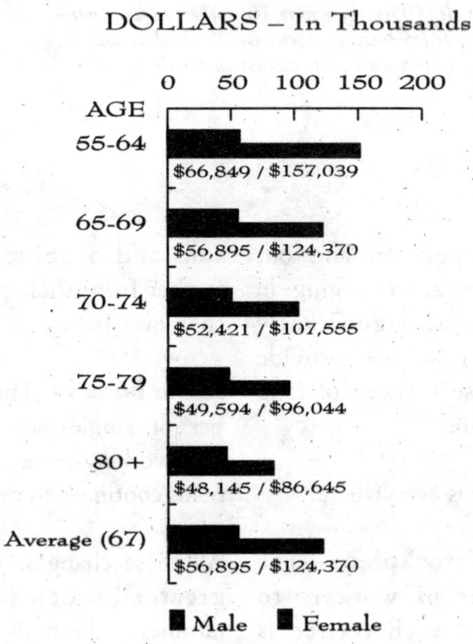

Long Term Care Costs – 1995

The average American man can expect to spend $56,895 on long term care. The average woman will spend $124,370.

SOURCE: Lifeplans Inc.

pay for their care. Medicaid is a federal-state program that provides health care to people who are impoverished. Medicaid was designed to help the poor, not the elderly. But Medicaid has become our nation's long term care system by default.

Problem: Millions of people who worked all their lives and paid taxes have been impoverished because they got sick and needed long term care. Millions more face the same fate unless the system changes. For the elderly to qualify for Medicaid, they must spend all of their life savings until they meet the state-determined poverty level. Thus, the need for long term care forces the middle-class elderly onto welfare to receive care.

United States

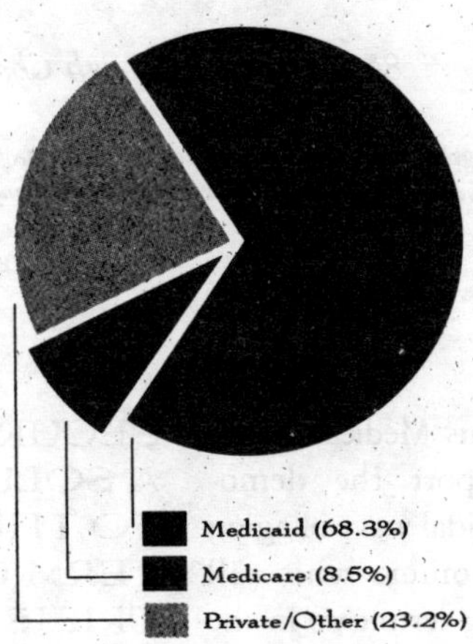

Residents by Primary Payer Source – 1996

More than 1 million people rely on Medicaid to pay for their nursing home care.

SOURCE: Health Care Financing Administration

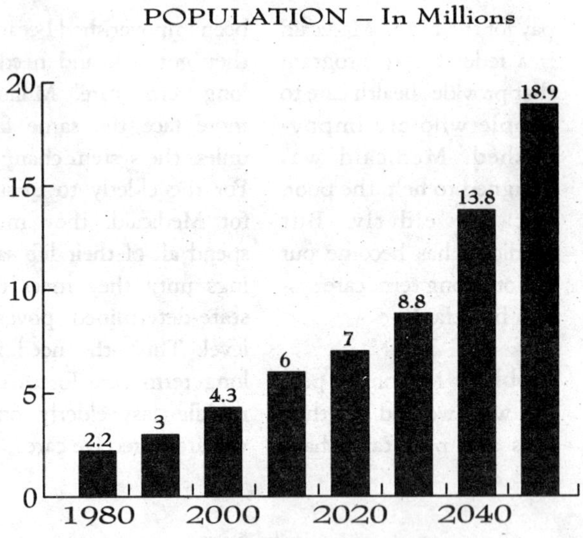

85-and-Older Growth Chart

The fastest growing segment of our population is people age 85 and older. People in that age group are the heaviest users of long term care services.

SOURCE: U.S. Bureau of the Census

Problem: Medicaid cannot support the demographic tidal wave of aging baby boomers who will need long term care in the next century. Most states are struggling now to meet their Medicaid budgets. The demand the elderly will place on Medicaid soon will outweigh Medicaid's ability to meet the elderly's long term care needs.

SECURE CARE: A SOLUTION TO THE LONG TERM CARE CRISIS

The long term care community is committed to progressive and compassionate reforms that will enable our nation to meet the long term care needs of all Americans.

We call our approach *SecureCare.* It is built on four principles designed to solve our nation's long term care crisis while preserving the safety net for America's poor elderly and disabled.

Solution: Transform long term care from a welfare program to a health care program.

The elderly are not forced to impoverish themselves to get hospital or physician services. They should not be required to become poor because they have medical conditions that require long term care. Fundamental compassion and fairness demand shifting our nation's long term care financing system from the Medicaid welfare program to the mainstream of our nation's health care financing system.

Solution: Coordinate long term care private resources with Medicare and Social Security.

Health care policy should support integration of hospital, physician, and long term care into a seamless system that provides all Americans with the personal security, health, and long term care services they need and deserve.

Solution: Encourage personal and family responsibility for long term care.

The government's capacity to pay for long term care is decreasing. Families and individuals must have the information and tools they need to plan for their long term care needs. Consumers should learn about and use new resources such as private long term care insurance.

Solution: Maximize quality and control costs through market competition and consumer choice.

To provide individuals with care that is efficient and cost effective, the federal program for acute and long term care coverage must be funded through a consumer-driven, competitive insurance market. Insurers and providers must be held accountable for the quality of the care they provide. Consumers and their families should be free to choose where they receive their care.

THE TIME FOR CHANGE IS NOW

Our nation is not prepared to care for its aging population. We must replace the existing long term care system with a new system that is designed to meet the long term care needs of our grandparents, our parents, and ourselves before the current system collapses.

Elderly and disabled Americans deserve quality long term care. It is what each of us wants for our loved ones and ourselves. If we are to ensure that quality long term care is available to all who need it, the nation must work together for change. *SecureCare* is that change.

Mr. CASHDOLLAR. Thank you, sir. Basically what this SecureCare program would do, is create an integrated program of long-term care and acute care under the Federal Government jurisdiction. But it would leave a significant role for private sector resources so that the Federal Government would not have to foot the entire bill for long-term care or acute care. It would establish the appropriate incentives for individuals and families to plan ahead for acute care and long-term care coverage.

Regarding quality, the current regulatory approach to quality in long-term care is all stick and no carrot. The current system registers only deficiencies and offers no recognition or rewards for improvement. We all know from personal experience and from what we have heard about other industries and endeavors that such a negative approach is not the best way to pursue quality.

Indeed, the current regulatory system has serious negative consequences for the morale, motivation, and retention of long-term caregiver staff. More of the same—pushing still harder on the current regulatory apparatus—can only yield marginal benefits at best. It is time for the nation to try a new approach to long-term care quality improvement.

Long-term care residents would be better served by an approach that focuses on improving key measures of well-being and satisfaction over time. Appropriate and consistent quality measurement is crucial to the ability of long-term care providers to understand central quality issues, to learn from mistakes, and to improve.

The State of South Dakota has asked HCFA for a waiver to demonstrate an alternative system for measuring and improving quality in that state's long-term care facilities. This system, which would run parallel to the current system, would facilitate the comparison between nursing facilities on key measures of resident well-being and satisfaction. It would also, of course, allow a facility to compare its performance on key measures of quality over time.

The Nevada Health Care Association and the American Health Care Association strongly urge Nevada senators and members of the Senate Aging Committee to take an active role in helping such a demonstration go forward in South Dakota or perhaps in Nevada.

Senator, again, I appreciate this opportunity to speak on behalf of long-term caregivers and those for whom we care, and I would be happy to answer any questions that may follow. Thank you.

Senator REID. We will have some for you.

[The prepared statement of Mr. Cashdollar follows:]

NHCA

Mailing address; PO Box 3226
Carson City, Nevada 89702
(702) 885 - 1006

Statement
of
Winthrop Cashdollar, Executive Director

Nevada Health Care Association

The Many Faces of Long-Term Care: Today's Bitter Pill or Tomorrow's Cure?

Hearings of the

United States Senate
Special Committee on Aging

January 12 & 13,1998

NEVADA HEALTH CARE ASSOCIATION

Good morning, Senator Reid, and representatives of the Special Committee on Aging. I am Winthrop Cashdollar, Executive Director of the Nevada Health Care Association (NHCA), an association of Nevada's long term care providers. NHCA is affiliated with the American Health Care Association (AHCA), a federation of 50 state health care organizations which represents more than 11,000 assisted living, nursing facility, and subacute long term care providers nationwide. Thank you for the opportunity to speak to the U.S. Senate Special Committee on Aging on behalf of long term caregivers and those for whom we care. In my testimony at these hearings, I would like to combine a Nevada perspective with a national perspective and, in so doing, to draw upon some forward-looking work and ideas of the AHCA.

The Nevada Perspective: Challenges We Face May Make Our State a Bellwether

Nevada is unique in many respects. Our state's population growth is the fastest in the nation. The state's economy has developed around a booming gaming industry and rich mineral wealth. Our intergovernmental arrangements are also unique. When it comes to long term care, however, Nevada faces the same challenges as the rest of the nation – only in more concentrated form. Nevada's unique demographics, fiscal circumstances, and state and local government roles can make it a bellwether – or a canary in a silver mine – for the nation's long term care policy.

Demographic Factors

According to information recently publicized by the State of Nevada, our state continues to have the fastest rate of population growth in the nation. With statewide population growth now at 5.5 % annually (6.8% in Clark County), Nevada's population is projected to top two million in 1999. Nevada's elderly population is also growing rapidly, driven not only by overall population growth, but also because the state's beauty, climate, recreational opportunities, and tax structure make it a desirable state in which to retire. U.S. Census data from the 1990 census indicate that Nevada had the greatest percentage growth in population over age 65 between 1980 and 1990 (94%). This continuing growth in the state's elderly population will require a very substantial increase in long term care capacity, workforce, and spending in the coming years.

Fiscal Factors

Nevada levies no state income tax. The state and its counties rely heavily on revenue from gaming and mining. Although these are generally rich sources of government revenue, they leave state and local treasuries subject to boom and bust. Indeed, gaming tax receipts are currently lagging state projections and the price of gold has fallen below $300 an ounce. The rapid growth and development of the state also brings intensified competition for public funds for education, infrastructure, and other needs. Although all states should anticipate an increased fiscal burden for long term care, changing fiscal circumstances in Nevada could intensify budget problems in relatively short order.

Leading the Way to Tomorrow's Cure?

If necessity is the mother of invention, then Nevada must become inventive – and soon. The state's demographic, fiscal, and intergovernmental circumstances are likely to test the limits of the current long term care system sooner and more severely than other parts of the nation. This means that Nevada may need to address access to services, long term care workforce, and financing issues very soon. Although I believe that the nation as a whole needs to move faster on real long term care reform, I would also suggest that Nevada could take a leading role as a site for demonstrating the national reform proposals that follow in this testimony.

The Need for Change in Access to Long Term Care Services

The current governmental division of responsibility for acute health care and long term care for the nation's senior citizens is confusing; places beneficiaries more according to program rigidities than clinical needs; and causes too many of our frail elderly to fall between the cracks of the system. One of the most common complaints about our current government long term care system is that it steers the vast majority of beneficiaries and resources to institutional long term care.

The differences between Medicare and Medicaid are confusing to elderly Americans. Most Americans do not make the distinction between acute care and long term care that our government programs do – an accident of legislative evolution. In order to rationalize access to the full continuum of acute care/long term care services, it is time that we better integrate acute care and long term care for America's senior citizens. This will require a restructuring of the current division of labor between the federal government and the states.

The Need for Change in How We Pursue Quality in Long Term Care

Our long term care system has evolved a very extensive and complicated regulatory apparatus to pursue the safety and well-being of the nation's long term care residents. Ten years after the enactment of the Nursing Home Reforms of the Omnibus Budget Reconciliation Act of 1987 (OBRA '87), however, there remain serious misgivings about the quality of care in the nation's long term care facilities. Long term caregivers have gotten scant credit for their efforts to realize the promise of the OBRA '87 reforms. Many in the Congress, the state legislatures, and the public want to apply still stronger doses of the same medicine.

However, more of the same – pushing still harder on the current regulatory apparatus – can only yield marginal benefits at best. It is time for the nation to try a new approach to long term care quality improvement.

The current regulatory approach to quality is all stick and no carrot. The current system registers only "deficiencies" and offers no recognition or rewards for improvement. We all know from personal experience, and from what we have heard about other industries and endeavors, that such a negative approach is not the best way to pursue quality. Indeed, the current regulatory system has serious negative consequences for the morale, motivation, and retention of long term caregiver staff.

Long term care residents would be better served by an approach that focuses on improving key measures of well-being and satisfaction over time. Appropriate and consistent quality measurement is crucial to the ability of long term care providers to understand central quality issues; to learn from mistakes; and to improve. If quality measurement is not consistent; if it dwells too much on factors not relevant to resident well-being; if it focuses on fault-finding rather than improvement; then it is not conducive to enhancing quality of care.

The state of South Dakota has asked HCFA for a waiver to demonstrate an alternative system for measuring and improving quality in the state's long term care facilities. This system, which would run parallel to the current regulatory system, would facilitate the comparison between nursing facilities on key measures of resident well-being and satisfaction. It would also, of course, allow a facility to compare its performance on key measures of quality over time. The NHCA and AHCA strongly urge Nevada's Senators and Members of the Senate Aging Committee to take an active role in helping such a demonstration to go forward in South Dakota – or even in Nevada.

The Need for Change in How We Pay for Long Term Care

Our society has not made adequate provision for financing the costs of long term care. Individuals and families are not saving for, or insuring themselves against, the costs of long term care. The demographic tidal wave of Americans who will be elderly in the coming decades will stretch Medicaid beyond its capacity.

Most elderly Americans are unaware of the magnitude of long term care costs and of the limits of government assistance. Most Americans do not foresee needing long term care. Most do not realize how costly months or years of long term care can be. Many Americans wrongly assume that government programs or their general health insurance will cover the costs of any long term care services they might need. For all these reasons, individuals and families face long term care costs for which they have not planned and which they cannot afford.

The costs of long term care can quickly wipe out the assets even of those who have worked and saved for a lifetime. The average cost of nursing home care is now approximately $41,000 per year (according to the AHCA). While the single greatest risk of catastrophic health care cost facing the elderly is the cost of nursing home care, the nation's current long term care policy does not promote personal planning, saving, or the purchase of insurance against the risk of long term care costs. Nor does the nation's

government sector provide comprehensive social insurance against the financial catastrophe of long term care costs. Only after a long term care recipient has been impoverished does government assistance become available through Medicaid – a welfare program.

In recent decades, total Medicaid payments (state and federal) have seen tremendous growth. Although Medicaid spending growth has leveled off in the very recent past, total Medicaid spending tripled during the first half of this decade -- from $54.5 billion in federal fiscal year 1989 to almost $160 billion in fiscal year 1995 (HCFA data). Under current policies, demographic certainties -- with or without an economic downturn – will bring a return of rampant Medicaid growth in the years to come.

Without fundamental long term care financing reform, our growing elderly population will come to rely much more heavily on Medicaid to pay for long term care. According to the Health Care Financing Administration (HCFA), Medicaid was the source of payment for more than two-thirds (68.3%) of nursing facility residents in 1996. U.S. Census Bureau projections show that the fastest growing segment of our population is people age 85 and older – the age group which needs long term care the most. **Today's long term care financing system cannot meet tomorrow's long term care needs.**

An Alternative: Integrate Acute Care and Long Term Care for the Elderly

The nation created Social Security and Medicare because Americans did not feel it was right to let old age, disability, or the costs of health care bankrupt senior citizens after a lifetime of work, taxpaying, and self-sufficiency. Yet Medicaid requires that those who have worked and paid their own way for the whole of their adult lives must lose everything (or legally hide everything) before they can get help with long term care. It is a welfare program. It is time to change this – time to move long term care from welfare to health care. **Congress should transform government programs to make a federal long term care program – along with Social Security and Medicare – the third pillar of security for America's senior citizens.**

Many reject the idea of "federalizing" long term care out of hand because they believe it would inevitably cost incalculable sums of taxpayer money. A new federal entitlement would indeed cost untold billions if it were developed as an entirely federal benefit merely added to Medicare coverage. The new benefit can be made quite fiscally responsible, however, if it is conditioned on a prior exercise of responsibility by beneficiaries. For example, government long term care coverage could be extended only after an individual purchases an appropriate long term care insurance policy.

This is not a new idea. Rather, it is a combination of several ideas already proposed or in practice. The idea of federalizing Medicaid long term care can be credited largely to former Senator Nancy Kassebaum (R-KS). During the 104th Congress, Senator Kassebaum introduced legislation that proposed dividing the Medicaid program. Her legislation would have sent the component of Medicaid that provides acute care to the poor (along with Food Stamps, AFDC, and the Supplemental Feeding Program for Women, Infants, and Children) to the states and would have sent responsibility for long term care for the elderly to the federal government. Such an arrangement would allow states to take undivided responsibility for the welfare population, which would facilitate consolidation and coordination of all the various programs that serve this population. Meanwhile, the federal government would have sole responsibility for the elderly, facilitating the integration of acute health care, long term care, and income security programs.

The idea of establishing federal long term care coverage that follows a period of personal responsibility dates back almost ten years to legislation introduced by then Senator George Mitchell (D-Maine). Senator Mitchell's "Long Term Care Assistance Act of 1988" would have put in place federal long term care coverage beginning after a two-year period, during which an individual would have been responsible for his or her own long term care. Individuals would have been expected to cover themselves during this period of personal responsibility with savings or long term care insurance if they could afford it.

A variation of this proposal is already in practice in New York State. New York currently extends Medicaid long term care coverage to those who purchase qualified long term care insurance policies even if they have considerable assets. Under this program, designed and supported with the help of the Robert Wood Johnson Foundation, an individual who purchases a policy that meets all the requirements of the program qualifies for New York's relatively generous Medicaid long term care coverage when the benefits of the private insurance policy are exhausted. (Connecticut, Indiana, and California have similar programs.) Such a program offers a responsible alternative to the practice of using legal loopholes to qualify for Medicaid coverage by hiding assets. This same approach could be adopted nationwide and linked to the Medicare program.

SecureCare: Principles for Long Term Care Reform

The American Health Care Association is working to move forward with reforms to address the long term care access, quality, and financing needs of America's senior citizens. As the nation's largest association of long term care providers, AHCA is committed to leading efforts to bring about progressive and compassionate reforms that will enable our nation to address the problems of the current health care system for those in need of long term care services and to meet the demographic, political, and fiscal challenges on the horizon. I would like to take this opportunity to present to the Senate Aging Committee AHCA's SecureCare principles for long term care reform.

- **Transform long term care from a welfare program to a health care program.**

  Fundamental compassion and fairness demand that we end a policy that requires Americans to bankrupt themselves and become welfare recipients in order to receive needed long term care services.

- **Coordinate long term care private resources with Medicare and Social Security.**

  Health care policy should support the integration of physician, hospital, and long term care into a seamless system that provides Americans with the health care, long term care, and financial security they need and deserve.

- **Encourage personal and family responsibility for long term care.**

  The government sector should not be expected to – and will not be able to – pay for all the long term care that a growing population of elderly will need. Families and individuals must have the information and tools they need in order to plan for their long term care needs. Consumers need to learn about and use new resources such as private long term care insurance.

- **Maximize quality and control costs through market competition and consumer choice.**

  To provide Americans with care that is efficient and cost effective, the federal program for acute and long term care coverage must be funded through a consumer-driven, competitive insurance market. Insurers and providers must be held accountable for the quality of the care they provide. Consumers and their families should be free to choose where they receive their care.

AHCA is working to turn its SecureCare principles into a more detailed proposal for long term care reform. I invite Members of the Senate Aging Committee and other interested parties to contact the AHCA – or me – for more information on the SecureCare proposal.

Conclusion

Although the nation's demographics and fiscal forecasts make long term care a daunting issue, lawmakers dare not shy away from it. If neglected or mishandled, the long term care issue could haunt us for a very long time. Only if we take timely steps on a path that will lead long term care policy in a new direction will we avoid the problems that plague current entitlement programs for the elderly. The Nevada Health Care Association commends Senator Harry Reid for holding these hearings and for his work to address long term care issues.

Senator REID. We will now hear from Donna Shilinsky. She is a registered nurse. She is the Director of the Community Care Associates. Please proceed.

STATEMENT OF DONNA J. SHILINSKY, R.N., M.S., COMMUNITY CARE ASSOCIATE

Ms. SHILINSKY. Thank you, Senator Reid. It is exciting to see Nevada in such a visionary role. We are indeed in need of a progressive community-based long-term care plan. Also, we need to be reminded that aging is not an illness, nor is it a disease; yet, many people who are aging have severe medical and mental disabilities.

As the Senator said previously, Nevada has one of the highest suicide rates in the country. We also have an aging, homeless population which few think or care about. Yet, there is little valid data about specific cohorts. Calls for assistance and information are received by many service providers and information referral organizations, but no centralized data collection is done.

A central repository is necessary for effective planning. Many working in the aging services see the following as key community-based long-term care challenges. Low cost housing is a great challenge. A housing the elderly report in November of 1997 indicates that the move to senior housing is primarily need-driven.

Lower income seniors are less likely to have resources to pay for services that enable them to keep living in their own homes as they age, and as a result are more likely to move to senior housing.

There is a widening gap between the financially secure and the aging poor. Many people now working cannot afford the savings or 401(k) plans as proposed in a recent congressional bill. These individuals will most likely be the lower income seniors as described in the report.

Several states have low cost senior housing complexes which provide support for activities of daily living and more. The existing PACE program that Dr. Weiss alluded to is another model of care. I also encourage Nevada Medicaid to consider establishing a long-term voucher program which pays for assisted living. Thirty states have already done so.

Home health and hospice programs are essential in providing for a continuum of care between the institution and the community. Home health criteria for coverage of services is limiting and expansion of the definition of home health care to include custodial support needs consideration.

Individuals living alone need more support and services than is offered under the current regulations. Families are the largest group of caregivers. Affordable respite care programs are essential for both the caregiver and the care receiver. We need tax relief for family caregivers, tax incentives to remain living in the least restrictive environment, and programs which pay for care outside of a nursing home.

The government needs to foster public and private partnerships for affordable housing and for assistance with independent living skills and household activities. Connection with the community is critical in maintaining one's sense of belonging. Small neighborhood, intergenerational social and meal programs to which a person could walk or the availability of affordable and reliable transportation would go far to reduce isolation and fears of people living alone.

Affordable day care programs, 24 hours a day, 7 days a week are needed to support the working families and to reduce isolation. Community-based care coordinators are needed to provide for a continuum of care and a seamless care delivery system.

As the prevalence of Alzheimer's and related dementias increase, the community needs to adapt to the changing needs of its citizens. Lack of preventive care in the generally uninsured 60 to 65-year group portends for crisis management. President Clinton's proposal for coverage of this group is both pragmatic and visionary.

Insurance companies as well as Medicare need to place more emphasis on the social needs of its beneficiaries. High risk screening and support for custodial care can potentially improve outcomes.

Finally, there is a critical shortage of manpower for community-based care. Public and private partnerships need to be developed to train a potential work force. Establishing volunteer programs with schools and civic organizations can provide for support for frail and challenged individuals.

Public and private partnerships, private enterprise, civic groups, and volunteer organizations are all part of the community that must come together to address community-based long-term care issues and develop models of support which will serve us in the next 20 years. Thank you.

Senator REID. Thank you.

[The prepared statement of Ms. Shilinsky follows:]

December 30, 1997

The Honorable Charles E. Grassley, Chairman
United States Senate Special Committee on Aging
Dirksen Senate Office Building, Room G-31
Washington, D.C. 20510

Dear Senator Grassley:

Thank you for requesting my input regarding the community-based long term care issues of the future as they relate to Nevada. It is exciting to see the State of Nevada participating in this visionary role. We are in need of a progressive and aggressive plan for our older citizens as we enter the next millennium. However, we cannot expect the federal government or the regulators to enact legislation controlling programs or activities which are the communities' responsibility. Government's role is to provide incentives to private enterprise and to redefine public entities mission. Private enterprise is not the enemy yet it is suspect thereby complicating the partnership process which when embraced yields excellent community service.

The future, near and not so near, involves individuals who are currently entering their late 60's and early 70's and the baby-boomers.

Northern Nevada demographics for 1996 by age groupings:
Source: Population Characteristics: Official Nevada Estimates (1996) and Projections (1997+)

65-74	-	37,466
75-84	-	34,499
85 +	-	5,054
Total	-	77,019

As one looks at the needs and issues related to aging in our society we need to be reminded that aging is not an illness nor a disease. But one must be cognizant that many individuals who are aging have severe physical and mental disabilities. This is a population that has challenges in which the professionals working in aging services have yet to address.

Aging is a natural progression which everyone experiences. How we age is very individualized and is primarily dependent not upon our chronological age but on our genes, our lifestyle choices and our earlier health related problems. We will not all be healthier in the future but many of us will because we practice preventative health. Even with preventative health practices many of us will not be able to eliminate the chronic conditions which presently effect so many. We will be able to reduce the adverse effects and extend our life span but obviously disease and social dilemmas will not go away. How we live our future lives is primarily dependent upon how we lived in our earlier years. If our lifestyle choices have been compromising to a healthy lifestyle in the past this will effect the aging process.

Nevada has many varied lifestyles which has been well documented over the past few years. It also has one of the highest suicide rates in the country.

Age breakdown of actual suicide in Washoe County (11.5 mo. 1997): Source: Washoe County Coroner-Medical Examiner.

* total deaths include 8 who were residents out-of-state.

Total	90 *
61-70	8
71-80	12
+80	5

Another issue which is less talked about is the older homeless person. There is little data about the impact of the elderly homeless and their specific needs. Lifestyle and social ills will compound the issues touched on previously. The challenges we face as a compassionate yet pragmatic society in developing aging policy for the future are not easily solved nor are they simple. Complex issues face us as we are complicated human beings affected by changes we often cannot control. There is no cookbook approach.

Policy makers have a difficult job to do. It is impossible to address the care needs of the entire population but you are being expected to do just that. There is always a trap in combining cohort groups into one or two categories and frequently this is done by using raw chronological age and illness/death statistics then anticipating outcomes based on previous experience. This forecasting methodology has its flaws and will not be successful

47-539 98 - 11

in the future. It is essential to have a central repository for data gathering of requests for service, specific cohort demographics that will enable programs to be developed according to actual instead of perceived needs.

We have never experienced more cohesive yet diverse groups. Generally, we are healthier than our predecessors due to medical miracles and technology, more educated due to access to formal and informal learning systems, more aware of our environment and how we effect its balance. Yet we are more cynical about the future, distrusting of outside influences and have social ills which many choose to ignore. Individualism is paramount in our behaviors. Many elders whom I have worked with do not acknowledge their chronological ages as a defining indicator. They do not want to be subjected to being with "those old people". They struggle with a independence/interdependence role.

This makes an approach to our retirement and aged years very complex. Many will fight to retain their individuality no matter what the consequences, many will not ever accept the premise that they are as old as their peer. They see ageism in every experience with formal providers of care and strive to resist the stereotyping which is so prevalent. Others desire the security of support systems and ease of access to services they choose to accept. Policy makers must be sensitive to the needs of these as well as other groups not described here. How can this be done?

You are probably thinking to yourselves at this point - oh my, I heard this before. Unfortunately, human factors have no place in policy making.

Many, working in "aging services", see the following as the key community based long term care challenges facing Northern Nevada.

CHALLENGES

HOUSING

A Housing The Elderly Report (November 1997) indicates that the *"demand for senior housing is still strong; low income, active seniors underserved"*.

Housing must be adequate and available to meet the individual's needs and desires.

"The move to senior housing is primarily need driven. Lower-income seniors are less likely to have the resources to pay for services that will enable them to keep living in their own homes as they age and, as a result, are more likely to move to senior housing." (p.1)

Crisis Call Care and Share (CCC&S) has received 43 queries about assisted living and 88 calls about low-income housing in 5 months.

ISSUES: Individual housing remains primary choice.
Respite for caregiver and care receiver.
Foster care for short-term crises.
Affordable/low cost residential care.

Institutional care -(intermediate & skilled).

RECOMMENDATIONS:

Provide tax incentives for elders to remain in least restrictive living situation with support systems and services appropriate to needs.

Foster private enterprise to establish partnerships with public entities to offer affordable, quality services using trained and properly screened employees.

Areas to consider:

1. School training programs to address non-hands on or supervisory care needs on a volunteer/grade attainment basis.
2. Public school free education/training of mature adult in caring for person needing assistance - custodial care. Lower level of training than a certified nursing assistant.
3. Reduce expenses of bureaucratic paperwork but do not reduce oversight responsibilities. Focus on service not reporting.
4. Community network of trained personnel and regulated respite/foster care private homes for short term placement with minimal notice. Use

child foster home concept.

According to the Housing the Elderly Report (November 1997) *"Through the Medicaid long-term care voucher program seniors in 30 states can already use Medicaid funds to help pay for assisted living"*

1. Nevada Medicaid must consider offering this voucher program to low income seniors.

Support private enterprise (non- or for-profit entities) in establishing low cost, affordable services to maintain achievable level of independence.

Services to be considered are:

1. Housekeeping/ grocery/ yard & building maintenance.
2. Assistance with activities of daily living and Instrumental activities of daily living. *CCC&S has received 72 calls inquiring about homemaker services.* Affordability is the primary issue.
3. Small intimate intergenerational socialization and meal programs in individual's neighborhoods to which persons could walk.
4. Congregate housing concepts for the mentally or physically challenged individual currently residing in a supportive supervised environment who will also be experiencing the problems associated with aging.

Additionally, many low income elders do not have access to a personal automobile and live outside the designated areas for the established transportation system. Isolation is increased. *CCC&S has received 62 calls regarding need for transportation in the past 5 months.*

RECOMMENDATIONS:

1. Encourage private enterprise to establish comprehensive transportation systems. Reduce the disincentives to implementing such a plan.
2. Provide tax incentives for private/public partnerships.
3. Encourage a user friendly system for all potential users not just impaired elders.
4. Allow system to generate revenue to offset expenses while encouraging low income sliding scale.
5. Provide incentives to insurance companies to offer low cost liability insurance for this enterprise.

SUPPORT SERVICES

ISSUES:

Adult day care programs presently meet some needs in the community. Available programs are too few and too limited. *CCC&S has received 15 calls for day care information in the past 5 months.*

Adult day care for many adults is a logical and cost effective program of care to support individuals in their desire to remain in their own or their children's home.

Community-based care coordination is essential to support people remaining in the least restrictive living situation. Care coordination must be seamless throughout the entire health and social care spectrum and must be proactive rather than reactive in its approach.

Alzheimer's Disease is predicted to affect more than 50% of the over 65 population by 2040. Obviously, this is another primary consideration in planning community based services. Early detection and prevention of the debilitating symptoms could extend the chronicity of this disease and enable people to live in a supportive, structured community which is able to adapt to the changing needs of its community.

Respite care for family caregivers is essential. *CCC&S has received in the past 5 months 29 calls for respite* and the Alzheimer's Association receives many more.

CCC&S reports that 55 calls were received in the past 5 months inquiring about home delivered meals. Home

Allocate a certain amount of federal monies for HUD housing to be used for low income, affordable group/congregate care. Houses must be built to American for Disabilities Standards.

TRANSPORTATION

ISSUES: Reliable transportation systems continue to be a primary need for our citizens. It is devastating for one to lose a license or to choose to stop driving a personal vehicle due to decline in reflexes and/or vision as well as ability to make good judgement decisions. Many persons feel they cannot relinquish their license even though they may know that their driving skills are compromised. We have a culture that equates owning and driving a personal vehicle with personal freedom and independence. As one begins losing the skills which enables him to drive safely, the loss of ability to be able to get where one needs to go is a critical loss. Without adequate and efficient transportation systems in the entire metropolitan and rural area many individuals are forced to drive or remain isolated at home.

delivered meals, at this point, do not address the need for special diets. The current service area in Reno area is too limited for the community at large.

RECOMMENDATIONS:

1. Community-based Geriatric Care Coordinators educated with advanced degrees in the health care profession and experienced in medical and psychosocial/spiritual issues and counseling and in working with the population they serve are essential to assure a continuum of care and a seamless delivery system.
2. Proactive care coordination rather than episodic, fragmented and reactive. Prevention focus is essential to minimize the effects of adverse changes in an individual.
3. Insurance companies including Medicare to place more emphasis on the social problems which create the medical emergencies. High risk screening by independent care managers to identify actual or potential problems such as: malnutrition frequently associated with an underlying depression, loneliness, inadequate financial resources and functional losses.
4. Volunteer opportunities for the non-employed who

Choose to occupy their free hours providing community service.

5. Partnerships with child day care centers to provide for a cross-generational approach to care needs in the community.
6. Community centers which can meet the varied needs of the citizens without forcing adults into situations which are not comfortable for them.
7. Partnership to establish 24 hour a day centers for the family who work off shifts. Sleeping accommodations for the person who is staying overnight.
8. City and county commissions who redesign their communities to meet the needs of the person with evolving dementia. Some examples: modify signal lights to enable a mobility impaired person to cross streets safely. Eliminate left turns after stop to allow for pedestrian safety. Safe and lighted bus or transportation stops. Large street signs which enable a person with impaired vision to see more adequately. A community which honors its older persons rather than treating them with disdain and indifference.

HUMAN RESOURCES

ISSUES: **Manpower is a critical problem in the helping professions. Non-institutional care needs more employees as it generally is a one-to-one caregiving relationship. There is a need to address the contributions of the family caregivers as well as the paid non-family caregivers.**

Quality employees who are truly caregivers are essential to provide services and support to a most vulnerable population. Potential for abuse and exploitation is ever present even with the most sophisticated screening. The cost of screening prospective employees needs to be reduced and more timely. Law enforcement reports must be completed and returned in a short time period to prevent people from being hired because the need is so great that the recipient of care cannot wait or he will be more compromised.

There is an increase in calls to the Crisis Call Care and Share line about desire for employment opportunities from persons in the community who are over 70. *CCC&S received 65 calls in the past 5 months*. Employment opportunities within an

individual's abilities and interests must be made available.

RECOMMENDATIONS:

1. **Standardize prospective employee screening for behavioral traits and felony or misdemeanor convictions. Give priority to law enforcement screening, set a realistic response date and adhere to it.**
2. **Establish public/private partnerships to train mature workers; to establish volunteer programs with schools and service clubs to provide care for persons who need it urgently thereby preventing institutionalization.**
3. **Provide tax incentives for adult family caregivers. More openly define family than just nuclear and biological.**
4. **Educate the public and private enterprise to the value and work ethic of mature workers.**

HOME HEALTH AND HOSPICE

ISSUES:

Skilled home health has evolved over the last 15 years and will continue to do so. As hospitals continue to recognize the value of an individual recovering from an illness in their own home they more readily work with

physicians to early discharge to home health. Home health employees must be ever refining their skills and insurance programs including Medicare must change their benefit structure to promote early institutional discharge.

Home Health no longer is a "luxury" care level. It is the least restrictive care level for acute illness recovery. At times, continuous care is absolutely essential. Other times, custodial care is more important to keeping a person out of the hospital. Compromised individuals who are feeling poorly or are medicated have impaired learning and memory. Medication mis-management is a primary reason for hospital readmission.

Current concerns raised by many Medicare recipients is the potential for Medicare co-pays and lack of support systems to promote their recovery. When we look to the future we must address the payment issues in a forthright and constructive manner. I know of many Medicare recipients who verbalize unwillingness to accept home based care because they have to pay for it. Wrong or right, it is reality!

RECOMMENDATIONS:

1. Develop criteria when continuous care and custodial care is appropriate in caring for a Medicare or an insurance beneficiary.
2. Provide incentives to home health and hospice to move toward quantifiable and qualifiable outcome based care and away from fee-for-service care.
3. Consider phasing in co-pay so that the frail elderly who are in need of home health and hospice services can access care without burden of co-pay but the younger Medicare recipient recognizes his responsibility in paying for services rendered.
4. Provide for comprehensive education about consumer responsibility before enacting co-pay system for Medicare.
5. Research feasibility of covering custodial care in the home in certain circumstances that would benefit the recipient and be more cost effective than institutional care.

In summary, Hillary Clinton has coined the phrase "It takes a village to raise a child". We believe that it takes a village to support its older citizens so they can maintain dignity and self-esteem which they richly deserve.

Public/private partnerships, private enterprise, civic groups and volunteer organizations are all part of a community that must come together to address the community-based care needs of its citizens and develop models of care which will serve us into the next twenty years.

Community-based long term care can be seen as an umbrella which protects its citizens from the debilitating effects that social and medical problems can cause thereby improving one's quality of life.

Thank you!

Respectfully submitted,

Donna J. Shilinsky

Donna J. Shilinsky, RN, MS
Community-based Geriatric Care Manager
12/30/97

Senator REID. Dr. Steven Phillips, medical doctor, who is the Medical Director of the Social Health Maintenance Organization, Senior Dimensions, Sierra Health Services, with operations in Las Vegas, Reno, and the surrounding areas. Dr. Phillips.

STATEMENT OF STEVEN L. PHILLIPS, M.D., C.M.D., MEDICAL DIRECTOR, SOCIAL HEALTH MAINTENANCE ORGANIZATION, SENIOR DIMENSIONS, SIERRA HEALTH SERVICES, INC.

Dr. PHILLIPS. Thank you, Senator Reid and members of the field hearing committee. Long-term care must no longer be held synonymous with institutional care and/or spending one's final days, months or years in a nursing facility setting. The nursing facility represents only one discrete part within the continuum of care. The continuum of care is intended to unite all areas of health care into an integrated delivery system. These include, and are not limited to, independent living, group care, assisted living, rehabilitation, extended care services, skilled nursing, hospice, home health care, and acute care.

The common characteristics that unite these parts into a continuum of care are the primary care physician and/or equivalent. A continuum of care requires that a component management system be replaced by a more systematic approach. Component management focuses on only one aspect of the health care system at a time.

Inherent problems of component management include not recognizing health care as interrelated, all diseases tend to be treated the same, the factoring of treatment over prevention, and the inability to coordinate the delivery system. Therefore, there is no continuity of care. There is fragmentation. Weakening of the patient/physician relationship, and very important in this day and age, placing clinicians and administrators at odds with one another.

The discrete parts within the health care delivery model, as frequently occurs throughout the United States, has become very focused on what they do and how to maintain their own financial solvency. This has created barriers that must be appreciated and sensitively addressed in order that everyone feels comfortable working within an integrated system.

As others have said, the blending of private, public, entrepreneurial funds, can lead to an integrated system because without integration, the provision of quality-based services with associated cost efficiencies cannot occur.

The Social Health Maintenance Organization II, also affectionately known as SHMO II by many of us, is a designated Health Care Financing Administration (HCFA) demonstration project that is funded through a risk-adjusted payment mechanism. The intent of SHMO II is to address medical, psychological, functional, and social needs of seniors in a coordinated manner.

There are three components within the SHMO II demonstration, care coordination, extended care benefits, and a geriatric resource team. Care coordination is based upon the elements of screening for risk in all members, getting a little data by a lot of people; assessment of those identified to be at risk, getting a lot of information about a few people; development of a plan of care based upon identified risks; implementation of the plan of care; monitoring of that plan of care; reassessment of the patient at determined intervals; evaluation of the plan of care; and ultimately the reporting of outcomes.

Each element is critical to the overall success of adequately addressing the medical, psychological, functional, and social needs of the senior population that is being served. The extended care benefits are designed specifically to augment the health plan's existing benefits and community-based services.

They are made available through the care coordination process and are not an entitlement. Rather, they are determined by established criteria. They include such things as counseling for situational disorders, short-term institutional care respite, short-term group home respite, home safety, and a personal emergency response system.

The rationale behind the use of these services is to reduce the burden of disease while maintaining the member's health in the safest and most independent environment possible.

The final component of the SHMO II is the geriatric resource team. The GRT serves as an educational resource for the entire health care delivery system as well as clinical expertise. Within both traditional Medicare and Medicare Risk HMO delivery settings, knowledge of geriatrics is often lacking. For this reason, it has become part of the study design.

My recommendations for long-term care policy changes include emphasizing the entire continuum of care in all current and future Federal and state initiatives. Schools of medicine, schools of nursing, other allied health care professionals will develop curricula that foster an understanding and willingness to work within the continuum of care.

The institution of requirements that all health care professionals have a specified number of CME or other equivalent continuing education credits which pertain to the continuum of care.

Finally, the creation of a demonstration program that fosters a partnering of the multiple components of the continuum of care into a model program that incorporates all of the discrete parts into a united project with the common goal of maximizing the care of those they serve.

An example, the inclusion of the PACE program for all-inclusive care of the elderly with the Social Health Maintenance Organization model. I believe the State of Nevada is in a unique position right now to accomplish that. Thank you.

"The Many Faces of Long-Term Care: Today's Bitter Pill or Tomorrow's Cure?"

Testimony before the

Senate Special Committee on Aging
Field Hearing

12 January 1998
West Charleston Library
Las Vegas, Nevada

13 January 1998
Washoe Medical Center Auditorium
Reno, Nevada

Presented by
Steven L. Phillips, MD, CMD

Senator Reid and members of the field hearing committee. I am Steven L. Phillips, Medical Director of Senior Dimensions Extended Care a HCFA designated Social HMO demonstration project based out of Las Vegas, Nevada. As a Geriatrician who is actively involved in both the clinical and administrative roles of health care for older Nevadans I am truly honored to have this opportunity to address the future of long-term care and potential remedies for its current ailments.

The field of long-term care must no longer be held synonymous with institutional care and/or spending one's final days, months or years in a nursing home setting. The ware housing of those no longer capable of caring for themselves or without the necessary family and social support to remain in the community at large has resulted in today's bitter pill of long-term care. This may have been the case in the past but does not reflect the current and future direction of health care needs in the United States of America. The nursing facility represents only one discrete part within the Continuum of Care. A Continuum of Care is intended to unite all areas of health care into an integrated delivery system. The discrete parts within the health care delivery system are the various levels of care that meet an individuals needs. These include independent living, group care, assisted living, rehabilitation, extended care, skilled nursing, hospice, home health care, and acute care. The common characteristic that unites these parts into a Continuum of Care is the primary-care physician or equivalent.

A Continuum of Care requires that a component management system be replaced by a more systematic approach. Component management focuses on only one aspect of the health care system at a time. Inherent problems of component management include:

- -not recognizing health care is interrelated;
- -all diseases tend to be treated the same;
- -factoring treatment over prevention;
- -leading to an uncoordinated delivery system without continuity of care;
- -paying primarily for the most expensive services in the most expensive setting;
- -weakening of the patient-physician relationship; and
- -placing clinicians and administrators at odds with one another.

The discrete parts within a health care delivery model have become very focused on what they do and how to maintain financial solvency. This has created barriers that must be appreciated and sensitively addressed in order that everyone feels comfortable working within an integrated system. Without integration the provision of the most cost-efficient and quality-based services cannot occur.

Traditional Medicare fee-for-service provides greater incentives for a component management approach to health care delivery. This has created an emphasis on acute care intervention rather than prevention. For those clinicians that have identified someone that requires skilled nursing and/or rehabilitative services not available or reasonable to provide in the home or outpatient setting they must place this person in an acute care hospital. This is frequently an unjustified use of acute care services and exposes that patient to an environment which may lead to adverse outcomes. This system of care prevents health care providers from proactively meeting the needs of those they serve in the most appropriate care setting.

Medicare Risk HMOs have been given more flexibility in the manner in which health care is delivered to those they serve. These HMOs are paid a fixed amount per enrolled member per month (PMPM) that is a calculation that reflects the average adjusted per capita cost (AAPCC) of a traditional Medicare recipient within a specific county or region served. The AAPCC varies significantly from state to state and even county by county. By receiving payment in an up front manner the HMO can theoretically allocate resources to preventative care activities and allow for the movement of patients to the most appropriate level of care. This requires the development of an integrated delivery model that supports the Continuum of Care. Few Medicare Risk HMOs have truly been successful in aligning the health care delivery elements with those financial aspects required to maintain those they serve in the most appropriate setting, based upon true need.

The Program for All-Inclusive Care for the Elderly (PACE) has recently been moved from demonstration status to programmatic status. The PACE model allows for the blending of Medicare and Medicaid dollars for those individuals that are found to be eligible for placement within a nursing facility setting. The objective is to provide all needed services that will allow the PACE members to remain in the most independent setting possible. This model relies upon the creation of health care teams that assess and manage member needs in a coordinated fashion relying heavily upon an interdisciplinary team approach.

The Social Health Maintenance Organization II (SHMO II) is a designated Health Care Financing Administration (HCFA) demonstration project that is funded through a risk adjusted payment mechanism. The intent of SHMO II is to address medical, psychological, functional, and social needs of seniors in a coordinated manner. There are three components within the SHMO II demonstration: Care Coordination; Extended Care Benefits; and a Geriatric Resource Team.

Care Coordination is based upon the elements of:

- -screening for risk;
- -assessment of those identified to be at-risk;
- -development of a plan of care based upon identified risks;
- -implementation of the plan of care;
- -monitoring the plan of care;
- -reassessment of the patient;
- -evaluation of the plan of care; and
- -reporting of the outcomes.

Each element is critical to the overall success of adequately addressing the medical, psychological, functional, and social needs of the senior population that is being served.

The Extended Care Benefits are designed specifically to augment the health plan's existing benefits and community based-services. They are made available through the Care Coordination process and are not an entitlement, rather they are determined by established criteria. These benefits include:

- -counseling for situational disorders;
- -nutritional services;
- -transportation;
- -personal care;
- -homemaker services;
- -adult day care;
- -in-home companion;
- -short-term institutional care;
- -short-term group home care;
- -maintenance therapy;
- -home safety; and

-a personal emergency response system.

The rationale behind the use of these services is to reduce the burden of disease while maintaining the member's health in the safest and most independent environment possible.

The final component of the SHMO II demonstration project is the Geriatric Resource Team (GRT). The GRT is represented by multiple health care disciplines that assist in further clarification of the needs of high-risk member's. The GRT provides intervention recommendations and assists the primary care providers with reassessment and evaluation as needed. In addition to its clinical role the GRT serves as an educational resource for the entire health care delivery system. A core knowledge of geriatric expertise is often lacking with both traditional Medicare and Medicare Risk HMO delivery settings. For this reason the SHMO II demonstration incorporated the development of a GRT into the study design.

Presently there are a total of six (6) Medicare HMOs that have been selected by HCFA to participate in the SHMO II demonstration. Due to the complexity of this program only one (1) of the selected participants is operational at this time. That HMO is Health Plan of Nevada and has truly placed the state of Nevada squarely in the forefront of senior health care in the United States. The SHMO II demonstration is available through Senior Dimensions Extended Care (SDEC). SDEC began on November 1 ,1996 in Las Vegas, Nevada and is scheduled to be offered in the Reno/Sparks area by March 1, 1998. Over the next several years, Care Coordination, Extended Care Benefits and a Geriatric Resource Team or their equivalents are likely to become a standard of practice within all Medicare Risk HMOs. This demonstration has allowed for the creation of a true Continuum of Care directed and coordinated through a long-term care initiative that ensures the appropriate utilization of resources based principally upon the needs of the members served. At the end of our first twelve months, we have been successful in maintaining 85 percent of our at risk members for nursing home placement in a less restrictive environment. As an advocate for improving senior health care the SHMO II demonstration truly enhances my ability to address the medical, psychological, functional, and social needs of those patients I serve.

Recommendations for Long-Term Care Policy

1. Emphasize the entire Continuum of Care in all current and future Federal and State initiatives.
2. Schools of Medicine, Nursing and other Allied Health Care Professionals will develop curricula that foster an understanding and willingness to work within the Continuum of Care.
3. Institute requirements that all health care professionals have a specified number of CME, CEU or other equivalent continuing education credits which pertain to the Continuum of Care.

4. **Eliminate impediments that inhibit health care professionals and organizations/institutions within the Continuum of Care to deliver the most appropriate care based upon an individuals needs and personal desires.**
5. **Create a demonstration program that fosters the partnering of the multiple components of the Continuum of Care into a model program that incorporates all of the discrete parts into a united project with a common goal of maximizing the care of those they serve.**

Senator REID. Dr. Phillips, tell us a little more about this study. These studies are not going on all over the United States. Aren't we one of the unique places that is allowed to test this?

Dr. PHILLIPS. Thank you, Senator. With 5 minutes, I had to reduce a little. I appreciate the opportunity. There have been six identified HMOs in the country for the SHMO II demonstration. At the present time, only one is operational. It is the Health Plan of Nevada since November 1, 1996. It will be operational in Reno on March 1, 1998. So at the present time, sir, there is only one that truly puts Nevada squarely in the forefront of the future of health care delivery for seniors.

Senator REID. And you have a number of years left in the proposal before final results are evaluated. Is that not true?

Dr. PHILLIPS. Yes, sir. It started out as a three-year demonstration. At the end of the first year, Congress saw fit to actually extend it another year, so we have until December 31, 2000.

Senator REID. Dr. Phillips, I do not think we will hear as much here as we did in Las Vegas yesterday about managed care. I do not think it is an exaggeration to say that we had some people who had some very serious questions yesterday about managed care. As you know, there is a large segment of the people in Clark County who are treated with different managed care entities.

In fact, the percentage in Clark County is larger than any other place in the country, as I understand it. But it does not matter where you go. I travel around the country a little bit and no matter where you go, there are jokes made about managed care. There is a general feeling of concern because managed care has changed the traditional way of health care delivery in America.

My question to you, your being the medical director of one of the largest HMOs in America, tell me what is being done on the national level, state level, local level, and by the private sector to make people feel better about managed care.

Just let me say before you answer the question, as you know, the President has suggested a bill of rights for people who go to HMOs so they can make a more wise choice, just as we talked to a number of the other panelists about people who are putting one of their loved ones in a rest home. They need more information. So in short, how are we going to solve this public relations dilemma we are in now about managed care?

Dr. PHILLIPS. Well, Senator, I fully support the President's recommendation for the bill of rights. As a matter of fact, the American Association of Health Plans endorsed a bill of rights approximately 2½ or 3 years ago.

I think there certainly is a lot that is positive about organized care. I personally wish they would do away with the term "managed care" and call it more organized care or some delivery model that is integrated. But be that as it may, at the national level quality programs are ongoing such as the National Committee for Quality Assurance, in which health plans pursue accreditation through the NCQA.

There are also appeal rights within Medicare HMOs that do not exist for your traditional recipient, if you will, of health care through Medicare. In other words, if someone is having problems within their health plan, whether it is in Nevada or in another state, they have the ability to request evaluation of their case on an individual basis first by the plan.

That is called initial determination by the health plan, and if the member or loved one, guardian, is not pleased with that determination, they can request in writing that that be referred on to a national review panel out of Rochester, NY called Network Design Group.

They then have the ability to go through six levels of appeal in order to hopefully get resolution of their concerns.

Senator REID. I do not know how many heard the news this morning, but the statistics are out showing that health care costs rose the smallest amount since they started recording health care costs this past year. So one reason that Congressman Gibbons and I can stand up here and brag about all the good things happening in the economy is one of the reasons is health care costs have gone down.

Now, a lot of people can take credit for that and I do not know all the reasons, but I think one reason is that Congress and the administration has been more actively involved in trying to figure out ways to get rid of fraud, waste, and abuse, and also respond to the health care givers.

You know, it is easy to continually beat up on doctors and hospitals and I have done my share over the years, but I think we also arrive at a point where we have to make sure that they also are well taken care of. While we may not like to acknowledge it, doctors need to make some kind of a decent living because the average cost of a doctor getting out of medical school, the bills they owe is well over $100,000.

That is if you do not go into some of the other speciality programs. I also say to Mr. Cashdollar and Ms. Simons, you know, I think it is important that we have representatives here during these hearings of the private sector because it is a very fine line that we have to balance as policy-makers.

That fine line is how much control are we going to order in the system from the Federal and state levels, and in ordering different regimens, what are we going to do to the people, the capitalists out there trying to make a living doing health care?

It is a very fine line. My personal feeling is we have got to be very careful. I want to make sure that the system is one that runs well. We have a continuum of service. I think that is a great program that Dr. Weiss has talked about and Dr. Phillips and Ms. Shilinsky also talked about it. We need to make sure that there is care at all levels and it does not stop and start.

But we also have to make sure that those people who are in the free enterprise system can make a go of it. Mr. Cashdollar is relatively new in this state, and I have been on his case since he got here making sure that we get information about the rest home industry, the convalescent care.

We need to make sure that we have adequate controls but yet folks are able to make a living. It would be the worst of all worlds if you all went out of business because the State of Nevada and the Federal Government would then be forced to take care of everything and we are not equipped to do that. That is an under-statement.

So I would like to hear comments from anybody on the panel that would like to react to my somewhat too long statement.

Mr. CASHDOLLAR. Senator, if I may, thank you for the remarks you just made. The United States, unlike some other nations, such as Britain for instance, England, Britain, and some other nations, has chosen to meet a large part of its health care needs through the private sector, or rather a partnership between the private sector and the public sector.

Senator REID. I would interrupt here. This is a tremendous jump forward for England who principally was a socialized medicine country just a few years ago.

Mr. CASHDOLLAR. So we have this mixed private/public health care system and we need to pursue the policies that make it work in the best way possible. Now, a lot of people are uncomfortable with the proximity of profit and health care or profit and long-term care. We have that connection in the United States so we need to join it with appropriate market motivation and also appropriate regulation.

I agree with everyone here that we need to have a government role, a Federal role and a state role, in overseeing the frail elderly and residents of long-term care. Everybody agrees on that. Mr. Panelli spoke about the system in some detail.

Now, one of the things he said was that 75 percent of facilities in the United States are "not in substantial compliance." I believe he also said that something like 100 percent of Nevada facilities, at some time, are not "in substantial compliance." I would suggest then that this is not very helpful information.

The phrase, "not in substantial compliance," really does not offer the public the kind of information that it needs to understand what really is going on in long-term care. First and foremost, I would like to suggest that that terminology be changed to differentiate between facilities that you would not want to put a loved one in and facilities that are "out of compliance" just on some technical or trivial matters.

We need to differentiate between the bad, the good and the better that and I believe you spoke to that yesterday, Senator. We could do much better to have the public understand quality and ways to improve quality and the relative quality of long-term care providers. That would also tie back into the market motivation, because when people know what is good and what is not good, they will always choose what is good.

I say again, we in the industry have been working on an alternative quality system that would focus on, as Mr. Panelli said, actual resident outcomes, the well-being of the residents. We think that we can figure out which things matter and how to compare them over time within one facility or between facilities and come up with something that really makes sense to the public.

Senator REID. Anyone else care to comment on that or has it been fairly well covered?

Ms. SIMONS. It has, Senator. I would like to follow on the heels of some of your suggested comments and that is allowing private enterprise to continue forward in private enterprise. I think most service providers in the health care industry today are somewhat entrepreneurial, whether they are a home health agency, whether they are a skilled nursing facility, or an assisted living center.

I think one of the main reasons we are seeing assisted living explode nationwide has been from the consumer emphasis of what they would like to see occur. However, assisted living must not sit back and say, "We have got a free rein to run forward without anybody overseeing some of the controls and some of the disclosure issues that you are now hearing nationwide in the industry."

However, continuing to allow for creativity and cautioning against focusing on black and white tangibles, as I suggested, such as room size, physical plant, things that really have nothing to do with client service and client care is what has to happen across the spectrum of service. No linear thinking, but a lot of collaborative effort.

Senator REID. What I would like to do is have you, Ms. Simons, and you, Ms. Shilinsky, tell us about your areas of business. What do they do? Why do patients come to you? What do you do for them?

Ms. SHILINSKY. I am a community-based geriatric care manager. I do not work in a facility. I work with families and older individuals who presently are living at home but are experiencing declines in their functional abilities.

Senator REID. You help people make choices?

Ms. SHILINSKY. Yes, I help people make choices by giving them all of the information about what is available in the community and guiding them as to what is most appropriate for them given their current situation.

Senator REID. We have an interesting situation. We have too few beds in southern Nevada and we have adequate beds in northern Nevada. Tell me, Ms. Shilinsky, I think your program is wonderful and we have heard the need for this, the counseling, so that the people feel better about what they are going to do with their loved one.

But do you have adequate resources to cover all the people that need to be visited with?

Ms. SHILINSKY. Do I have adequate resources? I do not provide the services that I recommend. What I do——

Senator REID. No, I know. I mean counseling services.

Ms. SHILINSKY. In the community?

Senator REID. Yes.

Ms. SHILINSKY. No, there is not adequate resources. We are always struggling to find live-in help, which is absolutely impossible to find quality live-in help; custodial care; group care homes that are quality.

Senator REID. Tell me about your operation. How many people are there?

Ms. SHILINSKY. We are three geriatric care managers at this point.

Senator REID. And we have tens of thousands of people literally that need your help.

Ms. SHILINSKY. Yes.

Senator REID. What is your area of jurisdiction? Is it mainly Washoe County? Is it part of Washoe County, the City of Reno? What is it?

Ms. SHILINSKY. I look at where the need is and whether I can respond to the needs. I will go all the way down to Carson City if I need to out to Fallon if I need to. Washoe County is fairly extensive. There is a geriatric care manager in Winnemucca, and then I believe there is a geriatric care manager in Las Vegas, and there is one in Minden.

Senator REID. So it is fair to say that more of you would allow people to make better choices?

Ms. SHILINSKY. Yes.

Senator REID. Would you, Ms. Simons, tell us what you do and what you do for your patients?

Ms. SIMONS. Residents. Senator, thank you for the opportunity——

Senator REID. Residents.

Ms. SIMONS. That is okay, because we are not a medical facility. Before I answer that remark, I would just like to share an excitement that I am seeing, having been involved in long-term care situations since birth. I think we are truly a blessed state. I cannot help but remain extremely excited when I sit here and look at this room and see many individuals who I have come to know over the last 30 years of my conscious involvement and how we cannot be extremely proud of our state and the accessibility within our state as we develop new programs and new courses for where we are going to go.

Senator REID. If I could interrupt, also, I am really impressed with the people still standing.

Ms. SIMONS. Awesome. You guys are great.

Senator REID. We have been going now for more than two hours.

Ms. SIMONS. Thank you. Senator, as I said, I was born into this. The longest I have had a resident live with me is 29 years. Average length of stay in my previous facilities was 8 to 15 years; that becomes family. But aside from that, I, too, was a caregiver of an elderly mother who pioneered this and then had a massive stroke and I took care of her at home for 9 years and had to do the nursing home placement issue and dealt with the gut-wrenching feelings of guilt and am I doing the right choices and what is out there.

In 1981, there was not near the access to sources, resources, and programs that there is now and that is why as an advocate for seniors, I remain continually encouraged at where we are going to the future with regard to what we do.

As far as what I do personally, I have an assisted living facility for seniors that I built completely differently than anybody else has built in the United States and it still remains unique. I took a risk. It was a good risk, but it was a devoted risk based on what my seniors told me and that was they did not want to be with a bunch of old people.

So consequently, they are not with a bunch of old people, although there are 60 of them and we have a lot of fun and we are able to encourage abilities and enhance capabilities and overcome a lot of the myths of aging, notwithstanding that if you are going to be a grumpy, unhappy, miserable older person, then I cannot help you with that.

But the one thing I can promise and I think that we all need to continue to commit to and everybody who knows me knows this is a personal commitment and that is of high touch care and not high tech care. So I look forward to my 60 hugs every day and I do my hugometers to assess health.

I realize it is not a scientific method, Senator, but it does work and it gives me a barometer for depression and all kinds of things beyond what we can analyze on pressure scales. I remain committed as an individual in the industry to make myself available, accessible, and open to sharing my concepts and thoughts and future wishes for our senior population.

Senator REID. Dr. Weiss, I would like to hear from you, and first what I want you to do is tell us a little bit about the Sanford Center on Aging. We have heard this word thrown around in the last couple days. Give us a little bit of the history of the center, how it got started, what it does now. I think we would all appreciate that. We heard your testimony; it was very lucid. I have heard it twice now and am very impressed with what your goals are, but tell us about the center.

Mr. WEISS. The Sanford Center for Aging started actually from an anonymous donation by Jean and Graham Sanford who came from the Carson Valley.

Senator REID. It was not so anonymous then, was it?

Mr. WEISS. I'm sorry?

Dr. PHILLIPS. It was anonymous that day.

Mr. WEISS. Initially. [Laughter.]

To the university to do something in the aging field, primarily because Jean Sanford was caring for her elderly mother in the Carson Valley and was in a nursing home and did not like the alternatives. With that, the university—this is way before I came—did some very good stuff with the gerontology and geriatric center. Because of that, Jean Sanford willed at least 80 percent of her estate to the university.

Senator REID. How do you work with the medical school?

Mr. WEISS. We are co-sponsored by the School of Medicine and by the School for Human and Community Sciences.

Senator REID. So you and Dr. Bernick are partners, not competitors?

Mr. WEISS. Absolutely. We formed a Geriatric Medical Advisory Committee that consists of all geriatricians throughout the state. It is a statewide organization and we hope to touch every older adult throughout the state. Senator, if I may add one thing about the assisted living movement? It is the fastest-growing health care movement in this country and it is primarily because it is providing some viable home-like personal care services juxtaposed with the housing services.

We need to find, and what I did not hear from Wendy, is that it is a private pay service. There is not public funds to pay for this service. We need to find some ways of funding people who make under $2,000 a month or so to be able to pay for this kind of service.

Senator REID. Dr. Weiss, you brought up a point that we did not discuss and we should before this hearing ends and that is, who is going to be responsible for the continuum of care? Is it going to be all the Federal Government? Are we going to give the state all the responsibility?

Are we going to dump it off onto the major cities in this country? Or are we going to include government with a partnership with the insurance industry and the health care providers? I think that is where we have to go and I have given some of my reasons for that earlier.

I had a meeting last week in Carson City where a couple—I went to a senior lunch program there. I went to a couple at a table and they said, "Senator, you know, we have been paying for many years on an insurance policy to take care of us for the time when one of us cannot take care of the other. We checked just the other day and it pays $280 a month."

They wasted their money. They might just as well have bought clothes or another car which they could have afforded over those many years. We need to make sure that there is adequate controls over the insurance industry to make sure they do not deceive those purchasing insurance.

The Kennedy-Kassebaum legislation, which is now law, we hope, will be a step in the direction that will set some guidelines for extended care insurance. I also think that if we in Washington try to protect one industry or another industry, we are in trouble. I think we have to have an integrated system where we have programs like Ms. Simons that people can look to with some degree of help.

Now, Dr. Weiss, you mentioned yesterday, or Dr. Phillips, I do not remember which, that California, New York, Iowa, a number of States reward people for sacrificing. Assume that couple, in good faith, bought that insurance policy and they come to their declining years and one of them needs help.

We would recognize, under the California, New York, and Iowa plan, that they have made some sacrifice and they would have some benefits under Medicaid. Is that right? Who helped with that?

Mr. CASHDOLLAR. I mentioned that yesterday. It is one form of private/public partnership that is already working in the United States and I would suggest that it could work in the entire United States. In regards to the insurance product itself, it shows how the state of, say, California or New York or Iowa, can set standards which the consumers can use and buy a policy that meets those standards.

Those policies would pay significantly more, of course, than $280 a month. Those are good policies that would cover the cost of good long-term care. The way it works is, if a person purchases one of these policies and uses all of the policy benefits, then the person will have long-term care covered by Medicaid without having to go bankrupt; without having to go on welfare; without having to sell the house and lose everything.

I agree with you that we should have a long-term care policy that does not require an elderly person to become bankrupt after a lifetime of self-sufficiency.

Senator REID. And one of the sad things, and there are people in this room, in fact, most everyone because many are government officials or representatives, people who volunteer their time for various organizations that deal only with seniors, we have all had experience with very proud people having to, in effect, say, "OK, I have to go on welfare." That is really tough.

Now, the chart that we have behind us indicates that over half the people in extended care facilities are there after having been declared indigent. They are there because of Medicaid. That is all Medicaid will cover. Medicare covers only 9 percent; private insurance, 2 percent; the VA covers 4 percent.

We really have to do a better job and, of course, 33 percent is paid for people like Mrs. George yesterday who, in effect, has bankrupt herself already. She has sold everything she has for her mother. I think I started this hearing talking about Hubert Humphrey. We may disagree with some of the things Vice President Humphrey said over the years, but I think we would all agree with the statement he made that people in their golden years, no matter where they find themselves in the spectrum of health, we have some obligation to make sure that they are still living with dignity.

I think, as much as I do not like to acknowledge it, that is not really the case all the time now. So I appreciate very much the testimony we have heard today. If you will remain where you are, and if the witnesses down below, we have a series of questions that have come from all over the state that we are going to attempt to answer now, and I do mean attempt because some of them are addressed to me.

"Medicare fraud, waste, and abuse is of major concern. What can we do as individuals to help solve this problem?" We held hearings in Washington last November to talk about fraud, waste, and abuse in the system. We certainly proved that there was fraud, waste, and abuse in the program. Some said as much as 15 cents of every dollar spent in health care. That may be a little high, but it is high regardless.

There is a program in Pennsylvania that we looked at that is really promising. That program takes retired accountants, nurses, doctors, lawyers, people who had been in the health care field and, in effect, has them as volunteers to look over some of the questionable bills.

Then after they look these over, they have a number they can call that is a real person, not somebody who has one of those digital voices that infuriates us. We think this is a step in the right direction. We are going to try to have a number of programs around the country based on this model. So I have only mentioned one of the programs.

Don Lahey from Carson City also noted here, he was glad to hear about Restore Trust and that is a program we have talked about at some length here today. Dr. Bernick, if you do not mind coming forward, I have got a question for you. Oh, there is a microphone down there for you? Good. We will just ask you this question.

"Can most of the aged be expected to develop Alzheimer's disease? Shouldn't younger people, ages 20 to 50, be made aware of the disease as they plan their lives in the event that they become victims?" I do not know how the rest of you feel, but I think I will wait to find out.

Dr. BERNICK. Even at best, the prevalence of Alzheimer's over age 85, 20 percent is due to the disease. In those between the 65 and 75 age group, it is really 2 percent of the population. Between

75 and 85, it is 20 percent. So it is true that the older you get, the higher your chance of getting the disease.

Senator REID. Doctor, I would also say that Alzheimer's is not the only disease we get as we get older. Prostate cancer, we have learned, becomes a problem.

Dr. BERNICK. There are many diseases, but I think what frightens many people is the prevalence of Alzheimer's disease because that is the way they are going to end their life and that is not necessarily true.

Senator REID. And as I mentioned before and I will mention again, we are very fortunate that there are people like Dr. Bernick who is spending his time in academia. He is not out trying to figure out how much money he can make, and there is nothing wrong with that if he makes that decision, but we have many outstanding physicians in America today who are involved in medical research and we are very fortunate for that.

I have previously introduced legislation to make sure that those people who are trained, who want to do medical research get forgiveness of their loans if they are willing to work at the National Institutes of Health. Right now we have many, many people who would rather work in those types of environments who cannot afford to because they all come out owing $180,000. They cannot handle that. This question came from Zelda Anderson in Sparks.

We have a question here from Elko, NV, through our fax machine. "Can Congress facilitate the integration of private and public dollars to finance research for the prevention and care of Alzheimer's and other diseases associated with aging?" Dr. Bernick?

Dr. BERNICK. Senator, could you repeat the question again?

Senator REID. Yes, be happy to. This is again from Elko. "Can Congress facilitate the integration of private and public dollars to finance research for the prevention and care of Alzheimer's and other diseases associated with aging?"

Dr. BERNICK. I certainly think that is a goal that a lot of people would like to see. Again, there is a vested interest in industry, in the pharmaceutical industry to look for treatments of Alzheimer's and other prominent diseases, and I think, of course, there is an interest on the Federal level to support research that will find cures for some of the diseases because the consequences will not be good if we do not.

Senator REID. Dr. Bernick, I believe that all research, no matter what basic science research we do, is good for us all. That is why when President Reagan came out in 1983 with his Star Wars program at the State of the Union message, I was one of the few Democrats to endorse his program. I never had great belief that the program would work as he designed it, but I knew that the research would be beneficial to us all and it has been with accelerators, with lasers, and all the many things that developed from that.

And so, I would say to the lady who asked the question that whatever research is done, we can certainly do a better job of coordinating it, but I am in favor of basic science research whether it is on science programs to find out what is in space or to discover what causes the many diseases that we do not have an answer to.

Mr. WEISS. Senator, may I make a comment?

Senator REID. Of course.

Mr. WEISS. I also fully encourage providing additional resources for applied research activities. I think we have attained a state in the scientific community——

Senator REID. Please tell us the difference, those of us who are not scientists.

Mr. WEISS. Applied research can be with the cooperation of consumers and providers, and the public actually experiment different types of services, whether or not they are effective, whether they provide better quality.

Senator REID. As Dr. Phillips' program.

Mr. WEISS. Exactly. And I think, actually, managed care may even provide a vehicle to that because of the kinds of rate structures that they have. It is not just a fee for service. It might be an alternative way. We can explore that.

Senator REID. One of the things we have not talked about here today and we should, yesterday in Las Vegas we had the state representative of the home health care industry testify. As you know, we just ran out of time to have everybody testify. These two ladies were unable to testify yesterday in Las Vegas.

What she said was surprising. She said home health care needs some significant changes. Right now in home health care, any bill you run up you get paid for. That is the way Medicare used to be. What she said, what we need is a prospective payment plan. We need to figure out a way to cut down on costs in home health care because it is such a great program and I want to make sure that what is spread across the record of this hearing is the fact that we have recognized the importance of home health care.

The next question is from Charles Dowd of Reno. "What is a qualified caregiver? What qualities are necessary? Age, education, training, personal health, availability? How does one become a qualified caregiver?" Mr. Cashdollar, please answer that.

Mr. CASHDOLLAR. Well, as you well know, Senator, the nursing home reforms that were enacted into law a little bit more than 10 years ago do spell out requirements, Federal requirements, for training of certified nurse aides, the most numerous caregivers in nursing facilities. They are under a Federal requirement for extensive training, 75 hours of training, which includes testing.

The Nevada Board of Nursing oversees that and the Nevada Health Care Association does work with the Board of Nursing on related issues. The administrators of nursing facilities also are under a requirement for education and training and also continuing education.

Senator REID. And you support that?

Mr. CASHDOLLAR. Of course, of course. For instance, in the State of Nevada, an administrator's license has to be renewed every two years and that administrator needs to undergo 40 hours of continuing education in order to get that license renewal. The process to get a license initially is very extensive and includes testing.

Senator REID. And that is what we were told yesterday by Mr. Panelli who said one of the big problems he has is enough people to make sure when there is a new institution he can do it quickly. He does not have the manpower to do it now.

Mr. CASHDOLLAR. And I would be remiss if I did not say, of course, that nurses are the backbone of the caregiving staff in long-term care facilities, registered nurses, and in some cases, LPNs. For most of these positions, there is a continual struggle to find and train and recruit enough of them and the problem could get worse without concerted effort.

Senator REID. We have here a beautiful pin that someone lost. Jerry Reed will have this if someone wants to claim it.

This question is from Winnemucca and this is for you, Dr. Phillips. "Has anything been done to get an HMO or senior-type insurance like Reno or Elko has? It seems those of us in the center of Nevada are left out of these types of care. Six months ago I talked to the ombudsman from Elko. Nothing has happened. This would help."

Dr. PHILLIPS. Yes, there have been efforts by several of the HMOs licensed in the State of Nevada, which have looked in Elko, Winnemucca, other parts of the state. Some do offer in the rurals right now, but I will tell you where a major problem exists. Look at Carson City where the HMOs are unable to, at least from a Medicare standpoint, provide the kinds of services that are needed in Carson, Minden, Gardnerville.

I am sad to say that one of the hindrances, a major hindrance is the medical community. The physicians have not been able to come to the table, with the health plans to negotiate for a Medicare Risk HMO in those areas. As we have heard from several of us, there is a true triad for providing health care to Nevada seniors.

It requires health systems, whether it is Washoe Health System, other health systems in the state coming together with health plans and with the providers in the community. Until we have those three legs of a stool working together to keep everybody upright, we still suffer from lack of services in many parts of the state.

Senator REID. We are going to now go and direct this to Wendy Simons. "Do we have statistics on the number of assisted living centers in the United States? If so, is that number on the rise, or how does Nevada compare nationally?" This is from Pam Gaines, who is a registered nurse in Elko.

Ms. SIMONS. That is an excellent question. Unfortunately, Elko is one of the areas that does not have an adequate supply or source of residential care or assisted living and has been in screaming need of that alternative up there for a long time.

In the last, I guess it is 6 or 7 years, assisted living as an entity unto itself began to evolve in the United States under the guise and guidance of a gentleman named Paul Klausen who started the Sunrise Properties based on a European or Norwegian model of care.

In answer to the question directly, Senator, yes, there is an increase that is beyond the imagination of assisted living in the United States. My own fear for my industry is that there is a lot of large corporations and large entities taking a look at this as a good alternative to a long-term care skilled nursing placement and it could create a monster.

However, the industry itself, under the guidance of the Assisted Living Federation of America, is taking strong initiatives to be very proactive, and you will be hearing some things quite proactive in

47-539 98 - 12

February from ALFA with regard to guidance of assisted living in the United States.

Residential care, which is considered to be the smaller residential group homes that we hear so much of, have been here since, in Nevada certainly, 1948, and we see those stay steady. Those are the areas that people have cautions because they tend to be the mom-and-pop insidious operations, many of which are exceptional, some of which are not.

But I think we see a balance of large properties and a good balance of small properties and we are just on the very beginning of a huge wave of this as a resource for long-term care.

Senator REID. We have a question here that is directed to the panel, but I will answer it. "As Medicare continues to limit the number of home health care visits per patient or illness episode, more patients will be forced into long-term care facilities either permanently or temporarily. What measures are being taken to assure that the needed beds will be available for Nevada residents and that the transfer between home and long-term care takes place as expeditiously as possible?" This is from Kay Ray, also of Elko.

We went into this at great length yesterday and sadly not much. We have to jump right on this as soon as Congress convenes to see if we can resolve some of these issues. Home health care is clearly a way of keeping people out of convalescent homes. It is a lot cheaper. We are going to do our best. Right now there is not much protection.

Dr. PHILLIPS. Senator, could I just interject if I may, please?

Senator REID. Please.

Dr. PHILLIPS. Along the lines of home health care and some of the restrictions in visits, there are other areas of the continuum that are definitely under the same target right now, and that is out-patient physical therapy, occupational therapy, communication therapy if it is not based out of a hospital setting.

I think for somewhere like Nevada, that is a critical issue considering the rural needs that we have. So I would request that they also be addressed when home health care is. Thank you.

Senator REID. We have a number of other questions that have come to us. Our time is gone. Everyone that submitted a question will be answered in great detail by me and the three men to my left. We have a record here. The questions and the answers will be made part of the record. We will have those answers completed by February 2, that is the date that we have set.

So we appreciate everyone's attendance here today. It has been a very good hearing. The problem is that we raise a lot more questions, as we did yesterday, than answers, but that is the way it is. I appreciate very much those who joined us from rural Nevada. We have a public policy challenge on the horizon.

I hope the Medicare Commission, of which Senator Breaux is a member, will be able to work with us on this. Exactly how our nation addresses its long-term care remains to be seen. The hearing stands adjourned. [Applause.]

[Whereupon, at 11:30 a.m., the committee was adjourned.]

APPENDIX

Elderly Long-Term Care Expenditures by Source of Payment, 1995 ($ in billions)

Nursing home care	
Medicaid	$24.2
Medicare	8.4
Other federal	0.7
Other state and local	0.6
Out-of-pocket payments and other	30.0
Private insurance	0.4
Total	64.4
Home care	
Medicaid	4.3
Medicare	14.3
Other federal	1.7
Other state and local	0.5
Out-of-pocket payments and other	5.5
Private insurance	0.3
Total	26.5
Total long-term care	90.9

Source: Office of the Assistant Secretary for Planning and Evaluation, DHHS. Totals may not add due to rounding.

Who Pays for Nursing Home Care?

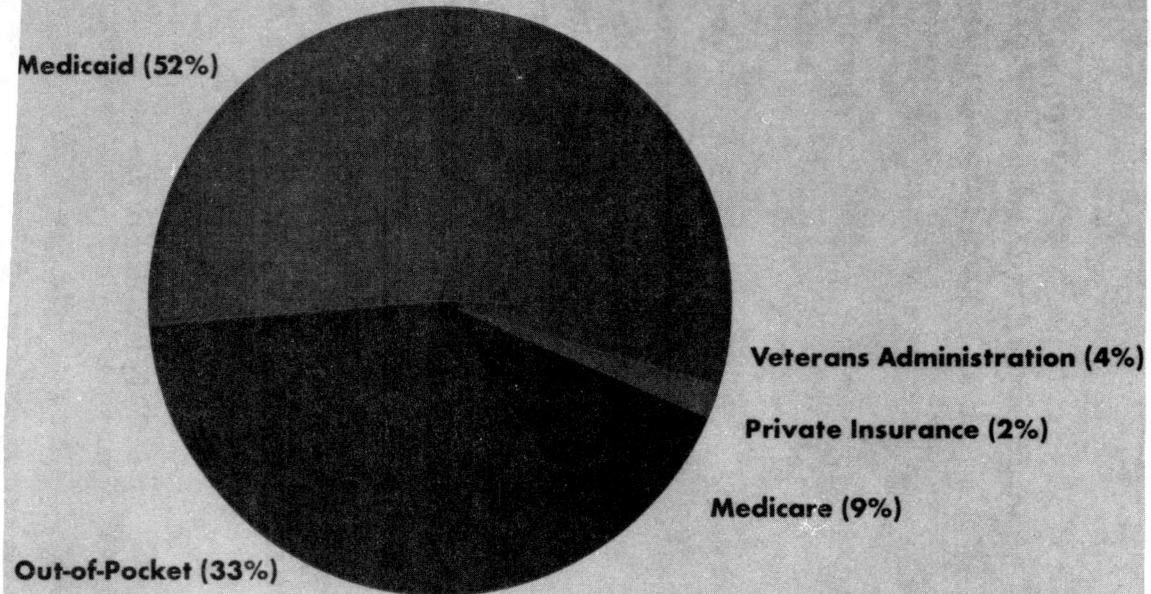

Source: Public Policy Institute, AARP. January 1995

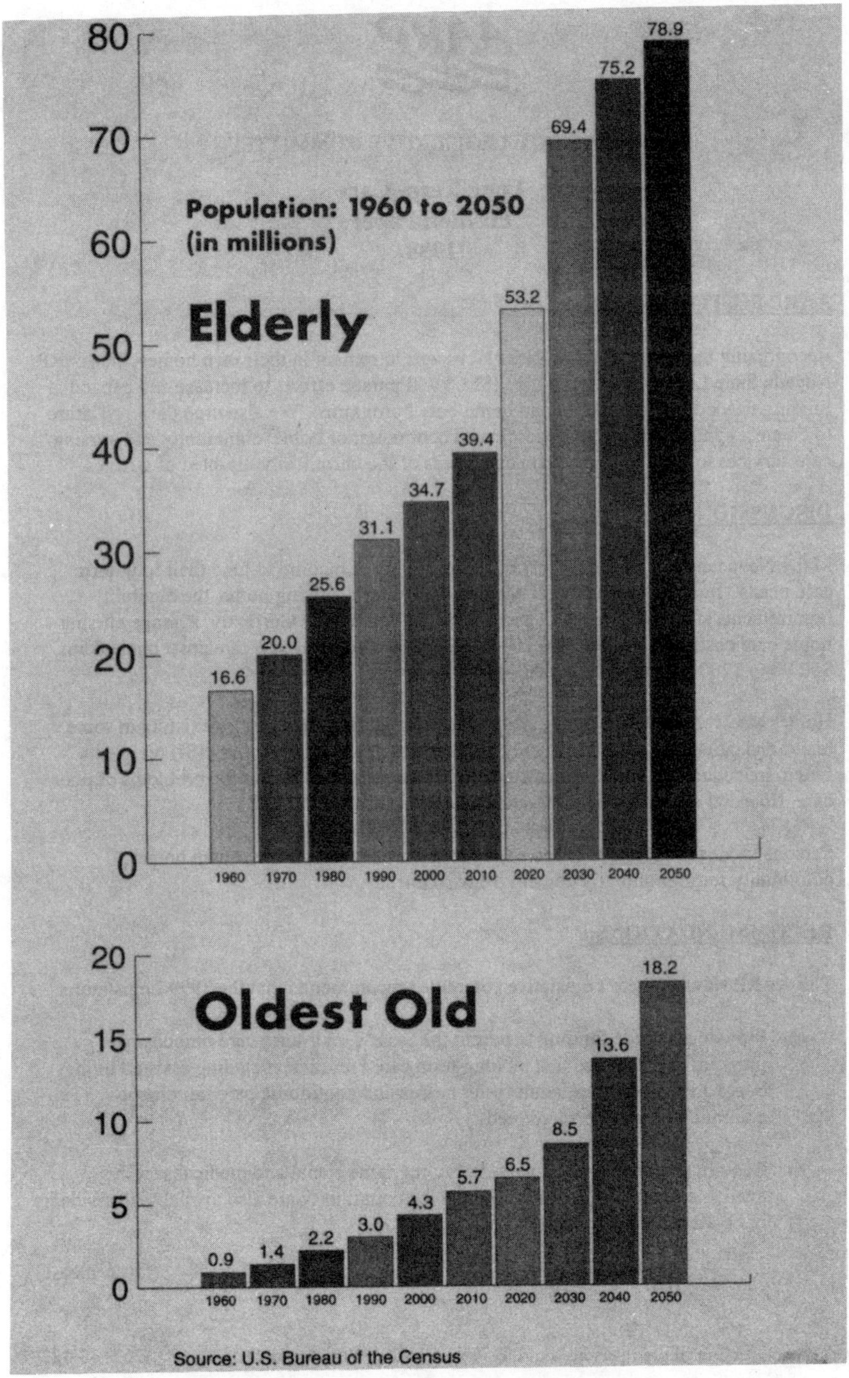
Population: 1960 to 2050
(in millions)
Elderly
80
70
60
50
40
30
20
10
0
16.6
20.0
25.6
31.1
34.7
39.4
53.2
69.4
75.2
78.9
1960
1970
1980
1990
2000
2010
2020
2030
2040
2050
Oldest Old
20
15
10
5
0
0.9
1.4
2.2
3.0
4.3
5.7
6.5
8.5
13.6
18.2
1960
1970
1980
1990
2000
2010
2020
2030
2040
2050
Source: U.S. Bureau of the Census

AARP

NEVADA STATE LEGISLATIVE COMMITTEE

Long-Term Care
Position Paper
1998

AARP POSITION:

Recognizing the desire of many older Nevadans to remain in their own homes, the AARP Nevada State Legislative Committee (SLC) will pursue efforts to increase and expand funding needed for community and home-based programs. We also urge the Legislature to create a comprehensive and coordinated continuum of home, community and nursing care services to meet the long-term care needs of the chronically disabled of all ages.

DISCUSSION:

Many Nevadans can no longer rely on their retirement income to fund their long-term care needs. In order to qualify for Medicaid, to enter a nursing home, the eligibility requirements state that almost all assets must be liquidated. Currently, average nursing home care costs are between $30,000 and $50,000 a year. Home care costs range from $50.00 to $200.00 per visit, depending on the level of care needed.

Homes also very widely in quality, with the most glaring deficiencies existing in some board and care homes serving mainly Supplemental Security Income (SSI) recipients. Often, inadequate regulations and funding have contributed to chronic problems of poor care, financial exploitation, abuse and neglect.

Persons of all ages <u>prefer</u> to receive long-term care services in their own homes, community settings and in a homelike environment.

RECOMMENDATIONS:

The AARP Nevada State Legislative committee recommends that the 1999 Legislature:

a) Provide adequate funding to permit the State's long-term care ombudsman program to expand so that all long-term care facilities, including assisted living, board and care homes, adult foster homes and continuing care retirement communities may be monitored.

b) Require public agencies to assure that the same social and medical services available to other persons residing in the community are also available to residents of board and care homes.

(Over, please)

American Association of Retired Persons 601 E Street, N.W., Washington, DC 20049 (202) 434-2277

c) Require nursing facility admission contracts to be presented, before signing, and to define what is covered by the Medicaid payment so that facilities deliver appropriate services and do not overcharge residents.

d) Increase the availability of home and community-based services by limiting the number of Medicaid-funded nursing homes through a Certificate-of-Need process thus shifting monies that would have been spent in nursing homes to home and community-based care programs.

e) Provide community spouses with financial protection by setting the highest "community spouse resources allowance" and "spousal maintenance needs allowance" under federal law.

For further information, please contact:

Joseph Fisher
State Legislative Committee Chair
4650 Rio Encantado Lane
Reno, NV 89502-5344
(702) 826-9513
(702) 826-9513 **FAX**

Doris Alcorn, Chair
Long-Term Care Subcommittee
9328 Sun Rose Ave
Las Vegas, NV 89134-6022
(702) 228-0261

Ed Fend
Capital City Task Force Coordinator
7201 Blue Falls Circle
Reno, NV 89511-1016
(702) 852-5993
(702) 852-2516 **FAX**

West Region Office
9750 3rd Avenue N.E.
Suite 400
Seattle, WA 98115
(206) 526-7918
(206) 523-8138 **FAX**

Adopted 11/12/97

AARP

NEVADA STATE LEGISLATIVE COMMITTEE

Medicaid
Position Paper
1998

AARP POSITION:

The AARP Nevada State Legislative Committee (SLC) supports the expansion of Medicaid coverage by utilizing all available federal, state and local public funds as well as private funds.

DISCUSSION:

The Nevada Medicaid Program is a critical part of AARP's 1998 Legislative Program seeking to assure that Nevadans have adequate and affordable coverage of high-quality health and long-term care, particularly for low-income elderly and persons with disabilities.

As Nevada's budget continues to be consumed by escalating health care costs for Medicaid, and access to care remains problematic for Medicaid beneficiaries, Nevada has looked to managed care as a means of controlling costs while improving access.

The Congressional Budget Office reports that the direct evidence does not yet give a clear picture of whether, or by how much, the use of managed care programs affects Medicaid costs. Other research evidence suggests that successful managed care plans can save between 5 and 15 percent over fee-for-service Medicaid. However, these savings have been produced through the enrollment of the least costly segment of the Medicaid population, children and families. When elderly and disabled beneficiaries become eligible for managed care, overall savings to the Medicaid program from enrolling elderly beneficiaries in managed care plans is limited.

Managed care is not an instant solution for improving access to health care or for saving dollars for the Medicaid population. Making managed care work in Medicaid requires considerable attention to understanding the needs, cultural preferences, and characteristics of poor communities. Adequate time and resources in program design, coupled with continuous monitoring and oversight of program implementation, are needed to ensure that the potential benefits of managed care are realized.

(Over, please)

RECOMMENDATIONS:

The AARP Nevada State Legislative Committee recommends that the 1999 Legislature take action to:

1. Ensure the provision of adequate state funding for the Nevada Medicaid Program.

2. Seek the broadest possible Medicaid waivers to expand health care coverage for the uninsured and under-insured.

3. Establish a foundation using private funds to expand health care for children.

4. Strengthen financial protections for Medicaid beneficiaries and their families.

For further information, please contact:

Joseph Fisher
State Legislative Committee Chair
4650 Rio Encantado Lane
Reno, NV 89502-5344
(702) 826-9513
(702) 826-9513 **FAX**

Joseph Fisher, Chair
Medicaid Subcommittee
4650 Rio Encantado Lane
Reno, NV 89502-5344
(702) 826-9513
(702) 826-9513 **FAX**

Ed Fend
Capital City Task Force Coordinator
7201 Blue Falls Circle
Reno, NV 89511-1016
(702) 852-5993
(702) 852-2516 **FAX**

West Region Office
9750 3rd Avenue N.E.
Suite 400
Seattle, WA 98115
(206) 526-7918
(206) 523-8138 **FAX**

Adopted: 11/12/97

AARP

NEVADA STATE LEGISLATIVE COMMITTEE

Managed Care Position Paper 1998

AARP POSITION:

AARP and the Nevada State Legislative Committee support state efforts to ensure that Medicare recipients have the opportunity to use a managed care organization if they desire. AARP encourages ongoing research to determine whether managed care organizations achieve savings and deliver quality care. Such research should investigate the impact of managed care by model types on individuals with chronic illness, age, income and disability.

DISCUSSION:

The passage of AB-156 (Managed Care Regulations) and AB-30 (Appeal Procedures) in 1997, has provided Nevada citizens with information and protection in the area of managed care. However, an on-going program of education for our senior citizens is essential to the success of this program. In addition, we must ensure that adequate competition exists and that the quality of care is satisfactory in the market place. At present there are only four managed care organizations that are federally certified in Nevada; this will have to be monitored closely to ensure all citizens have access to this vital service.

One of the main questions still to be answered is "will managed care reduce the cost of medical services?" This subject must be followed closely, for the rising cost of medical services remains a major problem in our state. Additionally, can managed care provide services such a prescription drugs, eyeglasses, diabetic self-management, as well as provisions for long-term care and still remain cost effective?

The SLC supports the availability of choices between fee-for-service and managed care for Medicare beneficiaries. In the context of mandated enrollment for Medicaid, great care must be taken to preserve the Medicare rights of the dual eligible. Those with dual eligibility should be able to choose from fee-for-service or managed care.

(Over, please)

American Association of Retired Persons 601 E Street, N.W., Washington, DC 20049 (202) 434-2277

RECOMMENDATIONS:

1. Require managed care organizations be fiscally sound, solvent and competitive.
2. Establish procedures to ensure quality assurance and improvement which includes internal quality assessment and external quality review.
3. Provide accessibility and availability of services in a timely manner.
4. Establish and publish grievance and appeals procedures, standardized data for evaluation, and consumer and quality assurance information, as outlined in AB-156.
5. Continue strong efforts to reduce the increasing cost of medical services for the State.

For further information, please contact:

Joseph Fisher
State Legislative Committee Chair
4650 Rio Encantado Lane
Reno, NV 89502-5344
(702) 826-9513
(702) 826-9513 **FAX**

Ed Fend, Chair
Managed Care Subcommittee
7201 Blue Falls Circle
Reno, NV 89511-1016
(702) 852-5993
(702) 852-2516 **FAX**

Ed Fend
Captial City Task Force Coordinator
7201 Blue Falls Circle
Reno, NV 89511-1016
(702) 852-5993
(702) 852-2516 **FAX**

West Region Office
9750 3rd Avenue N.E.
Suite 400
Seattle, WA 98115
(206) 526-7918
(206) 523-8138 **FAX**

Adopted 11/12/97

This field hearing is addressing and discussing how individual states can ensure that older citizens have available and affordable quality care. To expand on this it should address how the state plans to resolve issues concerning the geriatric psychiatric patient or the difficult to manage patient who needs Long Term Care (LTC) without having to place them out of state away from their loved ones and their support system. This is a hardship on the family and the patient. Thus, it should be a right of all resident's that these services are available within the State.

The OBRA regulations indicated under 483.45 Specialized Services state " If specialized rehabilitative services such as but not limited to physical therapy, speech-language pathology, occupational therapy and health rehabilitative services for mental illness and mental retardation, are required in the resident's comprehensive plan of care the facility must provide the required services; or obtain the required services from an outside resource from a provider of specialized rehabilitative services". The purpose of the Pre-Admission Screening and Annual Resident Review (PASARR) is to identify those residents who need specialized services for mental health or mental retardation and assure that they receive the appropriate care. Unfortunately, once a geriatric resident is identified as needing specialized mental health services for LTC, there are no facilities identified that specialize in providing this service in Nevada.

This problem is not going to disappear. Nevada must be willing to provide the geriatric psychiatric Long Term Care services or reimburse at a rate that will promote the development of facilities providing the needed services.

Is Nevada really ready to go into the next century and ensure accessible and affordable services including geriatric psychiatric care?

Carla A. Buckner LCSW
Contract Nursing Home Coordinator
VAMC, Reno

The Many Faces of Long-Term Care

Long-Term Care For Minority Elders

David C. Love, Executive Director
The Dr. A. Lois Harry Institute
Bethel AME Church
2655 North Rock Boulevard
Sparks, Nevada 89431

Concerns have been expressed by members of the minority communities that not only are their elders underserved, but they are uncounted, also. Many plans that have been made to serve the ever increasing elderly population do not make mention or take note of any special needs or services for the minority elderly. Little is known of them outside of the census data. However, it is well known, but not well understood that minority seniors do not make use of long-term care services in proportion to their numbers in the population. This could be due to discrimination, language, economic, financial or cultural barriers.

Persons over 65 years of age are the fastest growing group in the population of the United States. Minorities are the fastest growing group of any of the population groups who will be in need of facilities that will provide them Long-Term Care and Social Services at a reasonable cost. Therefore, many caregivers of minority elders leave their professional job to care for elderly friends or relatives due to the high cost of long-term care.

Elder care assistance should be of concern in the work setting and some type of long-term care should be included in the employers benefit package. Since personnel officers could probably point out that elder care programs such as long-term care have an effect on employee productivity when the individual functions in the dual role of caregiver

page 2

and employee. Many times such individual exhibits reduced productivity, suffers from low morale, often tardy or absent, take more unscheduled days off than their co-workers and tend to use company time for personal business when in the work setting. This happens because there is a need for employers to offer benefits either for child or elder care in long-term care facilities. On the other hand long-term care facilities could offer discounts on published rates or a flexible long term care benefit plan.

National studies on minority elders have have found that minority seniors are in the most critical need of services of any group in the population due to the cumulative effects of lifelong experiences of discrimination and lack of awareness of and sensitivity to the needs of minority elderly patients.

There is a need to develop and design long-term care services to meet the needs of the four federally designated minority groups(African Americans, Native Americans, Asians/Pacific Islanders and Hispanics).

Improving the Quality of Life - and Death - in America

Written Testimony provided to the

Field Hearing of the

U.S. Senate Special Committee on Aging

12 January 1998
Las Vegas, Nevada

On behalf of the

Hospice Association of Nevada

Presented by
Richard Fitzpatrick
President

Senator Reid, Assistant Secretary Takamura, members of the panels, ladies and gentlemen. I am Richard Fitzpatrick, Executive Director of Nevada Operations for VistaCare and President of the Hospice Association of Nevada. The fourteen hospices across our state appreciate the opportunity today to address the critical issue of adequate long-term care.

It is only appropriate that you focus on these national issues in our state with its incredibly fast-growing senior population. Also, there is probably no more diverse state in our country than Nevada. Some of us live in urban cities; some in suburbs, others in small towns and rural areas - a few live in remote frontier territories. A handful of our state's residents are very rich; while too many are quite poor; and most of us are in the middle. There is a rapidly expanding number of children and an ever-growing percentage of senior citizens. Some of us were born here; most of us weren't. In fact, there may be no single characteristic that we all share—but, the one common denominator of each and every Nevadan: we are all going to die. And that's where **hospice** enters the scene. We are that part of the health care continuum that deals with those who have life-limiting illnesses. When medicine cannot add any more days to an individual's life; we are there to add quality of life to those final days.

Hospice is a comprehensive, medically directed, team-oriented program of care that seeks to treat and comfort patients and their families at home or in a home-like setting. It is a philosophy of care that accepts death as a natural part of life, and seeks to neither hasten nor prolong the dying process.

Hospice has a long and distinguished history in Nevada. The Nathan Adelson Hospice was one of the first such facilities in the country. Clark County Health District established one of the original county-based public hospice programs in the US. The Hospice of Northern Nevada was serving Reno's terminally ill long before most communities in this country had such programs. And in the past two years, eight new hospice programs have begun across our state. During this past year (1997), more than 2,000 Nevadans - and their families - faced the reality of death with the help of a compassionate and professional hospice team

In spite of this glowing report, there are two ominous facts facing us: 1) as we meet here today, there are thousands of people across this state who are in their final months, weeks or days of life are alone - without the support of a hospice team; and, 2) in reaction to the understandable fear of dying alone and in pain, a national movement calling for "physician-assisted suicide" as a solution, is getting established and growing in Nevada. I'm here today to let you know that our hospices are ready to help meet both of those challenges - but we need your help.

Nationally, and in Nevada, all of the hospice programs combined care for approximately 17% of those with terminal illnesses - meaning that more than four out of five people who could take advantage of these services—don't. They often die unpleasant and difficult deaths: alone in a nursing home; hooked up to tubes and machines in a hospital; in physical and psychological pain. And their loved ones stand by not knowing what to say or how to help.

Research has shown that, if given a choice, most terminally ill patients would choose to spend their final days surrounded by family in an atmosphere filled with love, comfort and care. Unfortunately, many people in Nevada like in other parts of the country -- are not aware that such an option is available to them. We are working with key state officials and the legislature on specific proposals that the state government can undertake that could make significant progress in increasing access to quality end-of-life care for our citizens.

On the federal level, there are three significant steps you could take to improve access to hospice care:

First, the Medicare Hospice Benefit was created more than 15 years ago when the hospice movement was in its infancy and there was little factual data to go on. Today, there are more than 3,000 hospices operating and hundreds of thousands of Americans have been aided by these program. This is a good time to step back and review its effectiveness and how the structure of the hospice benefit could be changed to make it simpler to use and capable of providing valuable – and cost effective -- services to more people at the end of their lives.

Second, the ability to die in one's own home is attractive to most people. Unfortunately, not everyone has a home environment that makes that possible. Therefore, many find themselves at the end of life in institutionalized care. This concept – and the government funding that supports it – needs to be broadened to allow people to choose assisted living, group homes and special hospice homes.

Third, many of those who are nearing the end of life are the men and women who fought to defend this country in military service. Many of them are counting on the Department of Veterans Affairs for support. There needs to be a specific program that allows veterans to have access to community-based hospice care. There is no rationale for the VA to attempt to replicated what is already in place across our country – and this state. It should be given the clear direction to contract with local hospices to provide care for veterans in and out of VA medical centers. Nevada has the fastest growing veteran population in the country – with some of the most minimal of services. This is the ideal place for a pilot project to demonstrate how such a collaborative effort would work.

As one who has been involved with the hospice movement since the early 1980's, I find it most fascinating to finally see the media paying attention to end-of-life issues. Sadly, it isn't the good that the 3,000+ hospice programs around the country do every day that has been making the news - but the quirky actions of one misguided doctor in the back of a rusting van in Detroit.

While we appreciate the recent focus on these critical issues, we are most frustrated - even angered, by the stark, incomplete picture of the end of life that they present. The perception seems to be that patient must choose between :

- A painful existence devoid of value - aggressive treatment until the bitter end **or**
- asking a Doctor to purposely end your life.

Although the question has often been framed as an issue of choice - the debate misses the most rational option: -- the one that's in between the two extremes: that choice is hospice.

But in spite of the offensiveness of the physician-assisted suicide concept; the disturbing fact is that it is has substantial public support. Why?

Research shows that there are a number of fears people have about becoming terminally ill:

- the perception that there is a significant financial, emotional and physical burden that they, as a patient, would place on their families
- they would loose control over the medical services being provided to them
- they will be abandoned by the health care system
- they will die in pain

Unfortunately, as the results of the multi-year SUPPORT study of patients in hospitals showed, the public has every right to be concerned. And the problem it is not just in hospitals. It may be less documented but we know the health care system has also failed to meet the needs of terminally ill individuals in nursing facilities, adult care centers and those who are left in their own homes without adequate support.

While these are the sort of fears that could drive a patient to consider physician-assisted suicide - and a state's electorate to consider voting for such an option - they are also the sort of fears that hospice care is uniquely structured to allay.

The answer lies with multi-disciplinary palliative and hospice care. But, as I said earlier, we are seeing, at best, 1 of 7 hospice-appropriate patients. Even then, after many have needlessly suffered for weeks and months without hospice—waiting for the physician to become more certain that the patient will die within 6 months -- 25% are referred with less than 2 weeks to live.

The real issues that we need to address are: a patient's rights to obtain adequate pain and symptom control; more frequent and earlier referral to a hospice; an elimination of impediments that inhibit the ability for organizations to delivery high quality hospice care in the home and home-like settings; and the establishment of a society that views death as a part of life, not as a failure.

Senator Reid, we deeply appreciate today's discussion; and we invite your attention the 3 specific proposals we offer. In addition, we draw your attention to the excellent work and recommendations of Nevada Attorney General Frankie Sue Del Papa and the *Death with Dignity and Caring in Nevada* project. Their Report, issued in January 1997, expands upon these and other important issues. The Hospice Association of Nevada stands ready to be the a part in the effort to ensure an adequate quality of life—and an adequate quality of death—for all of our citizens.

For more information: contact Richard Fitzpatrick 702.734.0307

Senate Special Hearing on Aging
Field Hearing
January 12, 1997
Las Vegas, Nevada
Prepared by Roberta Skelton, RN, Administrator/CEO
Home Health Services of Nevada
Elko, Nevada

Honorable Senator Harry Reid:

Mr. Chairman:

On behalf of Home Health Care Association of Nevada (HHCAN) and its member it is an honor and a pleasure for me to be able to sit on this most prestigious panel in which you and your staff have engaged.

It has been very interesting to me in my career as a professional nurse for over 40 years in the great state of Nevada to observe first hand the ever changing health care scene. Many plans have been worked on and shelved. However, probably the most significant plan that was passed is the Medicare insurance program for older Americans. This was a monumental undertaking and hailed as the answer for the senior citizen. Now, nearly 32 years later it is in or will be in financial crises according to Congress. As with all government programs, opportunists push the lever to see how far they can get to retrieve the almighty dollar before the hammer comes down. This attitude alone causes havoc and grave concern to companies who try to live by the rules. As a result of this, Congress passes punitive legislation to come down hard on providers of home health care.

Ironically, the news media picks up on the bad guys and runs with it. However, this panel knows full well there are a lot of good folks out there providing service to our elderly population.

Home Health Services of Nevada, in my book, is of the good agencies. It was established in 1961 in Elko, Nevada as a non-profit corporation by a group of concerned citizens who saw a need for homemaking service in Elko County. The agency then went on to become Medicare certified being one of the first in the state of Nevada. Today our corporation serves 13 rural counties with 10 branch offices. We have a staff of over 200 employees. We go as far east as Wells, Nevada and south to Pahrump, which is northwest of Las Vegas.

I have some real concerns regarding certain methodology which Congress and the President have signed into law. Our corporation is a free standing home health agency committed to serving the elderly in rural Nevada. We realize we cannot serve everyone wherever they choose to live. However, at this point in time we have been able to provide care to the majority of referrals received.

Cost shifting will <u>not</u> solve Medicare's problem. If a homebound patient cannot receive a certain amount of care in the home, then they will be back in the hospital. Some will go to long term care or skilled nursing facilities, but again, in my opinion, this is cost shifting. Again, does America want to institutionalized the aged into skilled nursing facilities? It is a well known fact costs are less by keeping the patient in the home. Our agency has a well rounded program whereby we work with the Division of Aging Services under the CHIPS program and Title III B. Therefor, the patient has continuity of care available.

In lieu of hospice, our company provides pain management since we are not a Hospice certified Medicare agency. We have looked into this but the numbers are not there in calculating the per diem rate. With all the new regulations it is even more apparent we could not financially afford hospice.

For free standing home health agencies such as ours, bonding is a critical issue. The state of Nevada passed legislation in which the Division of Aging Services holds in their name of $100,000. Medicaid is also going to bond home care along with Medicare as a requirement. We are deeply concerned with the pending Medicare bond as to what their demand will be. Since these are non-reimbursable costs to a non-profit company, I beg the question, where does the money come from? Home Health Services of Nevada already is bonded and also carries all the required insurance for liability and non owner's auto insurance.

I do not believe enough grass roots input was generated even though we sent much correspondence to National Association of Home Care (NAHC) and our congressional delegation opposing much of the legislation which was passed. I really think Congress forgot the little guy out there.

Presently there is so much confusion at the federal level, quite frankly, I am not sure when providers and their fiscal intermediaries will be able to do a cost report which will be acceptable.

We are very concerned with the capitalization plan. No bank in their right mind is going to reserve a line of credit for 6 months operating expenses on an operation such as ours. We have a line of credit to be used when the PIP check or checks from other payor sources are late. Good business practices is a must. Non profits have a difficult time in generating any reserve since there is no profit built into Medicare. Being rural there is not much in the way of other sources of income to generate monies. (I guess we could sell shoes.)

As it stands now, if our agency is forced to close due to lack of funds with the new costs caps, we will displace over 200 employees and 1194 unduplicated patients generating approximately 90,000 visits with a net revenue of 4.5 million dollars. My statistician has provided me with what our cost report will look like.

Mr. Chairman, you have a major, major issue with health care. However, I don't believe in punitive legislative such as just passed, by reducing our cost is the answer. I would entertain that Congress look at the average cost per visit by discipline by region and provide a direct payment method to the provider. The payment method can be contracted out thus I believe millions of dollars could be saved. Perhaps this is just too simple of a method.

I have attached a statement of what will happen to Home Health Services of Nevada with implementation of the IPS program initiated in October of 1997 in which I will take a moment to read into the record.

My Director of Professional Services has written a statement as to why venipuncture should not be deleted from home care, at least in the rural areas of our nation which I will also read into the record.

Also included are attachments prepared and presented by Ann Howard, Executive Director of the American Federation of

Home Health Associations which I feel the Senator will find very interesting. These attachments show how negative HCFA is treating its providers regardless of the good guy/bad guy.

On behalf of my Board of Directors, I thank you for allowing time to present rural home care to be added to the congressional record.

Submitted by:
Roberta K. Skelton, RN
Administrator/CEO
Home Health Services of Nevada

Attachment A

Financial Impact of the "Interim Payment System" on Home Health Services of Nevada

Reimbursement rates are based on reasonable rates up to the lower of:

	HHSN Amounts
(1) Aggregate Medicare Visit Limit (estimated by region)	$ 5,734,962.00
(2) Aggregate Medicare Cost (actual reported for 1996)	$ 5,239,196.00
(3) Aggregate Medicare Patient Limit*	$ 5,166,749.00

* Calculation of agency-specific per beneficiary cap, lowest of above:

+ 75% of HHSN average cost per patient based on 93-94 cost reporting-reduced by 2% and increased by a 3% regional adjustment.	$ 3,033.65
+ 25% of Census Division average cost (Mountain Region)-reduced by 2% and increased by a 3% regional adjustment.	$ 1,1126.99
= Calculated agency blended limit	$ 4,160.64
x Multiplied by projected unduplicated patient census	1,1194
= Aggregate per beneficiary limit (reimbursement limit)	$ 4,967,804.16

When the aggregate limit is compared to total Medicare costs using the 1996 cost report, the projected loss would be:	$ 5,239,196.00 ($ 271,391.84)

While HHSN's per patient cost of $ 4387.93 is below the regional per patient cost of $ 4466, we would experience a reduction of $ 60.93 per patient if the above methodology were applied to our agency. In addition, this reduction does not include factors for inflation, or changes in growth and patient mix which have taken place over the past two years.

The Interim Payment System

	Reimbursement Per Person	Reimbursement Per Visit	Visits Per Person Served
West South Central	$5,877	$57.51	102.1
AR	$3,586	$47.14	76.0
LA	$6,700	$53.19	125.8
OK	$6,035	$57.04	105.7
TX	$5,977	$61.36	97.4
Mountain	$4,050	$63.52	63.7
AZ	$3,932	$70.00	56.2
CO	$4,091	$68.38	59.8
ID	$3,347	$61.92	54.2
MT	$3,052	$59.37	51.6
NV	$4,466	$65.62	68.1
NM	$3,355	$60.03	56.0
UT	$5,481	$55.46	98.4
WY	$4,309	$56.00	77.0
Pacific	$3,862	$86.84	44.5
AK	$4,336	$99.28	43.4
CA	$4,075	$88.39	46.1
HI	$3,549	$85.79	41.0
OR	$3,188	$80.75	39.7
WA	$3,951	$79.46	38.4
Outlying	$1,658	$45.24	36.6

Source: Health Care Financing Administration. Health Care Financing Review Medicare and Medicaid Statistical Supplement. 1996

Prepared by NAHC

Calculations of Cost Limits, Per Beneficiary Limit, and Reimbursement
NAHC - Modeling Reimbursement Under the New Interim Payment System (8/15/97)
Limits, update factors, & census division data are estimates subject to change.

Estimated Per Visit Cost Limits	RURAL Estimated National Limit	Labor Portion 77.668%	Labor Portion w/Wage Index	Labor Portion w/Budget Neutrality	Non-Labor Portion	Total Labor & Non-Labor	Estimated Cost Limit w/cost repl adjust
Adjustment Factors			0.8775	1.078			1.0247
Skilled Nursing	$98.36	$76.39	$67.03	$72.26	$21.97	$94.23	$96.55
Physical Therapy	$105.57	$81.99	$71.95	$77.56	$23.58	$101.14	$103.63
Occupational Therapy	$111.84	$86.86	$76.22	$82.17	$24.98	$107.15	$109.79
Speech Pathology	$110.17	$85.57	$75.09	$80.95	$24.60	$105.55	$108.16
Medical Social Service	$149.87	$116.40	$102.14	$110.11	$33.47	$143.58	$147.12
Home Health Aide	$42.33	$32.88	$28.85	$31.10	$9.45	$40.55	$41.55

Calculation of Agency-Specific Per Beneficiary Annual Limit

1994 Total Medicare Visit Costs	$3,454,735.00
1994 Total Cost Limit	$4,186,860.00
1994 Total Reasonable Visit Cost	$3,454,735.000
1994 Total Medical Supplies	$31,524.00
1994 Total Reasonable Cost	$3,486,259.00
1994 Unduplicated Medicare Patients	870
Avg. Cost per Medicare Patient	$4,007.19
98% of Avg. Cost per Medicare Patient	$3,927.05
Market Basket Update	1.0300
Updated Avg. Cost per Patient	$4,044.86

	Census Division	Agency-Specific	Agency Blended Limit
Census Division Avg. Cost per Pt.	$4,466.00		
98% of Census Division Avg Cost/Pt.	$4,376.68		
Market Basket Update	1.0300		
Updated Census Division Avg. Cost/Pt.	$4,507.98	$4,044.86	
Blend	25%	75%	
Agency Blended Limit	$1,127.00	$3,033.65	$4,160.64

1994 Base Year Information	1994 Cost per Visit	1994 Medicare Visits	1994 Avg. Visits/Pt.
Skilled Nursing	$85.38	22,260.0	25.59
Physical Therapy	$99.92	4,008.0	4.61
Occupational Therapy	$116.76	620.0	0.71
Speech Pathology	$92.48	87.0	0.10
Medical Social Service	$90.82	116.0	0.13
Home Health Aide	$33.24	32,374.0	37.21
Total		59,465.0	68.35

Estimating Reimbursement for FY beginning on or after 10/1/97 Using Agency Projections

Projected Unduplicated Medicare Pts.	1,194
Aggregate Per Beneficiary Limit	$4,967,804.16

	Projected Cost per Visit	Projected No. of Visits	Projected Avg Visits/Pt.	Projected Cost per Discipline	Estimated Cost Limit	Projected Cost Limit Per Discipline
Skilled Nursing	$86.19	31,930	26.74	$2,752,046.70	$96.55	$3,082,841.50
Physical Therapy	$92.78	6,013	5.04	$557,848.27	$103.63	$623,127.19
Occupational Therapy	$89.33	314	0.26	$28,049.62	$109.79	$34,474.06
Speech Pathology	$89.87	681	0.57	$61,201.47	$108.16	$73,660.15
Medical Social Service	$100.40	144	0.12	$14,457.60	$147.12	$21,185.28
Home Health Aide	$33.66	51,355	43.01	$1,728,609.30	$41.55	$2,133,800.25
Total		90,437	75.74	$5,142,310.96		$5,969,078.43
Medical Supplies				$96,885.00		$96,885.00
Total Visit & Medical Suppy Cost				$5,239,195.96		$6,065,963.43

		Per Patient
Reimbursement	$4,967,804.16	$4,160.64
Total Cost	$5,239,195.96	
Breakeven (Loss)	($271,391.80)	

Note: This information can only be considered for illustrative purposes due to the limitations of the estimates

Home Health Services of Nevada

Attachment B

EFFECTS OF CHANGES IN MEDICARE ON RURAL NEVADA

Medicare's changes are probably feasible and somewhat cost effective for urban areas. It is evident that not a lot of consideration was given to rural areas.

Take the provision that states venipuncture is no longer a qualifying service for home health. HCFA's opinion is that a tech from the laboratory can go to the patient's home and draw the required blood specimen. In some rural areas it is not unusual for a home health employee to travel 100 to 200+ miles round trip to see a patient. The laboratory may be another 40 to 100 miles from the home health office. Obviously, the laboratory is not going to send a tech that distance to draw blood. Therefore, the patient's family must take the patient either to the laboratory or to the physician's office, which may be even further away than the laboratory. This requires that these homebound patients, with health problems, must travel in adverse weather conditions. In southern Nevada this means summer temperatures above 100°, and in northern Nevada sub-zero temperatures in the winter.

It would be more prudent to allow the venipuncture benefit to continue, but limit what other services could be provided in conjunction with that benefit. For example, if venipuncture is the only skilled service the patient requires, then do not allow CNA, Medical Social Worker or Occupational Therapy to be initiated.

As changes occur in the home care industry, the amount of patient/nurse contact will decrease. This will make it more difficult for the nurse to assess the patient's condition. Home health care is frequently the only consistent medical contact that many patients in rural areas have. Without home health care these patients will be faced with the prospect of placement in long term care facilities. This creates another hardship for the patient as there are not enough long term care beds in rural areas to accommodate the population. This means that patients would have to be placed in facilities outside of their communities. The next nearest facility may be four hours or more from the patient's community. It is evident that HCFA does not care if this type of situation occurs. A spokesperson for HCFA said as much at a conference in Baltimore this past summer when presented with the above scenario. However, this type of placement is not in the best interests of the patient, as they will not have the benefit of familiar surroundings or their family/support system.

HCFA has put pressure on the fiscal intermediaries to decrease the money spent on home care. This is being done very effectively through the focused medical review process. This is almost a no-win situation for home health agencies. As an agency corrects paperwork problems that are pointed out by the FI, the FI finds "new problems" that were never addressed before. For example, denying a visit for placement of a PICC (peripherally inserted central catheter) line because the order did not read "*Skilled Nurse* to place PICC line," rather, it read, "Place PICC line." According to the FI the visit would have been "medically necessary," but was denied due to the verbage used in the order. HCFA has been clear in the past that disciplines must function within their scope of practice as outlined by their state credentialing boards. The only disciplines that are allowed to place a PICC line in the state of Nevada are registered nurses or physicians. With the shortage of physicians in rural areas, if a physician had the time to place a PICC line, he would do so in the office or hospital to gain the reimbursment. It is not a procedure that a nursing assistant, social worker or physical, speech or occupational therapist would be allowed to do.

This type of tactic makes it almost impossible to guess what will be targeted next by the FI. As the FI denies visits that have been done by the home health agency, it saves HCFA money while placing a financial burden on the agency delivering the care. Agencies must pay their staff for the care delivered to the patient, and incur increasing administrative costs to keep paperwork problems to a minimum.

The changes in Medicare are meant to decrease the overall number of home care agencies, which in turn is supposed to decrease fraud and abuse. In urban areas this may not be an adverse event. In rural areas this is extremely detrimental. Rural areas are medically under served as it is and HCFA will decrease the patient's health care options even further.

Respectfully submitted by,

Wanda F. Paisano, R.N., B.A.N.

Director of Professional Services

Home Health Services of Nevada, Inc.

Elko, Nevada

December 24, 1997

Attachment C

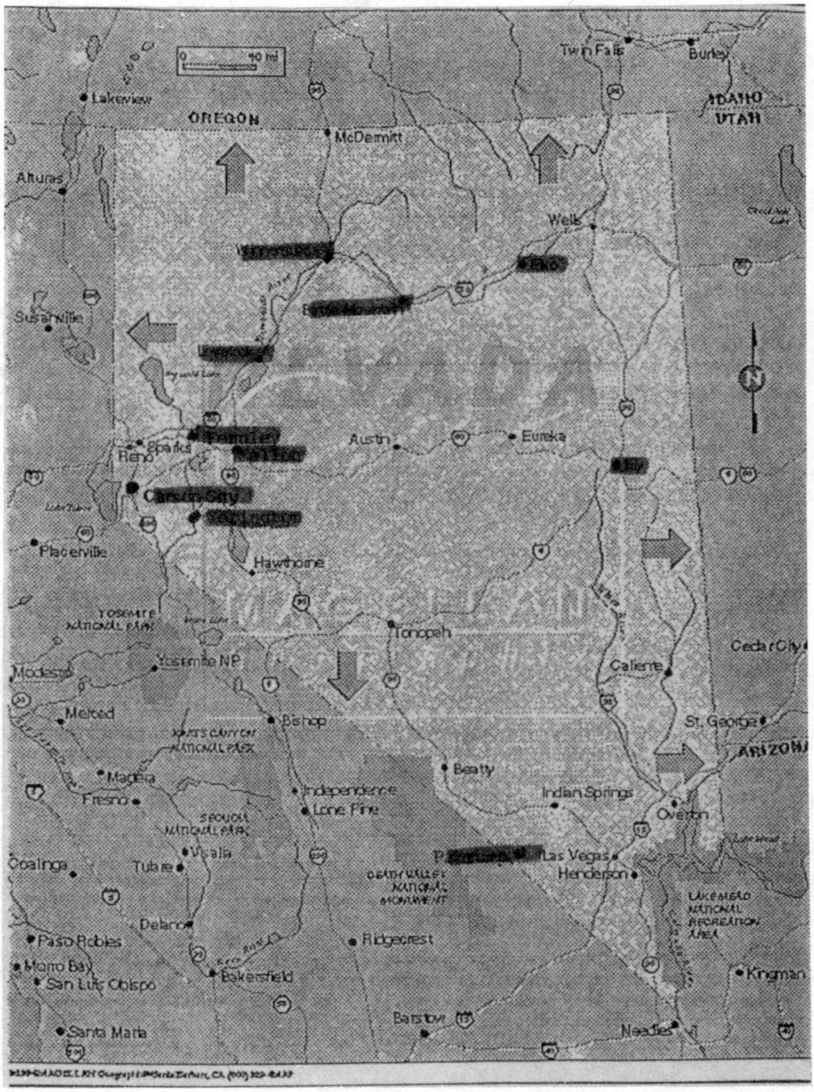

The locations of Home Health Services of Nevada's branch offices are highlighted.

Attachment D

THE BALANCED BUDGET ACT: HOME HEALTH BENEFICIARIES AT RISK

by
Ann B. Howard
Executive Director

As you know, Congress did not include a home health industry-initiated prospective payment system (PPS) proposal in the recently passed Balanced Budget Act (BBA) because the Health Care Financing Administration (HCFA) claimed that it could not implement it, especially within the timeframe specified.

During the course of the budget debate, the home health benefit came under a relentless barrage of negative publicity, including government studies, albeit flawed, and media reports alleging massive fraud, abuse, and overutilization. While there have been some providers who have abused the Medicare home health program, HCFA's exaggerated charges of fraud and abuse in the benefit have provided a fig leaf of legitimacy for punitive policies designed to ratchet down expenditures and eliminate providers from the program. The focus is on the bottom line, with no apparent consideration of whether or where disenfranchised home care patients will get care, or of the consequent cost of avoidable institutionalization for the American taxpayer.

Of all the negative provisions contained in the Balanced Budget Act, our paramount concern is the "interim payment system" which is effective for cost reporting periods beginning on or after October 1, 1997. Reimbursement rates are based on reasonable costs up to the lower of:

(1) cost limits reduced from 112 percent of the mean to 105 percent of the median, or

(2) an agency-specific per beneficiary cap based: (a) 75 percent on 98 percent of a provider's per patient cost of services in cost reporting periods ending in Federal Fiscal Year 1994, and (b) 25 percent on 98 percent of the regional average cost per home health patient in the base year.

The per patient cap, to be applied in the aggregate, will be based on old data from cost reporting periods ending from October 1, 1993 to September 30, 1994. For home health agencies without a 12-month cost reporting period ending in FY 1994, HCFA currently intends to set the beneficiary cap at the national median per patient cost during the base year. The legislative language does not require HCFA to apply a national rate. Newer providers in higher utilization states may be severely disadvantaged by such limits, while those in states with a low number of visits per patient will be handed a great competitive advantage.

This interim payment system is scheduled to remain in effect until HCFA develops and imposes a new PPS plan on October 1, 1999. But wait... if PPS is not ready, as mandated by Congress, HCFA will not suffer the consequences. The BBA stipulates an additional 15 percent reduction in home health reimbursement rates for FY 2000 if HCFA fails to meet its statutory obligation.

Beneficiaries with both the lowest and highest rates of utilization will be deprived of home care as a result of the Balanced Budget Act. Those who need only venipuncture services will no longer be eligible for the benefit as of February 5, 1998, while the sickest patients will find their access greatly restricted because the BBA will have the effect of reducing home health utilization to 1993-1994 levels.

It would appear that few home health agencies will be able to avail themselves of cost limits set at 105 percent of the median. They will be subject to the aggregate per patient cap instead. The Congressional Budget Office (CBO) scored the home health provisions at $16.1 billion in savings over Fiscal Years 1998-2002, starting with $1.5 billion in 1998. Congress was told that it was simply reducing the rate of growth of the benefit rather than cutting reimbursement from the current level of expenditures. If utilization rates are rolled back to 1993-1994 levels for the industry, this indeed will cause a significant reduction in visit levels and consequently in reimbursement.

Providers will find that they have to take drastic measures to bring their operations within their aggregate per patient limit. The very beneficiaries AFHHA sought to shield in the PPS plan -- and Congress said it wanted to protect -- are most at risk under the interim payment system. Many providers will be unable to accept the high intensity patients they have come to specialize in over the last four or five years. Taxpayers will end up paying more for institutionalization of vulnerable patients now being successfully cared for at home.

The Administration's opposition to the industry-initiated PPS plan, which was the only alternative on the table, is particularly troublesome because it would appear that HCFA knew all along that it could not implement the interim payment system by the effective dates or without massive disruption.

Now the home health industry faces administrative chaos, with new reimbursement methodologies and payment rates phasing in beginning October 1, 1997, when approximately 12 percent of providers moved onto the new system. These agencies know neither their per visit caps set at 105 percent of the median nor their agency-specific per beneficiary limit. What's more, they do not know which methodology will apply to them. The Balanced Budget Act does not require HCFA to develop caps at 105 percent of the median until January 1, 1998, or agency-specific per beneficiary limits until April 1, 1998.

HCFA may in fact be less able to implement the BBA provisions, which it vigorously sought, than the industry PPS proposal which it so adamantly opposed.

Anticipating a drumbeat for radical reimbursement changes, copayments, competitive bidding, and bundling, the industry did the responsible thing, working together for three years to develop a PPS proposal. Though the plan had flaws, it was a viable methodology and certainly preferable to the interim payment system we were finally handed by Congress.

A number of factors contributed in the end to the rejection of the proposal: relentless fraud and abuse reports emanating from HCFA, the General Accounting Office, and the Office of the Inspector General; dangerous rhetoric from home health agencies and associations seeking to advance specific policy proposals; and Congressional distrust of an industry which seems to be so distrustful of itself.

Ultimately, the discussion was never about older and disabled Americans and the value of the home health benefit in their lives. It was all about providers... and this is not the year of the provider.

AFHHA is currently analyzing HCFA databases and preparing a challenge to CBO's flawed scoring of the interim payment system, and also developing a legislative response to address the assault on the home health benefit.

* * * * * * *

47-539 98 - 13

HCFA NOT READY FOR INTERIM PAYMENT SYSTEM

by
Ann B. Howard

The information to follow is based on statements of HCFA officials at an October 3 meeting with representatives of the home health industry. You will note HCFA is uncertain about how it will implement the home health provisions of the Balanced Budget Act (BBA), though the new reimbursement system it so vigorously fought for went into effect for some providers on October 1, 1997.

Interim Payment System

* HCFA hopes to have per visit cost limits set at 105 percent of the median ready before January 1, 1998, the date mandated by the BBA. HCFA officials cannot give us any details on the methodology, for example, which outliers will be eliminated, since their actuaries are still working on these issues.

* HCFA also hopes to publish agency-specific per patient limits before April 1, 1998. Development of the new caps will require provision of additional, though currently unspecified, data from HHAs.

* HCFA believes that the BBA does not allow for any exceptions to lower reimbursement resulting from the new interim payment system. This means that an agency that has a more intense and high-tech case mix than it had in the base year -- causing it to exceed its new limits -- will not be granted an exception to the rates.

* The agency-specific per patient cap is based on a provider's unduplicated patient census. HCFA acknowledges a brewing problem based upon inconsistencies and inaccuracies in reporting a heretofore inconsequential, but now crucial, statistic. HCFA has not developed a process to sort out errors in reporting this critical number. A home health agency which counted admissions rather than unduplicated census will have an artificially low cap, with no apparent way to correct it.

* HCFA has not yet developed a methodology for tracking patients among home health agencies or for prorating payments under the per patient caps.

* Per patient limits will be calculated based on cost reporting periods ending in Federal fiscal year 1994 (from 10/01/93 to 09/30/94).

* Adjustments resulting from base year claims denials overturned by Administrative Law Judges and PRRB reversals of cost report disallowances will be calculated back into an agency's per patient caps.

* For newer providers and those without a 12 month cost reporting period ending in Federal fiscal year 1994, the beneficiary cap will be the <u>national median</u> per patient cost of home care services during the base year. The legislative language <u>does not require</u> HCFA to apply a national rate to newer HHAs. A national rate will create great distortions. Newer providers in higher utilization states may be severely disadvantaged by national limits, while those in states with a low number of visits per patient will be handed a great competitive advantage.

* For the purposes of calculating the 25 percent regional portion of the per beneficiary cap, HCFA could not tell us whether they will use census regions, HCFA regions, quadrants, or something else.

* Neither limits at 105 percent of the median nor per beneficiary caps will factor in cost increases which occurred between 1994 and 1996. The removal of two years worth of inflation makes the per patient cap, which does not reflect increases in utilization, even lower than it should otherwise be. The legislative language is ambiguous as to whether this provision applies to the per beneficiary cap, but it is no surprise that HCFA has determined that it does.

<u>Site of Service Billing</u>

* HHAs must bill for services based on where a patient resides rather than on the location of the agency for cost reporting periods beginning on or after October 1, 1997. HCFA is currently preparing instructions.

<u>Part A to Part B Transfer</u>

* The transfer of the bulk of the home health benefit to Part B, except for 100 visits following a three-day hospitalization, will entail some recordkeeping on the part of home health agencies. HCFA does not yet know what will be required and "hopes" that it will not be applied retroactively.

<u>Surety Bonds</u>

* HHAs must secure surety bonds of at least $50,000 by January 1, 1998. HCFA hopes to issue regulations by December 1. (Reports from knowledgeable sources indicate that HCFA is contemplating bonds equal to 15 percent of Medicare reimbursement.)

To avert a crisis for the home health industry, we believe that HCFA must:

* Publish its methodology and all calculations of limits set at 105 percent of the median for analysis by the home health industry.

* Have an outside objective entity attest to the validity of the methodologies and rates developed under the interim payment system.

* Develop an exceptions process for the new interim payment system.

* Use regional rather than national rates for calculating the per beneficiary cap for newer home health agencies.

* Hold providers harmless for not meeting requirements of the Balanced Budget Act, which HCFA itself is not prepared to implement. Provide a grace period after the effective date for HHAs to adjust their operations and develop new systems for reporting data to HCFA.

* Develop a process at the FI, HCFA regional, and HCFA central office levels through which HHAs can reconcile their records with the FI's, correct errors, and ensure that overturned disallowances are credited to their base year.

Attachment D.I

* **Suspend application of the new reimbursement system until all methodologies and reimbursement rates are developed and providers have been adequately notified.**

* * * * * * *

THE BAD NEWS INTERIM PAYMENT SYSTEM

based on writings by
Ted Sleight
AFHHA Treasurer

Under the interim payment system created by the Balanced Budget Act (BBA) for cost reporting periods beginning on or after October 1, 1997, home health agencies will be reimbursed the lower of:

1. reasonable costs incurred;
2. aggregate cost limits set at 105 percent of the median; or
3. agency-specific aggregate per beneficiary caps.

Currently, home health cost limits are set at 112 percent of the mean or average, and applied in the aggregate. In addition to reducing the caps to 105 percent of the median, Congress has added a per beneficiary cap. This new limit will have a very detrimental impact on home health agency operations and beneficiary access to services. HCFA will base reimbursement on an agency's average cost per beneficiary for cost reporting periods ending in FY 1994 (October 1, 1993, to September 30, 1994). A 75 percent weighting is given to this number, and 25 percent to the regional average per beneficiary cost in the base year. The two amounts are added, reduced by 2 percent (a provision added to achieve greater savings), then increased by the home health market basket for two (not four) years (approximately 1.07 percent). This represents an agency's per beneficiary limit. The provider multiplies this amount by the unduplicated census to calculate its maximum aggregate reimbursement.

The per beneficiary cap hurts providers who experienced growth in volume and costs since 1994 because of consumer and physician demand, expansion of the type and level of service they offer, and/or from opening new offices. Our computations indicate that these agencies will incur dramatic costs in reimbursement. One provider now $5 million under her cost limits anticipates she will exceed her new caps by $3 million. Another agency is looking at actual cuts of $6 million, approximately half of its billings for 1997.

Use of 1993 data for calculation of beneficiary caps represents a reduction of approximately 30 percent in utilization rates. In 1993, the average number of visits per beneficiary was approximately 56 visits; by 1996 the number of visits had increased to 79 per patient. Growth in the industry which occurred after the base year is thereby discounted.

<u>Sample Computation of Aggregate Per Beneficiary Cost Limits</u>

Assume that Provider A's actual cost per visit in 1993 was $60 per visit, based on an unduplicated census of 1,000 patients, and 60 visits per unduplicated census. In 1997, because of expansion and increased utilization as discussed above, the cost per visit has increased to $70 per visit, the patient census has increased to 1,200, and visits per unduplicated census has increased to 80 visits.

Under the base year, the per beneficiary cost limit would be $3,600. (Assumes that the provider-specific and the region averages are the same.) This amount, updated by the computation spelled out by HCFA, would be $3.775. However, based on the current cost per visit of the agency of $70 per visit, instead of providing the patient with 60 visits as in the base year, the agency would only be able to provide 48 visits ($3,775/$70 per visit).

Aggregate Effect

With the updated per beneficiary cost limit of $3.775, and an unduplicated census of 1,200 patients, the maximum reimbursement for this agency (assuming that the aggregate per beneficiary cap is the least of the three measurements) would be $4,524,000. In the most current year, based on the $70 per visit and 80 visits per patient, with unduplicated census of 1.2000, the actual costs incurred during 1997 would be approximately $6,720,000. This provider would be forced to cut $2,196,000 (or a 33 percent reduction) in expenses to meet the aggregate cost limits.

Tracking of Patients' Expenditures

Because of the way that the law is written, an agency must be very cautious in accepting a patient who has been in another agency's service within the year, since the per beneficiary cap is an aggregate expenditure to be shared among all agencies serving the patient. Upon admission, the provider may have to obtain financial information (from HCFA or the fiscal intermediary) regarding expenditures that have already been made on the patient's behalf. Ultimately, this will require agencies that have historically provided service to more critical patients to cut back on serving those beneficiaries. They will focus instead on patients who require a limited number of visits, and count on the unduplicated census. An agency will have to balance the low users with the high utilization so that the average expenditure per patient does not exceed the per beneficiary aggregate cap.

Where Does the Interim Payment System Lead?

Will we see a massive bidding war for those patients who need only one or two home health visits? Will hospitalized patients go to the hospital-based agencies, under pressure from administrators to keep them within the system so that more overhead can be shifted? Fewer agencies will be able to serve the intense, difficult, and high-cost patients, who will be:

* forced into nursing homes or other skilled facilities, at a significantly higher cost;
* readmitted to the hospital again at a significantly higher cost;
* forced to go without care, eventually requiring them to be hospitalized; or
* forced to pay for services out of their own pocket, if they can afford to.

Agencies have little time to prepare to implement the above changes, but in preparation, we should be educating our patients to the fact that Congress and the Administration:

1. are reducing the amount of home health services that we can provide to them; and
2. are in effect telling beneficiaries that the government would rather they received no services or else obtained care in a hospital or skilled nursing facility.

We will need to work with our legislative representatives and with our national organizations to start the ball rolling on getting this changed. Otherwise, we will have to cut patient services, employee jobs and benefits, and other expenses as well.

The BBA Calls for Payment Based on
Where Service Is Rendered

The BBA codifies HCFA's policy of paying HHAs on the basis of where visits are performed rather than on the location of the agencies. HHAs will have to track and report visits performed in different MSA and non-MSA areas and enter this information onto the cost report separately. Reimbursement rates will likely vary among MSAs. HHAs should perform an analysis of the changes in their reimbursement limits based upon where services are rendered, as well as on the interim payment system of the BBA.

(Please see Attachment #1 for HCFA's instructions to FIs for implementing the new payment system. See Attachment #2 for HCFA's home health rural and MSA codes.)

* * * * * * *

SURVIVAL TACTICS WITH IMPENDING INTERIM PAYMENT SYSTEM REDUCTIONS

by
Ted Sleight

The new interim payment system (IPS) which is to become effective on October 1, 1997, brings with it significant reimbursement reductions to all home health providers. In this short time before the plan takes effect, providers must examine the ways in which they do business, and identify areas of cost-savings that can be implemented to remain below the revised IPS cost limits. It is clear that HCFA wants the providers to focus on the six basic services, and is not willing to pay for other ancillary services.

Benjamin Franklin is credited with the following quotation:

> "There are two ways of being happy -- we may diminish our wants or augment our means -- either will do. The results are the same. It is for each man to decide for himself, and do that which happens to be the easiest.
>
> "But if you are wise, you will do both at the same time, young or old, rich or poor, sick or well, and if you are very wise you will do both in such a way to augment the general happiness of society."

Diminish Yours Wants

Following are a few suggestions that might be used to reduce a provider's individual cost per visit, avoiding cutting employees or wages until the very last.

* Many providers have used operating leases to provide computer equipment, furniture and fixtures, fax and phone systems, and photocopiers for their businesses. Many of these providers have opted for three-year useful lives on the equipment, with a fair market

buyout at the end of the lease, where the asset could, at the option of the provider, be purchased at the current value of the equipment. HCFA assigns a 10-year life to photocopiers, and 20 years to telephone systems. Computers are assigned a five-year life. The provider should examine all such leases and contemplated leases to lower the payments and still remain within the definition of an operating lease.

These criteria are:

1. The lease does not automatically transfer ownership of the asset at completion of lease term.
2. The lease period is less than 75 percent of estimated economic useful life.
3. Interest rate comparable to other borrowings.
4. Fair market buyout at the end of the period or the option to return the assets upon completion of the lease term (with no bargain purchase price -- i.e., a one-dollar buyout at the end of the lease).
5. Future minimum lease payments equal less than 90 percent of the fair value of the leased property at the inception of the lease.

* Providers in areas where managed care is abundant may consider converting their health care policy to a managed care program, which claims to reduce costs to the policyholder. The provider must weigh the effects on their employees of converting to a managed care policy. Will the savings outweigh the negative feelings of the employees in having to meet stricter criteria under managed care?

* With increasing premiums on health and dental insurance, many providers are opting for a partially or totally self-insured program, rather than a strict premium service.

* Reduction in "nice-to-haves" must be made. Those that are ancillary and not critical to the operations of the company will have to go. Providers can somewhat mitigate the effect of this action by out-sourcing such activities as continuing education and safety to specialized companies focusing on these areas.

* Even though management services companies are drawing fire right now, it may be advantageous to join forces with other providers, moving the overhead costs and direct costs of such areas as budgeting, finance, legal, regulatory compliance and reporting to a management services company. These services would then be billed to the individual companies on an as-needed basis, rather than each provider shouldering the entire cost for the full year. This would also allow for specialization, where for example an individual could develop expertise in cost reporting, while another handles the day to day operations of the general ledger. The key to this out-sourcing to a related party is that the provider cannot own more than 10 percent of the entity, or else the charges to the provider must be reduced to cost. Therefore, a provider would have to set up the management services group with a group of providers or unrelated entities to get to the less than 10 percent ownership.

* Consider withdrawing from HCFA studies in which your agency participates. Currently, providers under the OASIS program are participating in a study to measure patient outcomes. These providers entered into this program, knowing that they had sufficient cushion in their cost limits that additional costs incurred could be covered through the Medicare program. With reduced reimbursement, the provider may have to choose between participating in such programs and surviving as an entity.

* Eliminate equipment that is non-essential. This may mean that a lease for an automobile must be cancelled, with the provider paying the penalty fees for early termination, and any additional differences between the fair market value of the vehicle and the leased value as computed by the lease company.

* Providers are entering a phase where a make-do attitude must be adapted. This means that no longer will the provider be able to trade in fax machines every three years for newer technology. Instead, innovative ways of upgrading existing equipment must be explored to keep the provider from falling too far behind on the technology curve.

Augment Your Means

A provider must examine areas where growth or expansion may result in a reduction in their per-visit costs. HCFA is making this increasingly difficult, with rumblings about revisions in the interpretation related to branch offices, licensure, new Conditions of Participation, etc. A provider may have the ability to expand services to under-served or unserved areas while utilizing excess capacity (although I am not sure that any home health agency operates with excess capacity). The provider would need to identify its fixed and variable costs, and judge the increase in incremental costs that would be incurred by adding an additional visit, thus spreading the fixed costs over a larger number of visits. If the provider can increase visits without increasing fixed costs, then it will come out ahead.

Many providers are looking into acquisitions of other entities that have lower operating costs, adding volume to their business at a lower incremental cost. Providers must be weary of purchasing an agency, however, and examine all cost reports and documentation to ensure that no non-allowable costs are hidden in open cost reports. The provider must also look at the quality of the people and processes of the acquired entity, to ensure a proper fit of vision and purpose from the employees and management of the acquired company.

As discussed above, the formation of a management services company can also augment the means of an agency, through gaining access to other providers who might have individuals with expertise it needs. Since a service, such as defense of denials, has already been set up and paid for, implementing the defense program through the management services company would be more cost effective than developing one in-house.

Joining a network could provide similar results, but successful networks are relatively new to the industry. Texas has recently seen the establishment of a home health network, but the benefits are still to be seen.

Do Both

As Franklin noted:

> "But if you are wise, you will do both at the same time, young or old, rich or poor, sick or well, and if you are very wise you will do both in such a way to augment the general happiness of society."

If possible, providers must engage in both of these processes at the same time. If done properly, the outcome will augment the survival the provider, as well as the survival of the Medicare benefit and its continued availability to Medicare beneficiaries.

Ann Howard's cover letter.

January 13, 1997

Dr. Bruce Vladeck, Administrator
Health Care Financing Administration
314G Hubert H. Humphrey Building
200 Independence Ave. S.W.
Washington, D.C. 20201

Re.: Post Payment Statistical Sampling
Revision to Chapter X of Intermediary Manual No. 3 (Claims Process)
Comprehensive Medical Review (CMR) Procedures for Statistical Sampling and Projection of MR Results to the Claims Universe
Reference: BPO-B12

Dear Dr. Vladeck:

As Treasurer of the American Federation of Home Health Agencies (AFHHA), I am writing this letter is to express my concern about the current Health Care Financing Administration's proposal to implement post payment statistical sampling on home health agencies' activities. I recently reviewed the proposed HCFA regulations on statistical sampling and projection of the results to the claims universe. I received and reviewed a copy of a letter that Ms. Ann Howard, Executive Director of AFHHA wrote, addressing issues of AFHHA members with the implementation of post payment statistical sampling.

The use of statistical sampling is valid when used correctly and can provide a statistically valid projection of an error to the population tested. However, the incorrect application of statistical sampling, the incorrect evaluation of sampling results, or the incorrect projection of sampling errors to the claims universe can be detrimental, as well as expensive to both the Medicare Program and the home health care provider when subsequent costs of defending an incorrect audit finding are incurred.

Recent trade publication articles indicate that HCFA/OIG/ORT auditors are attempting to utilize statistical sampling in their Comprehensive Medical Review audits. However, the articles indicate that the auditors are not truly implementing statistical sampling as it is outlined in the proposed regulations (related to statistical sample selection, sample evaluation, etc.). Rather, it appears that the auditors are short-cutting the process, using the results of their pilot samples (which are intended to identify the coefficient of variation and determine the actual sample size), and are then projecting an error to the entire case universe based on the results of testing the pilot sample instead of the results of the proper sample.

Any mis-use of statistical sampling could have extremely adverse effects on providers who then must repudiate the findings in order to maintain their earned reimbursements for costs already incurred on behalf of the Medicare Program. My concern regarding the use of sampling is also heightened upon my increased awareness of sampling currently being used in other sectors of the health care industry, such as in the PATH (Physicians at Teaching Hospital) sampling. Based upon reports from trade publications, the sampling used in the PATH hospital Medicare Part B audits appears to mirror the proposed sampling methodology for home health.

My comments in this letter will reference three articles from separate trade publications (see attached Exhibits) which indicate that the sampling methodology set forth in the proposed regulations is not being followed.

Statistical Sampling Background and Training

For reference purposes, my background in sampling techniques is based upon twelve years of public accounting experience, and the hands-on use of statistical sampling with the international accounting firms of KPMG Peat Marwick and Grant Thornton. Both firms' statistical sampling programs were primarily developed by Mr. Stephen Yates who is a partner in the National Office of Grant Thornton. Mr. Yates is Grant Thornton's National Director of Advanced Audit Techniques, specializing in Quantitative Methods and Modeling. These statistical sampling programs were developed and tested under the respective accounting firms' quality assurance programs, and are supported by and based upon statistical theory. Mr. Yates has also consulted with me as to the content of this letter, and has provided information that has been included in this letter related to the use of statistical sampling.

Sampling Approaches Available

Basically, there are two different approaches to sampling that can be used to accomplish HCFA's goal to reduce the cost of audits while still obtaining an accurate estimate of overpayments or underpayments with relation to claims processing. The first approach, which has been adopted by the accounting profession, is hypothesis sampling. This sampling approach was adopted for use by public accounting firms because it fits better into their audit risk model, wherein the firms were trying to assess, measure and limit the risk that the audit samples were not statistically valid. This sampling methodology is tied to an understanding and reliance upon the internal control structure.

The second approach is known as estimation sampling. This method ignores the internal control systems of a provider, and "independently" estimates the amount of overpayment or underpayment in a given population. While this method is still statistically valid, it does not take into consideration the internal control structure of the provider, the internal control systems and their effectiveness, and other controls in place that could reduce the amount and scope of the audit sample. In reading the proposed revisions to Chapter X of the Intermediary Manual, since there is no reference to an evaluation of internal controls, it would be my assumption that HCFA is relying on estimation sampling in their testing. However, under Section 3940.2, HCFA attempts to target providers for CMR based upon an error rate in claims submission, problems with documentation, etc. In effect, HCFA is stratifying the population of providers through this selection of providers, and drawing the assumption that the internal control systems of the providers identified are either weak or non-existent.

Selection of a Statistical Sample

Probability of selection: To have a valid statistical sample, a probability sample must be used. As detailed in Section 3940.6, Part B, Definitions, Number 3, Sampling is defined as "... the process of sample selection which is random, but insures that each unit in the universe has a known nonzero probability of selection...." In other words, there must exist the possibility that each unit of measurement (claim, dollar, etc.) has a probability of being selected for testing (none of the population is excluded from the probability of being selected).

Number 6 of the Definitions Section indicates that samples may be stratified to segregate dissimilar items into sub-groups, but the probability still must exist for each unit to be selected. Stratification should be used "... whenever it is believed that it would help the precision of the estimate or whenever there is a need to ensure that certain classes of sampling units are appropriately represented...."

My understanding from the proposed regulations is that HCFA recommended the use of statistical sampling in order to be able to "measure" the sampling error. The use of a probability sample permits the measurement of this sampling error. If a probability sample has not been selected (the sample was judgmentally or haphazardly selected), then projection of the error from the sample is possible, but measurement of the sampling error (as defined under Number 13 in this section) is not possible.

Random sample selection: Based upon press reports, another perceived flaw in the sample selection process is the actual selection of the sample. As discussed above, a probability sample should be used when sampling in order to ensure that measurement of the sample results can be statistically validated.

The trade association publications report that the claims selected for testing may have already been identified prior to the auditor's arrival at the location based upon certain issues noted on the claims during the claims review process by the intermediary. If this is the situation, the sample is not random, as it has been skewed, and each unit of the claims universe no longer has a nonzero probability of being selected. Ultimately, the sampling process has been prejudiced and slanted to produce the desired results that the auditor seeks, but such skewing could invalidate the measurement of the results of the sampling.

In the proposed regulations, HCFA recommends the use of RAT-STAT or the use of a random number generator to select the sample items from the claims universe in order to avoid invalidating the sample measurability. Other methods used by public accounting firms include dollar-unit sampling or systematic interval sampling with a random number used to establish the starting point. Both of these methods still provide that there is a nonzero probability that any item would be selected.

The practice of the auditors as reported indicates that the proper use of these tools to select a true random sample may have not been followed in the performance of their audits.

Usefulness of the sample: One risk in selecting a small sample size is that the "usefulness" of the sample and the results may be limited (i.e. the desired tolerance level, precision and confidence interval may not be attainable). The size of the sample should be large enough to meet the users objectives.

For example, a random sample of 30 items could be selected from a claims universe of 100,000 claims. Once the sample had been tested, the results of the sample could be projected to the claims universe, and be statistically valid. However, the confidence level that the projection of the error was within one standard deviation would be extremely low. Statistically, the auditor might only be able to conclude that there is a 10% probability that the projected error is within one standard deviation of the actual error. Such a low measurement or probability of accuracy would render the sample useless, as the margin for error is too great.

In the aforementioned articles, there was no mention as to the tolerance level and confidence level in the results of the sample. The Health Care Financing Administration, in Section 3940.7, requires a 95% confidence level be attained in order for the errors to be projected to the population for overpayment and underpayment estimations. With such small samples as mentioned in these articles, and the large amount and range of overpayments projected, I would seriously question whether the confidence level of 95% was attained.

Exclusion of High Dollar Items from the Sample

Normally, under statistical sampling, if certain items in the population are considered above the scope of materiality, these items are excluded from the sample, and tested completely. Because these items are tested 100%, any items identified as errors are not projected to the population. The statistical sample would then be extracted from the remaining population, and tested for validity. Any errors within these statistically sampled items could be projected to the population, exclusive of the high dollar items previously tested. However, if the identified error exceeds the boundaries of the statistical sample (the tolerable error is too high), then the sample cannot be accepted and the error cannot be projected to the population within the confidence level required, thus rendering the results of the sample useless.

Again, based upon the reported cases, there has been no indication of the stratification of the selected samples, and whether any of the claims exceeded the tolerable error in amount. If any of the claims exceeded the tolerable error, any errors in that specific claim should not be projected to the population.

Sample Size Determination

The proposed regulations circulated by HCFA related to statistical sampling for comprehensive medical review indicate the method of determining the appropriate sample size, through a formula outlined in item F of Section 3940.6.

Section 3940.6, Item F-1, Determining Sample Size, states:

"The coefficient of variation (CV) plays an important part in determining sample size. The size of the sample is a function of the amount of the variation in the universe under investigation, in this case the amount of overpayments. The larger the range of overpayments, the larger the sample has to be in order to achieve an acceptable sampling error. Use the CV to determine the sample size for specified levels of sampling error. As stated in the definitions section above (Section 3940.6.B), you must determine the CV either from previous sampling experience or by conducting a pilot study. These sources may include:

-- Previous overpayment samples (e.g., sample reviewed to confirm existence of a problem);
-- Prepayment reviews resulting in payment denials. These an be used to determine the potential overpayment amount and the CV of the potential overpayment;"

"If you do not have access to previous data that can be used to establish the potential overpayment amount and the CV, then draw a pilot sample. All strata/or samples should have a minimum sample size of sixty unless you have had prior consultations with CO staff, or unless the whole universe of stratum has been used. (No other claims remain.) The cases should be drawn for the pilot using the same sampling procedures and time period to be used in drawing the full sample. The sample does not need to be stratified. This pilot sample can be part of the full sample (see Exhibit 4 for procedure)."

An initial "pilot sample" of a minimum size of 60 items should be used to identify the coefficient of variation or CV, in order to determine the sample size to achieve a 95% confidence level. After that initial pilot sample had been tested, the results would be used to calculate the coefficient of variation. Once the CV has been determined, this would then be used to calculate the initial sample size.

In his review of the proposed regulations, Mr. Stephen Yates of the international accounting firm of Grant Thornton noted:

"To apply estimation sampling, the user needs to know a fundamental characteristic of the population sampled; the standard deviation. Once the standard deviation is known, then a sample size can be calculated that might meet the requirements of the sample (relative to confidence and precision) application. Without software, etc., the most common way to determine the standard deviation of the underlying population is take a "pilot sample." The government regulations suggest sample sizes of 60 to 100 items."

Based upon 3940.6.F, HCFA intends for the samples that are selected to have a confidence level of 95%. For a non-stratified sample, the auditor would determine the sample size based upon the coefficient of variation, the universe size, the tolerance level (or tolerable error), and the factor of the standard error used to determine the confidence interval. In the example included in this part of Section 3940.6, item F, the universe is 1,000 claims, and the estimated overpayment was greater than $50,000. The resultant sample was determined to be 312 claims, which exceeded 5% of the total claims. Because the sample size exceeded 5% of the total population, the sample was adjusted to 238 claims through an additional formula, as outlined in Section 3940.6.

For a stratified sample, additional computational formulas are provided. The regulations indicate that no resulting sample stratum should have less than 60 items (which correlates with the minimum pilot sample size identified in the proposed regulations). The example presented in the proposed regulations indicate a total population of 3,000 claims, and computes an initial sample size of 562 claims, which again is more than 5% of the population. The adjusted sample, using the same stratum, was calculated to be 478 items.

The methodology proposed in the revision to the Intermediary Manual, Chapter X appears to be statistically valid, based upon the reading of the regulations and relying on my previous sampling experience. However, in both the case of Thomas Jefferson University Medical Center and First American Home Health of Pennsylvania, the total of the sample was 100 items for each of the providers.

The size of these samples would lead one to believe that only the pilot sample to identify CV was used, and the sampling process was short-cut, without the resultant sample size computed and tested as outlined in Section 3940.6.F. Mr. Yates reiterated this opinion, stating:

"The results of the "pilot" sample are supposed to be used to determine the ultimate sample size. It appears that the individuals doing the sampling are stopping after the pilot sample and are not going further."

Had the sample size computations been applied to the population, the initial sample used by the OIG should have been significantly higher than 100 items.

Sample Evaluation

Upon the completion of the testing of the sample, the auditor should then evaluate the sample. If the projected error exceeds the targeted tolerance level (as discussed in INT3 3940.7) and the upper limit (as determined during the sample design process), then the sample estimates cannot be considered satisfactory, and the regulations require the auditor to contact the Regional Office of HCFA or a statistical expert. Ultimately, either the confidence level would have to be reduced (which is not allowed in the proposed regulations), the sample increased, or it would be determined that the sample could not be relied upon, and additional means of testing must be implemented.

In the cases discussed above, when the error was projected to the population based upon the initial sample size of 100 claims, it is doubtful that the 95% confidence level was attained through the computations as called for in 3940.6.F. However, the articles do not state that the auditors' findings disclose the information as called for in Section 3940.4.E, which calls for, in part:

"...an explanation of the sampling methodology, i.e., a description of the universe, the frame, and sample design; a definition of the sampling units, decisions concerning the sample selection procedure; the numbers and definitions of the strata and size of the sample, including allocations if stratified, the time period under review; the sample results including both the estimate of overpayment and the calculated sampling error as estimated from the sample results, any nonsampling error factors that might affect the validity of the results, the actual overpayment and underpayment amounts and the amount of the extrapolated overpayment...."

In the case of First American Home Health of Pennsylvania, the auditors claimed an overpayment of between $2.4 million and $5.1 million. The projected error obviously exceeds the tolerance level, and no confidence level was discussed. Similarly, the October 7, 1996 issue of the Medicare Compliance Alert discusses the case of Thomas Jefferson University Medical Center in Philadelphia, where the auditor's sample of 100 claims resulted in a projected recovery of $12 million. While the Medicare Compliance Alert does not identify the number of claims in the population, it would be reasonable to assume that the hospital, during the six years that the sample results are being projected, had billed more than 2,000 Medicare Part B claims, and that 100 claims did not represent 5% of the population.

In my opinion, considering the factors discussed previously, the sampling results would not be useable, as the confidence level most likely was not attained. In one such case, Palmetto GBA has admitted to Eli Home Health Care, in its December 1, 1996 issue, that "the small samples used in its pilot sampling project are not statistically valid..." but that "it will push ahead with the project anyway...."

Unless HCFA, the OIG, ORT and their auditors conform to the statistical sampling methodology as outlined in the proposed revision to the Intermediary Manual, the projection of errors cannot be relied upon, and claims for overpayment should not and cannot be supported as being in compliance with the proposed regulations, and are thus invalid.

Projection of an Error from One Population to a Broader Population

In the Thomas Jefferson University Medical Center case, all sampled items were selected for testing from 1994. However, the OIG's third party auditor then projected the error identified from a pilot sample of 100 claims tested during 1994 to the population of Part B claims filed by the hospital from 1990 through 1996, and requested $12 million in payments back to the Program.

The time period covered by the above sample represented 1990 through 1996. This extensive of a time frame contradicts Section 3940.3, which indicates that the period for review should be between "4 months up to 1 year." The coverage of such an extended period of time makes many significant assumptions, including the assumption that there were no significant fluctuations in volume of billings, no changes to the billing processes, no changes in the regulations and processes and procedures involved in the Medicare Part B billing process, and also no changes in the company's systems of internal accounting controls during the time period covered by the audit.

Since the period covered in the auditors' projection of the error was six years, to be statistically valid, the claims universe should have been split into six individual claims universes, each representing no more than a year period. Proper statistical sampling would require a determination of the coefficient of variation and the materiality level involved for each of these claims universes, assuming that the level of claims fluctuated from year to year. Items should have been selected from each year for testing, with a projection of an error identified in each sample limited to the population of claims for that individual year.

Consequences of Erroneous Application of Sampling and their Effect on Providers

According to an article in the December 1, 1996 issue of Eli Home Health Care (Exhibit 1), referring to Palmetto GBA, the intermediary openly admitted that their "...pilot sample size was not large enough to be statistically valid...." However, the intermediary was "...going to use those small sample sizes...." anyway. This apparent disregard for proper utilization of statistical sampling leads one to question whether providers can be assured that proper statistical sampling is being used when subjected to a CMR. Similar disregard is also reflected in the case of the Pennsylvania operations of First American Home Health discussed in the December 2, 1996 issue of ...home health line (Exhibit 2), wherein the OIG sampled only 100 out of a possible 15,959 claims, and then projected the error rate of 19% to the total population, claiming that the fiscal intermediary had overpaid the provider between $2.4 million and $5.1 million.

The proposed changes to the Intermediary Manual circulated on September 4, 1996 by HCFA address the specifics of statistical sampling to be applied to post payment comprehensive medical review. Here again, I am concerned that the cases cited in the trade publications indicate that the statistical methodology which is spelled out in the proposed regulations are being ignored, with erroneous assumptions being used in projecting the error rate to the claims universe. Where this application of sampling is especially alarming is the requests made to the provider to repay the money that was supposedly overpaid.

What has not yet been mentioned, but looms as a similarly significant threat, is the forward projection of the error to future claims filed by a provider. The proposed regulations provide for an administrative review and appeals process which providers would use in appealing any post payment medical review process. However, current practice finds that fiscal intermediaries have been holding back reimbursements due to the providers based on prior cost report audit findings, even though administrative review and appeals are pending related to those audit findings. The intermediaries have indicated that these holdbacks are founded upon their responsibility to not overpay a provider if there is a risk that the money cannot be recouped.

Since providers are operating on a cost reimbursed basis, not only the retrospective but also the prospective withholding of reimbursement payments for services that have been already been delivered always will adversely affect the providers' ability continue to provide service to the qualifying Medicare beneficiaries, who require the care, and on the home health agency's ability to continue as a going concern. The withholding of funds due to the provider would require the provider to defer the payment for goods or services received from either its employees or vendors, all of which ultimately requires additional financing with increased interest costs to the Program.

In the worst case scenario, such erroneous use of statistical sampling could result in the closing of the providers' agencies. The discharging of patients from home health agencies, with many of the patients either going without service or entering more costly programs such as hospitals or skilled nursing facilities, again will increase the financial burden on the Medicare Program.

In order to maintain the integrity of the provider/fiscal intermediary/HCFA relationship, I would hope that proper audit tools, combined with proper and adequate planning and adequate training of qualified auditors, would be an integral part of the examination of the operations of the provider.

Summary

The application of post-payment statistical sampling will greatly affect the reimbursement of each and every provider on which sampling is applied, and therefore, I believe that HCFA has a responsibility to set forth in the public record the methodology used in its sample selection, the determination of an acceptable error rate and tolerable error, the identification of its confidence level on its sampling process, and other pertinent information as called for in Section 3940.4.

Additionally, HCFA must require the ORT, OIG and fiscal intermediary auditors to comply with the statistical sampling methodology as spelled out in its regulations. If these regulations are not followed, HCFA should only legitimately request repayment from the providers for the actual error noted, and not the error rate projected to the total population of the provider.

Under the current method of reimbursement, the implementation of the post-payment statistical sampling for Comprehensive Medical Review (CMR) would be detrimental if it is implemented by intermediaries with the attitude expressed by Palmetto GBA. There must be responsibility and accountability on the part of HCFA, OIG, ORT and the fiscal intermediary. If audit tools such as statistical sampling are to be used, they must be used properly with consideration to all aspects of the audit tests, and in accordance with generally accepted accounting principles.

I hope that you consider the ramifications of any auditor inappropriately using an audit tool to arrive at an audit conclusion. I am aware that, in the public accounting realm, there have been lawsuits resulting from inappropriate audit findings and conclusions drawn from the incorrect application of audit findings.
I would also hope that HCFA would strive for excellence by ensuring that HCFA and its agent organizations properly implement and utilize audit tools, and not mis-use or abuse any audit tools. The improper use of statistical sampling is not a healthy solution to maintaining the solvency of the Medicare Program.

I would be happy to discuss my opinions concerning the proper use of statistical sampling further with you.

Respectfully,

Ted A. Sleight, CPA
Treasurer

Attachments
Ted A. Sleight, CPA
Treasurer
American Federation of Home Health Agencies

The attachments are not included on the AFHHA website. For a copy of the attachments, contact Robert Raible, webermensch.

Main menu

AFHHA documents

A Measurement of Customer Satisfaction

The Gallup Organization

Summary of Key Findings

INTRODUCTION

In 1996, the American Health Care Association (AHCA) commissioned the Gallup Organization of Princeton, New Jersey, to conduct a customer satisfaction survey for the National Center for Assisted Living, the assisted living arm of AHCA. The purpose of this study was to measure customer satisfaction among residents of assisted living facilities.

Questions included in the survey were mutually agreed upon by the Gallup Organization, AHCA and Gustafson and Associates. Gustafson and Associates was responsible for providing the initial qualitative information that was utilized in the development of the questions for the quantitative survey developed by the Gallup Organization. Gallup was responsible for ensuring that the questions were technically correct and without bias.

METHODOLOGY

AHCA contacted 1,200 assisted living facility members to request their participation in a nationwide customer satisfaction survey of assisted living facilities. Facilities that chose to participate in the study comprised the database for this study.

From April through October 1996, 300 residents of assisted living facilities across the continental United States were interviewed by telephone. Gallup used a three-callback methodology in which up to three calls were made to the same telephone number to eliminate bias in favor of those individuals easily reached by telephone.

As part of Gallup's quality control procedure, 10 percent of all interviews was checked by supervisory personnel to ensure that data were accurate and properly procured.
All interviews were conducted in Gallup's communication facility by professionally trained interviewers under the exclusive employment of the Gallup Organization.

The maximum expected error range at the 95 percent confidence level for a study of 300 respondents is plus or minus 5.7 percentage points. Stated more simply, if 100 different samples of 300 residents of assisted living facilities were randomly chosen from the population, 95 times out of 100 the total results obtained would vary no more than plus or minus 5.7 percentage points from the results that would be obtained if the entire population of assisted living residents was surveyed.

OBJECTIVES

Primary objectives of the AHCA Customer Satisfaction Survey for assisted living residents included:

1. Design an instrument to measure overall customer satisfaction in assisted living facilities.

2. Determine the themes of service that drive perceptions of overall satisfaction, loyalty, quality, value and price in assisted living facilities.

3. Determine the specific satisfiers within the themes of service that lead to increased customer satisfaction and sustained customer loyalty.

OVERALL SATISFACTION

Americans are living longer and expect appropriate levels of care throughout the aging process. This will result in an unprecedented demand for all types of long term care services. As this area of consumerism grows and customer expectations increase and change, the need for a reliable, accountable and consistent system for assessing and communicating the quality of assisted living services will increase.

In the following sections, discussion and recommendations will be given as to where emphasis should be placed to raise the overall satisfaction rating among assisted living residents. These concepts provide general direction for action and the necessary steps to pursue positive assisted living business outcomes such as the ability to attract and retain residents. The key to increasing these outcomes is a focus on building positive customer perceptions of overall satisfaction, loyalty, quality, value and price.

KEY THEMES

As part of this research, assisted living residents' perceptions of overall satisfaction, quality, value, loyalty and price were measured. The following specific areas of service or *key themes* were shown to drive those perceptions:

Management: Management that is friendly and caring and that runs a well-organized and operational facility.

Relationships: Providing the right atmosphere for developing and maintaining good relationships.

Meals and Dining Arrangements: Providing good meals that meet dietary requirements and are served in a pleasant setting.

Residents' Rights: The facility being viewed as an advocate for its residents' rights.

Living Needs: The facility handling residents' daily living needs properly.

Facility Structure: Providing a well-maintained facility with a pleasant ambiance that is easy to get around in.

Staff: Providing a high-quality staff that makes every attempt to meet resident needs.

Assistance in Transition: Providing good advice and assistance when choosing and moving into the assisted living facility.

KEY DRIVERS OF SATISFACTION

Key drivers of customer satisfaction (satisfiers) were identified for some of the above themes. Satisfiers are those behaviors or characteristics that lead to increased customer satisfaction and sustained customer loyalty.

Management
- keeping the facility organized and operating well
- having enough managers
- managers hiring enough staff to serve residents well

Residents' Rights
- not moving a resident out of the facility when death is imminent
- providing appropriate care
- allowing a reduced rate if a resident is hospitalized

Facility Structure
- providing a place to entertain friends and family
- providing a nice place to walk outside
- having the temperature set for the resident's comfort, not the staff's

Staff
- being well-educated about the elderly
- being around the residents unobtrusively
- being professional

Assistance in Transition
- helping the resident adjust to the facility
- helping the resident make new friends

RECOMMENDATIONS

Levels of overall satisfaction can be increased through the quality of service in key areas as delivered in the day-to-day interaction with assisted living residents. The research and analysis clearly show that for residents of assisted living facilities, the following should be emphasized:

- Provide an administration and management that are friendly and caring and that run a well-managed facility.
- Provide the right atmosphere for developing and maintaining good relationships with other residents.
- Provide good meals that meet residents' dietary needs and are served in a pleasant setting.
- Help residents handle their daily living needs properly.
- Provide a facility that has a pleasant ambiance, is easy to get around in, and is well maintained.
- Provide a high quality staff who make every attempt to meet the residents' needs.
- Provide good advice and assistance when choosing and moving into an assisted living facility.

A consistent focus in these areas is likely to result in the upward movement of overall satisfaction. The key to increasing perceptions of overall satisfaction, loyalty, quality, value and price is the relationships established between the residents, the management and the staff of the facility, and the responsiveness given to the residents' concerns and needs in these areas.

© 1997 The American Health Care Association

Federal Funds Supplement Assisted Living

States remain tentative in providing public funds for assisted living communities.

MARKIAN HAWRYLUK

The federal supplemental security income (SSI) program, which provides additional funds to low-income elderly and blind or disabled individuals, is becoming a growing source of funding for assisted living services.

States are finding that by supplementing the federal SSI benefit and combining it with Medicaid funds, they can reduce their overall Medicaid costs and provide a popular long term care option to low-income beneficiaries.

At the same time, states are wary of creating new entitlement programs. Many states have placed strict limits on their assisted living funding exposure. As a result, SSI payments account for only a fraction of assisted living funding today.

While states have had great flexibility in offering supplemented SSI funding for assisted living, states may use Medicaid funds only by obtaining a home- and community-based services waiver from the federal government. The Balanced Budget Act of 1997, however, streamlined the federal approval process for these waivers. As a result, states are expected to find the SSI-Medicaid option a lot more attractive.

Reviewing The Numbers

The maximum federal SSI payment to an individual in 1996 was $484 a month for an individual or $726 for a couple.

In 1996, 6.6 million individuals received a total of $24 billion in SSI payments. States also have the option of adding to the federal SSI contribution by providing state supplemental payments (SSPs). In 1996, the 6.6 million SSI recipients also received $3 billion in SSPs.

States also have the option of creating specific SSP levels for a variety of living arrangements, including assisted living. In 1996, 44 states were providing optional supplementation, including 38 that provided SSPs specifically for assisted living, according to a Social Security Administration report on SSP.

Nevertheless, public funding of assisted living services remains only a small percentage of the assisted living market. While a majority of states offer SSP funding for assisted living, the actual number of dollars being spent by states remains limited.

According to the American Health Care Association (AHCA) 1996 assisted living survey, only 40 percent of facilities had residents that received state reimbursement for assisted living services. Nationwide, less than 7 percent of assisted living residents received SSI payments, and less than 9 percent received Medicaid payments.

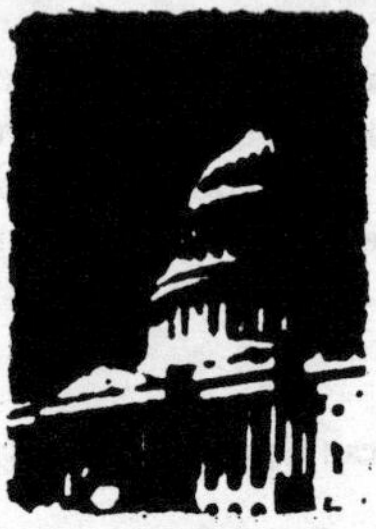

It is likely that there is a substantial overlap between the groups, the survey said. According to the Social Security Administration, slightly more than 250,000 individuals received SSI benefits under a state-sponsored assisted living arrangement.

Of the 38 states that have specific payment levels for assisted living, almost all have increased the maximum payment level since initiating the assisted living payment category. In 1995 maximum SSP payment levels ranged from $94 a month in Montana to $987 in Minnesota.

States have substantial leeway in defining the conditions and terms under which payments are made for each living arrangement under SSI. States can also tailor the living arrangement to a certain group of SSI recipients, such as the elderly. States commonly create a special category of SSP payments for residents of assisted living centers that relies on SSI and SSP to pay for room and board and on Medicaid to fund care services.

In Florida, for example, the SSI-SSP combination provides $586 a month for room and board, while the facility receives $750 a month for care services, for a total of $1,336.

In Massachusetts, the state's Division of Medical Assistance created a Group Adult Foster Care program under Medicaid to finance assisted living services. The SSI-SSP monthly payment totaled $575 in 1994 and was not considered adequate to cover the room-and-board component of assisted living. The Department of Transitional Assistance then created a separate SSI payment level for assisted living, providing up to $900 a month, and combined it with the Medicaid adult foster care payment of $1,020 a month, for a total of $1,920 a month for an assisted living resident. The program, however, was terminated in January 1995 until an analysis of the budgetary impact of the program could be completed.

Earlier this year, the Massachusetts legislature voted to fund the Department of Transitional Assistance to reinstate the SSI benefit category for assisted living in fiscal year 1998, which began July 1,

1997. The state is now working on the regulations needed for individuals to apply for this program, which are expected to take effect Jan. 1, 1998.

Like many other states, Massachusetts has set limits on its assisted living program. Although Medicaid spending has slowed over the past two years, state policymakers can still remember the double-digit growth in the program that ate up huge chunks of state budgets, says Steve Roizen, chief executive officer of The Whitney Place in Natick, Mass., and a member of the AHCA Assisted Living Committee. The assisted living option was created to help control Medicaid costs. Even with the federal SSI payment, policymakers were worried about creating a new entitlement.

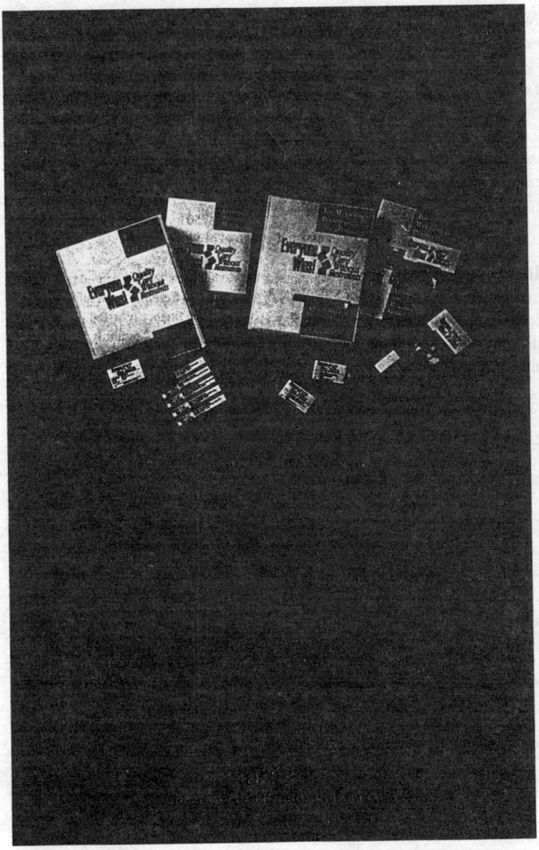

"The states are concerned about what this is going to do with the shift of demographics," Roizen says. "There is no certificate-of-need program for assisted living [in Massachusetts]. If you open this up to everybody that is eligible, you could have hoards of people."

Other states have created similar controls. Minnesota capped its payment for medical services at the state's share of the average monthly nursing facility payment for a particular case-mix classification. In fiscal year 1997, for example, the SSI and SSP payments totaled $589 a month, while service rates were capped at $654 a month to $1,519 a month, depending on case mix.

Using Program To Extend Benefits

While many states have looked to SSI and assisted living as a cost saver, others have seen SSI as a way to extend a long term care benefit to a low-income population. Iowa, which currently has no public funding for assisted living services, had been considering seeking a home- and community-based waiver to provide that option to those who cannot afford it.

"I think it's more what I would classify as a liberal approach that says that the whole concept of assisted living should be available to everybody," says Michael Hamm, administrator of the Hawkeye Care Centers in West Des Moines, Iowa, and a member of the AHCA Assisted Living Committee.

The push for public funding in the state, he says, has come from the Department of Elder Affairs, which he describes as having more of an advocacy-type mission, rather than the Department of Human Services, which provides oversight.

Assisted living has remained relatively regulation-free, allowing the residence to create a more homelike environment that appeals to consumers. While SSI and Medicaid payments may open the door to assisted living for many more low-income individuals, many believe public funding could also lead to increased regulation. ■

ncal
NATIONAL CENTER FOR ASSISTED LIVING

1201 L Street, NW
Washington, DC 20005-4014
Phone: 202-842-4444
FAX: 202-842-3860

ASSISTED LIVING

MEETING THE NEEDS OF A GROWING ELDERLY POPULATION

Fact: *The average ancient Greek lived until 18. The median life span of a Puritan was 33.*[1] *In 1991, the average life expectancy of an American male was 71.8 years and 78.9 years for females.*[2]

Fact: *In 1994, about one in eight Americans was age 65 and older. By 2030, one in five Americans will be a senior citizen.*[3]

Fact: *In 1994, 7.3 million Americans needed long term care services. By 2000, this number will rise to 9 million, and skyrocket to as many as 24 million by 2060.*[4]

INTRODUCTION

A combination of extended life expectancy and the graying of America is resulting in an unprecedented demand for a variety of long term care services.

A rapidly growing industry known as "assisted living" has emerged on the long term care spectrum between boarding houses for the elderly (where services are limited to housing) and skilled nursing facilities (which offer complex medical care).

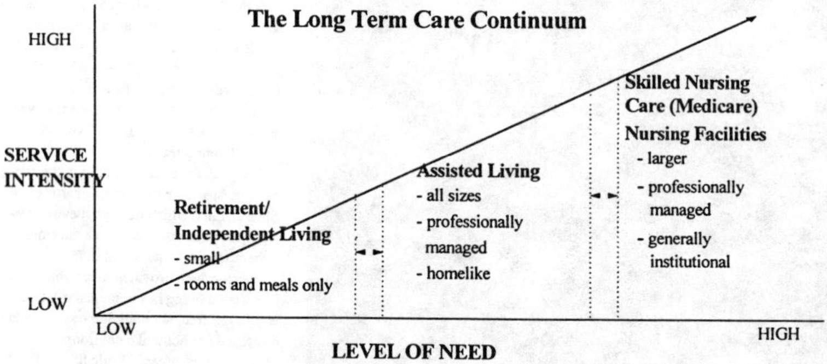

© 1997 by the National Center for Assisted Living

NCAL is the assisted living arm of the American Health Care Association, a federation of 50 affiliated associations representing more than 11,000 non-profit and for-profit assisted living, nursing facility and subacute providers nationally.

Based on a Scandinavian model for senior living, assisted living first emerged in America during the mid-1980s. The concept of assisted living is still so new that the businesses that offer it and the states that license it do not agree on a precise definition or name for assisted living.

Throughout the United States, assisted living is known by as many as 26 different names. Some of the most common are "residential care," "personal care," "congregate care" and "board and care."

In general, assisted living is not a substitute for, but a complement to, nursing facility care. Assisted living combines housing, personal services and light medical or nursing care in an environment that promotes maximum individual independence, privacy and choice. While assisted living residents may be too frail to live alone, they are too healthy to need most of the nursing services provided in a nursing facility. Assisted living residents share the risks and responsibilities for their daily activities and well-being with a residence staff geared to helping them enjoy the freedom and independence of private living.

Assisted living residences are not bound by federal regulation, which helps to keep costs down, as does the fact that assisted living residences generally do not offer the high-tech medical services available in nursing facilities. Whether proprietary or non-profit, assisted living residences serve mostly a private-pay clientele; therefore, consumer demand, not government mandate, is driving the industry's development in America.[5]

THE ASSISTED LIVING PHILOSOPHY

The philosophy of assisted living is to provide or arrange for supervision, assistance and limited health care services to relatively healthy senior citizens when needed. Residents can receive help with an array of personal activities, including: eating, dressing, bathing, transferring and toiletting, as well as meal preparation, laundry, housekeeping, recreation and transportation. While assisted living residences typically do not provide 24-hour skilled nursing care, help with daily tasks may include the supervision of medication by a qualified staff person.

The philosophy also emphasizes the right of the individual to choose the setting for care and services. The American Health Care Association's National Center for Assisted Living (NCAL) believes residents' rights should include the right to:

- Privacy
- Be treated at all times with dignity and respect
- Control personal finances
- Retain and have use of personal possessions
- Interact freely with others both within the home and in the community
- Practice religion or abstain from religious practice
- Control receipt of health-related services
- Be free from abuse and neglect

In the *1997 Facts and Trends: Assisted Living Sourcebook*, results of a NCAL national survey found residences had adopted policies addressing specific issues that many residents view as personal rights. Most residences placed no restrictions on visitors during the day, while 47 percent of the facilities allowed residents to have overnight guests.[6]

© 1997 by the National Center for Assisted Living

The survey also found that a majority of residences (70 percent) allowed the use of tobacco and (47 percent) the consumption of alcohol.

Consistent with the varying policies found in apartment living, the NCAL survey found 33 percent of residences allowed residents to keep small pets. Another 37 percent provided residence-owned pets for all residents to enjoy.

ASSISTED LIVING FACTS

- **Number of Residences** -- The absence of a common definition for assisted living makes it difficult to pinpoint the number of residences in the United States. Past studies put the range between 40,000 and 65,000 residences, housing up to one million people.[7] However, recent analyses by NCAL indicate that the number of assisted living residences is probably closer to 25,000, and that there are approximately 800,000 people living in those residences.

- **Resident Profile** -- The "typical" assisted living resident is an 82-year-old woman who is mobile, but needs assistance with one or two personal activities. Although most elderly assisted living residents are female, due to women's longer life expectancies, 29 percent are male. The "average" age of elderly residents, women and men combined, is 82 years according to NCAL's survey.

  The survey also found that while nearly one-third (31 percent) of all residents needed no help taking care of their own personal activities, others did in varying degrees. On average, assisted living residents needed help with 1.6 common personal activities.

Personal Activities	Independent	Some Help	Dependent
Bathing	34%	49%	17%
Dressing	58%	30%	12%
Transferring	78%	15%	7%
Toiletting	84%	10%	6%
Eating	88%	8%	4%

NCAL's survey also found a full 65 percent of assisted living residents needed or accepted help with housework, while 49 percent needed or accepted help with their daily medication.

Residents stay in assisted living residences an average of 3.3 years, and arrive from a variety of settings, according to the NCAL survey.

- 59 percent moved from their homes
- 14 percent came from a nursing facility
- 11 percent came from another assisted living residence
- 11 percent came from hospitals
- 5 percent came from other settings

© 1997 by the National Center for Assisted Living

Conversely, as needs change, elderly people leave assisted living residences. The NCAL survey found that a majority of residents left their assisted living homes because they needed a higher level of medical care.

- 14 percent returned to their homes
- 45 percent went to a nursing facility
- 12 percent went to another assisted living residence
- 11 percent went to a hospital
- 16 percent died
- 3 percent went to other settings

- **Costs** -- Costs for assisted living residences vary greatly and depend on the size of units, services provided and location. The NCAL survey found that 52 percent of all assisted living facilities charge between $1,001 and $2,000 in average monthly rent and fees. Another 20 percent charge between $2,001 and $3,000 and 4 percent charge more than $3,000 each month. A full 24 percent charge less than $1,000, with less than 1 percent charging under $500 per month.

DESIGN AND SERVICES

Assisted living services can be provided in free-standing facilities, near to or integrated with skilled nursing facilities, as components of continuing care retirement communities, or at independent housing complexes.

The NCAL survey found that residents typically can choose furnished or unfurnished studio or one-bedroom units with a private bathroom, though shared bathrooms are quite common. Living units can be shared with another individual. Assisted living residences can range from a high-rise apartment building to a three-story home.

The average size of an assisted living residence is 32 units. NCAL's survey found that 27 percent of residences had kitchenettes and another 14 percent offered full kitchens. Expansive common areas are typical of assisted living residences.

Because assisted living is an evolving long term care industry, the range of services offered by residences is wide. However, some generalizations can be made. Assisted living residences typically offer:

- 24-hour protective oversight and emergency response system
- Three meals a day plus snacks in a group dining room
- The provision and/or coordination of a range of services that promote resident quality of life, including:
  - Personal care, such as help with eating, bathing, dressing, and toiletting
  - Limited health care
  - Provision and/or coordination of required social services
  - Supervision and oversight for persons with cognitive disabilities
  - Social and religious activities

© 1997 by the National Center for Assisted Living

- Exercise and educational activities
- Transportation
- Laundry and linen service
- Housekeeping and maintenance

Assisted living residences generally offer more than basic services. Popular amenities can be available on site, particularly in larger assisted living residences. According to American Association of Retired Persons, a sampling of the various amenities offered includes: libraries; recreation rooms, sometimes with exercise equipment or pool table; cafes and shops; beauty parlors; and chapels.[(8)]

SERVICE AND STAFFING

When first arriving at an assisted living residence, each resident receives an individualized assessment to determine how the residence's services best can serve his/her needs. This service plan includes an assessment of the individual's physical and psychosocial capabilities. The individual, family, or a responsible party usually assists with the development of the service plan, which is reviewed and updated as needed.

Assisted living residences offer supervision and oversight of individuals with physical and mental impairments. Generally, assisted living residences adopt a philosophy of "aging in place" that allows individuals to remain at the residence as long as they are able to be supervised and maintained by the residence's staff.

The number and type of staff employed by assisted living residences varies greatly and depends on a number of factors, including state regulations, the number of people living in the residence and residents' service requirements.

Assisted living residences employ staff members directly or contract for services with outside providers. A residence staff may include: personal care attendants, nurses, activities coordinators, food service managers, administrators and maintenance personnel. Contract services frequently include: podiatrists, nutritionists, physical therapists, beauticians and physicians.[(9)]

LICENSURE AND REGULATION

Assisted living residences are not defined or regulated by the federal government. In the absence of federal regulations, most providers are subject to state and local laws. The NCAL survey found most assisted living residences (96 percent) were licensed by the states in which they operate. Residential care is the most common licensure term, followed by assisted living. But regulations between states vary regardless of the licensure term. As a result, competition between providers has become the catalyst for establishing levels of service, controlling costs, and maintaining a high quality of care.

WHO PAYS?

About 90 percent of assisted living services are paid for with private funds, making this market highly sensitive to economic forces.

© 1997 by the National Center for Assisted Living

The Supplementary Security Income, Older Americans Act, and Social Services Block Grant programs pay for some assisted living services, while about 22 states allow the federal Medicaid program to pay for some service components. States have the option to pay for assisted living under the Medicaid program by:

Including the services in the state's Medicaid plan. The Health Care Financing Administration (HCFA) has proposed expanding the Medicaid program to allow states to reimburse for personal care services in a variety of settings, other than the home, which may include assisted living residences.

Petitioning the Department of Health and Human Services for a home- and community-based services waiver under Medicaid. Several states are experimenting with expanding the availability of assisted living services through these waivers.

Other important funding facts to consider:

Assisted living is covered as an "alternative care benefit" in a growing number of long term care insurance policies. Since most elderly Americans do not carry long term care insurance, the majority of people in assisted living residences and/or their families still pay for the care themselves.[10]

Medicare does not pay for assisted living services under any circumstance. Medicare is limited to the provision of short-term, acute care for the elderly.

Managed care is not a significant factor in assisted living currently. According to the 1996 NCAL survey, 5 percent of assisted living residents pay for their care through a managed care program. However, as managed care grows and searches for lower cost alternatives, it is likely to play an increasing role in assisted living.

CONCLUSION

The scope of long term care services offered to the growing number of elderly Americans is ever-expanding. Assisted living, a relatively new and widely popular phenomenon, is on the forefront of this expansion, offering elderly clientele an attractive mixture of independence and personal care.

October 1997

© 1997 by the National Center for Assisted Living

SOURCES

(1) Williams, Doris K. Residential Care Services for the Elderly: Business Guide for Home-Based Eldercare 1991; 1.

(2) Frank B. Hobbs and Bonnie L. Damon. 65+ in the United States, U.S. Bureau of the Census. Current Population Reports, Special Studies, 3-1

(3) Ibid., 2-2

(4) U. S. Bureau of the Census. Statistical Abstract of the United States: 1995

(5) Kane, Rosalie A. and Karen Brown Wilson. Assisted Living in the United States: A New Paradigm for Residential Care for Frail Older Persons? 1993; preface.

(6) American Health Care Association's National Center for Assisted Living. 1997 Facts and Trends: The Assisted Living Sourcebook

(7) Lewin-ICF, Inc. Policy Synthesis on Assisted Living for the Frail Elderly November 9, 1992, II-2.

(8) Assisted Living in the United States, 21.

(9) Ibid., 30.

(10) "Assisted Living: New Thinking, New Model for Frail Elderly" Report on Long Term Care February 23, 1994.

© 1997 by the National Center for Assisted Living

Field Hearing of The
U.S. Senate Special Committee on Aging
Testimony Submitted By:
Michael Girard, Administrator Washoe Home Care
January 13, 1998
Reno Nevada

The Promise of Home Care:

There have been a number of studies and programs that have demonstrated that home care is a high quality cost effective alternative to institutional long term and chronic care.

- P.A.C.E programs have demonstrated that an expanded use of home care services, especially nurse aide and home maker services in conjunction with home based community case management can dramatically reduce total health care costs by reducing the utilization of hospital and nursing home costs.
- A case study of Indiana's In-Home/CHOICE Program conducted by the Hudson Institute, a conservative public policy research organization found that a broader use of home care unconstrained by the Medical model limitations traditionally employed by Medicare and Medicaid is cost effective and reduces high cost institutional care.
- In Nevada CHIP's a Medicaid waiver program is also demonstrating that expanding home care services beyond the Medicare skilled and intermittent model can prevent or delay institutional placement at a lower cost with increased patient satisfaction.
- The November 1995, New England Journal of Medicine published a study which concluded that a nurse-directed , multidisciplinary intervention consisting of comprehensive education of patients and families reduced hospital readmission rates and cost by $460 per patient.
- Nationally, statistical evidence reflects that as home health utilization has increased, Nursing Home Bed utilization has leveled off and even decreased.

These are but a few examples of how the creative expansion of home care utilization can reduce the social, commercial and personal costs of long term care. Not to mention that "home is where the heart is" and where patients and families want to be and stay.

In the greater Reno /Sparks area home health care of all types is greatly under utilized when compared to national statistics. Nationally approximately 10.4% of Medicare beneficiaries receive home health services and those patients receives approximately 76 visits. In Reno/Sparks approximately 7% of the Medicare beneficiaries receive home care services and those patients receive an average of 41 visits each. In other words, in the Reno/Sparks area approximately home care serves 33% fewer patient than the national average and those patients that do receive home care get 46% fewer visits than the national average.

Correspondingly, through reviews conducted by the health care actuarial and consulting firm of Milliman and Robertson on behalf of Washoe Health Systems it has been identified that there is an inordinately high incidence of rehospitalizations ond long term care utilization. Milliman and Robertson correlated these statistics with the low utilization of home care. Milliman and Robertson suggested that an appropriate and focused increase in home care utilization could reduce rehospitalizations and long term care while reducing total health care costs.

Obviously the expansion of the current paradigms of home care interventions can be a cost effective solution to our areas long term care challenges. However, the expansion of new paradigms represented by programs such as PACE, In Home/CHOICE and CHIPS can take the role of home care in solving long term care challenges even further.

Field Hearing of The
U.S. Senate Special Committee on Aging
Testimony Submitted By:
Michael Girard, Administrator Washoe Home Care
January 13, 1998
Reno Nevada

Home Care under the Balanced Budget Act:

Ironically, in spite of demonstrated high quality, high patient and family preference and satisfaction and cost efficiency the Balanced Budget Act of 1997 has taken home care in Northern Nevada a giant step backwards. The Balanced Budget Act represents a knee jerk over- reaction to incidences of fraud and abuse in home care that has rewarded the unethical high over-utilizers and penalized the responsible providers. In response to these incidences of fraud and abuse and over utilization congress passed a new home care interim payment system which was hastily devised based on preliminary HCFA projections. The new interim payment system was intended to reduce home care spending by$16.1 billion over five years. Now that HCFA has had more time, their latest projections indicate that their earlier projections were in error. The savings appear to have been under estimated by 125% . HCFA further admits that this estimate may still go up. Other estimates project the savings to be in excess of 250% and project savings of $40 billion instead of the intended target or $16 billion.

Tragically, it is further projected that 75% of the home health agencies currently have costs in excess of the limits imposed by the budget cuts. It is further projected that thousands of home health agencies will fail financially and close their doors. Ironically, the agencies facing bankruptcy are the good guys. These are the agencies that have operated honestly and did not over utilize services. These are the type of agencies that are in Reno and northern Nevada.

The Interim Payment System largely generates its cost savings by basing payments on 1993 utilization patterns. Agencies will have their payment limited based on the average number of visits it provided to patients in 1993. This method was chosen because it was felt that much of the fraud and abuse occurring in home care occurred by providing more visits than were necessary. Additionally, there was a significant growth in the number of visits per patient from 1993 to the present.

The reason this is a problem for home health agencies in Reno and northern Nevada is that this region of the country under utilized home care in 1993 and still does! Compared to the national average 30% fewer people receive home care services and those that do receive services receive 47% fewer visits. The evolution of the appropriate role of home care has occurred at different rates of speed and sophistication in different parts of the nation. The appropriate role of home care is to reduce health care costs. This is achieved by transferring the provision of care that from an institutional setting to the home. This transition requires medical communities to change from the comfort and security of caring for patients in a controlled environment to caring for patients in what is perceived as an uncontrolled environment. For these and other reasons Reno and northern Nevada served far fewer patients with home health and provided fewer visits to those patients than the rest of the country.

With the emergence of managed care in the Reno area the appropriate use of home care is just now being understood. It has been recognized that Reno experiences a higher than normal rate of re-hospitalizations and long term care utilization. It is beginning to be recognized that home care can reduce these two incidences and reduce health care costs. This means that more people will utilize home care and that some of them will need more visits. However, with the Balanced Budget Acts' Interim Payment System limiting home care to the archaic paradigm of 1993 utilization patterns the citizens of Reno have been sentenced to increased hospitalizations, re-hospitalizations and premature long term care placement at greater cost and suffering to themselves and society.

STATE OF NEVADA
DEPARTMENT OF HUMAN RESOURCES
DIVISION FOR AGING SERVICES
340 N. 11th Street, Suite 203
Las Vegas, Nevada 89101
(702) 486-3545 • Fax: (702) 486-3572

BOB MILLER
Governor

CHARLOTTE CRAWFORD
Director

CARLA SLOAN
Administrator

ADDRESS REPLY TO:

☐ ADMINISTRATIVE OFFICE
Mailing Address:
State Mail Room Complex
Las Vegas, Nevada 89158
(702) 486-3545
Fax: 486-3572

☐ 1665 Hot Springs Road
Suite 158
Carson City, Nevada 89710
(702) 687-4210
Fax: 687-4264

☐ 445 Apple Street
Suite 104
Reno, Nevada 89502
(702) 688-2964
Fax: 688-2969

☐ 850 Elm Street
Elko, Nevada 89801
(702) 738-1966
Fax: 753-8543

MEMORANDUM

DATE: February 24, 1998

TO: U.S. Senate Special Committee on Aging
Angela Hill, Hearing Clerk

FAX: (202) 224-8664

FROM: Carla Sloan, Administrator

SUBJECT: Response to Nevada Field Hearing Written Questions

Two written questions were forwarded to me by the Committee for reply following the Senate Special Committee on Aging Nevada Field Hearings held in January 1998. Response is as follows:

1. What is available for seniors who do not need skilled nursing care but require help and cannot afford the $125.00 a day charged by a private agency. I do have long term care insurance, but what happens in the interim?

Seniors capable of remaining in their own home with assistance in Nevada may be able to receive help through one of the following programs:

- Community Home-Based Initiatives Program (CHIP) – This program is a Medicaid waiver program administered by the Nevada Division for Aging Services. The target population includes persons age 65 and older who meet income and asset requirement, and who are at risk of institutionalization if services are not provided. Possible services include adult day care, respite care, personal care such as bathing and dressing, and homemaker services such as light housekeeping and meal preparation. Cost is based on the participant's ability to pay. There are income eligibility requirements for the program. To identify the Aging Services office in your area, call the Eldercare Helpline, 1-800-243-3638.

- Homemaker Program -- This program is administered by the Nevada Division for Health Care Financing and Policy. Persons living in the community who receive Medicaid to assist with their medical expenses may also be eligible for homemaker services which may include shopping, laundry, etc. The Eldercare Helpline, 1-800-243-3538, can help you to understand Medicaid eligibility requirements and/or refer you to the appropriate local Health Care Financing and Policy Office for assistance.

- County Assistance -- Some counties and/or senior centers are able to offer personal care and homemaker services at a low or no cost to eligible persons age 60 and older. Generally, eligibility depends on income and assets, and the inability of the person needing care to quality for state assistance. To determine if such assistance is available in your area, contact your county Social Services department, your nearest senior center, or the Eldercare Helpline, 1-800-243-3638.

- Non-Profit Services -- Private, non-profit agencies operating in some communities are able to assist eligible persons with low or no-cost service on a limited basis. For help determining if there is such a program in your area, call the Eldercare Helpline, 1-800-243-3638.

2. What do you foresee as a possible solution to the rapidly escalating 50-50 Medicaid Match cost to counties? Counties have no control of the numbers of patients or cost, and Lyon County has not had sufficient tax revenue to pay the total match for the last three years. Our 97/98 budget for LTC is $330,000 and we are currently anticipating match costs in excess of $575,000. What are options for counties?

The issue of escalating costs for county match for Medicaid institutional patients was addressed by the 1997 Nevada Legislature. Assembly Bill 183 provided for a change in statute so that the threshold income level was made a percentage of poverty rather than a fixed dollar amount. Accordingly, the burden of increasing long-term care costs will be shared between the counties and the state. Assembly Bill 183 also provided $300,000 to fund an account administered by the Nevada Association of Counties to deal with individual counties that are unable to pay the total match.

CC: J. Reed
C. Thompson

BOB MILLER
Governor

CHARLOTTE CRAWFORD
Director

YVONNE SYLVA
Administrator

VACANT
State Health Officer

STATE OF NEVADA
DEPARTMENT OF HUMAN RESOURCES
HEALTH DIVISION
BUREAU OF LICENSURE AND CERTIFICATION

☐ Health Facilities/Lab Services
1550 E. College Parkway
Suite 158
Carson City, Nevada 89706
(702) 687-4475
Fax: (702) 687-6588

☐ Health Facilities/Lab Services
4220 S. Maryland Parkway
Suite 810, Building D
Las Vegas, Nevada 89119
(702) 486-6515
Fax: (702) 486-6520

☐ Health Facilities/Lab Services
1475 Terminal Way
Suite D
Reno, Nevada 89502
(702) 688-2888
Fax: (702) 688-2898

☐ Emergency Medical Services
1550 E. College Parkway
Suite 158
Carson City, Nevada 89706
(702) 687-4475
Fax: (702) 687-6588

☐ Emergency Medical Services
550 Elm Street
Elko, Nevada 89801
(702) 753-1154
Fax: (702) 753-4112

☐ Emergency Medical Services
P.O. Box 1227
Tonopah, Nevada 89049
(702) 482-3722
Fax: (702) 482-6975

☐ Emergency Medical Services
1475 Terminal Way
Suite D
Reno, Nevada 89502
(702) 688-2888
Fax: (702) 688-2898

February 23, 1998

MEMORANDUM

TO: Angela Hill, Hearing Clerk
for Senate Aging Committee Field Hearings

FROM: R. J. Panelli, Bureau Chief

REGARDING: Senate Aging Committee Field Hearing Questions

Attached are the answers to the questions that were addressed to the panel in the Senate Aging Committee field hearings held in Reno and Las Vegas last month. If you would need additional information please contact me.

Reid.memo

Answers to questions from Senate Committee field hearings held last month in Las Vegas and Reno.

1. ***Private home providers should be required to have an R.N. to supervise medications, how the care is given, and the general performance of the home regarding food served, activities, etc.***

Although private home providers (residential facilities for groups) are not required by Nevada statutes and Nevada Administrative Codes to have a licensed RN on staff, some choose to do so. The regulations do however provide for regulatory oversight to ensure that staff members that do administer medications and provide care in the home of a license residential facility have received educational training on medications and are under the supervision of a license group home administrator. Facilities may also have licensed Home Health agencies come into their homes and provide skilled nursing services to those residents that may require such services in a home environment.

2. ***Can individuals phone licensing agency to inquire which health care faciities are in non-compliance?***

Individuals are encouraged to telephone the Bureau of Licensure and Certification, Health Division, and request information about the compliance history of healthcare facilities or any of the other facility types that are licensed by the Bureau; especially, when they are anticipating the use of one of these facilities for themselves or someone they are assisting in seeking services. The compliance history is public information and can be utilized when making those types of healthcare decisions.

3. ***You mentioned something about less documentation and focus on quality care. Can you go briefly over that?***

The statement of "less documentation and focus on quality of care" was in reference to the survey process of Skilled Nursing facilities (nursing homes). Since 1987, the Health Care Financing Administration has directed the survey process to gather information by actually assessing the quality of care and life of the residents and how the facilities handle resident's behavior issues instead of looking at written policies and procedures only. The State Agency staff conduct the survey process by observing the care of residents, interviewing residents about their life and care in the facilities, and for those resident that are unable to speak for themselves, interviewing their families regarding the care received and how the facilities accommodates their individual needs. Facilities who chose to participate in the Medicare / Medicaid program are committed to assist and care for the residents so the residents may attain their highest practicable physical, mental and psychosocial well-being. Survey deficiencies are based on "negative outcomes" for the resident when the facilities have not provided the care and services that have resulted in a lack of progress towards the resident's highest practicable physical, mental, and psychosocial well-being. Deficiencies are not written for lack of "documentation" only.

4. ***Is Federal and State licensing of nursing and assisted living facilities strict enough and enforceable?***

Federal Medicare / Medicaid certification for Skilled Nursing Facilities has over 500 regulatory requirements that the facilities staff must meet for each resident. These facilities are also mandated to have an annual survey by the State Agency to assure the requirements are being met. Resident, family members of residents, staff, or any concerned person may call the State survey agency or the State Long Term Care Ombudsman to complain about care and the complaint will be investigated. If the facilities are out of compliance a federal remedy can be imposed. If the facility does not come back into compliance they are subject to termination of the provider agreement in addition to the remedies.

The same can be said for State Licensure . If a facility does not maintain substantial compliance with the Nevada Administrative Codes and Nevada Revised Statutes, a state sanction can be imposed or/and suspension or revocation of their license.

Residential Facilities for groups (Assisted living facilities) are required to be State Licensed only because they are not certified by Medicare and the residents receive no Medicare funds for the services provided at these facilities. The State regulations were rewritten just last year and became enforceable last year. These regulations include many new areas and more specific regulations in the areas covering care, activities, environment and staff qualifications. The Health Division did this to assure the health and safety of residents entering these facilities.

Residential facilities are also subject to sanctions and/or suspension or revocation of their license if they do not remain in substantial compliance with the regulations.

5. ***As Medicare continues to limit the number of home health visits per patients or illness episode, more patients will be forced into long-term care facilities, either permanently or temporarily. What measures are being taken to assure that the needed beds will be available for Nevada Resident and that the transfer between home and LTC takes place as expediently as possible?***

In the past year there has been some needed changes to the Home Health Care requirements. Many have resulted from the large amount of fraud that was occurring in the home health industry. Patients are still receiving needed services if they are home bound. The Health Care Financing Administration which oversees Medicare wants the patients to stay in the home as long as possible because this is where the patients are usually the most content and have not limited those services.

There has been a tremendous growth in Adult Group Care in Nevada. These facilities have been able to met the needs of many residents of Nevada who required more continuous care than a home health agency can provide. This has made available some higher level of care beds available in Skilled Nursing Facilities. There also has been a tremendous growth in LTC beds along with the population growth in Nevada.

Community Care Associates

316 California Ave., Suite 130
Reno, NV 89509
Phone (702) 786-8288
Fax (702) 786-7574

GCM
National Association of Professional Geriatric Care Managers

February 20, 1998

Angela Hill, Hearing Clerk
United States Senate
Special Committee on Aging
Washington, DC 20510-6400

Dear Ms. Hill:

I am in receipt of a letter requesting response to questions raised at the Senate field hearing on January 13, 1998. As I just returned to the office, I only received this today. Please accept my apology for forwarding this by FAX.

Sincerely,

Donna J. Shilinsky

Responses to questions on community based care testimony at the January 13, 1998 field hearing in Reno, Nevada.

Who is the geriatric care manager in Winnemucca?

According to the 1996 directory compiled by the National Association of Professional Geriatric Care Managers, the person listed for Winnemucca is:

Jennifer Ranney, BA
702 623-2946

Feel free to contact the National Association for a more current listing of members. Their address is:

1604 North Country Club Road
Tucson, AZ 85716
520 881-8008

Will proposed voucher system be extended to pay for home care givers, homemakers and home health residential care along with assisted living?

The voucher system for assisted living implemented in 30 states is defined by the Medicaid system. We need to petition Nevada Medicaid to consider implementing such a program in the state and provide support for defining the various parameters. As yet, there is no definition within the state other than Adult Residential Care Facilities include both assisted living and group home.

If it gets to where I can't live alone and I must live with my daughter, will I be able to get the help I need?

There are many community based services and support systems available to assist older adults in their care needs. I can't say specifically what help you would get as I do not know your specific needs. A case manager through the senior center r the hospital can guide you in finding appropriate services and support systems.

I'm having difficulty in hiring a "caregiver" because of the salary and wages.

I am sorry, I don't have enough information in your comment to provide you an intelligent answer. Perhaps we can talk on the telephone and I can clarify your issues with you and provide you some guidance.

Donna Shibusky
2/20/98

Med Wise
Primary Care For Seniors

Laurence G. Gay, M.D., C.M.D.
Denver J. Miller, M.D., C.M.D., M.P.H.
Steven L. Phillips, M.D., C.M.D.

Angela Hill
Hearing Clerk, Special Committee on Aging
United States Senate
Washington, DC 20510-6400

February 20,1998

Dear Angela:

Here are my responses to the questions that were not answered during the field hearings. If you require more information please let me know.

1. My mother is presently housed (warehoused?) In a skilled care facility having moved from a hospital after surgery. She ill be able to move to a less care type or facility soon, but there is no mechanism for this. What can be done?

ANSWER: The skilled nursing facility is required to develop and implement a plan of care for your mother. Ask to meet with the care team in order to initiate discharge planning. Obtain a list of group care homes and/or assisted living facilities in your area to visit. The physical and occupational therapists at the nursing facility can provide you with the necessary information regarding your mothers short and long term needs.

2. Lack of sufficient care in long tern care facilities is not our only problem in care of the elderly. What can be done about the substandard bed side care for hospital patients? This seems to have come about because of the staff reduction policies of most hospitals-including St. Mary's Hospital and Washoe Medical Center.

ANSWER: When the reduction of staff in hospitals or other health care settings is shown to affect quality of care (adverse patient outcomes) and/or increase health care costs, changes will occur.

3. Will you explain "blending" of funds further?

ANSWER: The term "blending of funds" means the combining of a variety of payment sources to provide needed health care services. This can include Medicare, Medicaid and private dollars with the goal being to integrate acute and long term care.

50 Kirman Avenue · Suite 205 · Reno, Nevada 89502 · (702) 322-5050 · FAX (702) 322-6191

4. Has anything been done to get a HMO or senior type insurance like Reno-Elko has? It seems those of us in the center of Nevada are left out of that type of care. Six months ago I talked to the Ombudsman from Elko. Nothing has happened since. This could help elderly at home.

ANSWER: Please see my response on page 117 of the Reno testimony.

5. One of the problems in Medicare is the authority given to non-medical (not doctors) who determine the discharge of seriously ill patients in the hospital requiring hospital care. These persons are frequently untrained and are part time workers. How can this be corrected?

ANSWER: The role of Case Managers (usually Nurses) is definitely increasing in hospitals and other health care delivery settings. There is a need to assure that these Case Managers meet certain requirements to perform their duties. The use of a standardized test administered at either the state or federal level is one possibility. Under Medicare, the patient/family and/or physician have the right to appeal decisions to discharge.

Sincerely,

Steven L. Phillips, MD, CMD

UNIVERSITY OF NEVADA
SCHOOL OF MEDICINE

Dept. of Internal Medicine
Division of Neurology
901 S. Rancho Lane
Suite 105
Las Vegas, Nevada 89106
(702) 474-0532
Fax # (702) 477-0033

February 11, 1998

Special Committee on Aging
United States Senate
Washington, DC 20510-6400

Dear Committee Members,

This is written in response to the questions forwarded to me from the Special Aging Committee field hearing held in Nevada.

1. Q. Can most of the aged be expected to develop Alzheimer's Disease?
A. Though Alzheimer's Disease is not an inevitable consequence of aging, its estimated that between 30-50% of those over 85 years of age are afflicted with the disease. Greater awareness of this disease will allow younger individuals to make advanced financial decisions and determine the type of care they would want if they should eventually develop the disease.

2. Q. Can Congress facilitate the integration of private and public dollars to finance research...?
A. Currently, funding for research comes from several sources including the federal government, industry and private foundations/associations. As no single agency can realistically fund all the research necessary, partnerships between government and private industry must be encouraged in the future. Clearly, the ultimate means to deal with the public health problem of Alzheimer's Disease is to find ways to prevent or cure the disease.

3. Q. Upon what factors is the $12,000 for in home care estimate made?

A. This figure is based on the assumption that the individual is living with family and utilizes a resource such as adult day care for 8 -10 hours a day, 7 days a week. Given the customary cost of $35/day for day care, the per year cost would be close to $12,000. This figure does not include the family's fixed costs of utilities, food etc.

4. Q. Is anything being done about research for macular degeneration?

A. There is research being done in regard to macular degeneration. To obtain more information, one could contact the National Institute of Health.

I again appreciate the opportunity to participate in the Aging Committee field hearing and please let me know if any further information is needed.

Sincerely,

Charles Bernick, M.D.
Associate Professor of Neurology
University of Nevada School of Medicine

WITHROP CASHDOLLAR RESPONSES TO QUESTIONS

Question. Why don't they increase the ratio of employees needed in all departments of long term care? The current ratio is outdated.

Answer. Long term care providers can certainly understand why long term care consumers and their families might favor raising staffing requirements in long term care facilities. Most long term care facility administrators frequently find themselves struggling to find and hire additional nurses and nurse aides. However, it is not enough just to raise long term care staffing requirements.

Raising long term care staffing ratios requires that additional capable and qualified caregiver staff are available and that there are resources available to pay them. Therefore, any requirement for increased long term care staffing must also address long term caregiver workforce issues and the payment necessary to attract and keep them.

Question. Skilled nursing facilities are mandated to reduce medication for residents (i.e. a drug holiday). This is highly detrimental to the patients and leads to re-hospitalization. Are there efforts being made to rectify this problem? What about mental health? HMO acute care coverage?

Answer. Skilled nursing facilities are required to reduce the use of both chemical restraints (i.e. certain medications) and physical restraints in order to provide long term care facility residents with the greatest practical degree of dignity, comfort, and freedom. Restraint reduction can sometime bring increased risk of, for instance, injury from a fall.

Long term caregivers are also required to protect residents from falls, injuries, and other risks that might accompany restraint reduction. Therefore, long term caregivers must balance the benefits and risks of chemical and physical restraint reduction. This requires that restraint reduction be made only for those residents for whom it is appropriate and only to the degree that is safe.

There is no current effort to change the laws or regulations that require restraint reduction whenever feasible. Be assured, however, that Nevada's long term caregivers are working closely with the Federal and State officials who oversee restraint reduction. In January, the Nevada Health Care Association (NHCA) sponsored a Restraint Reduction Workshop in Reno, led by a representative of the Federal Health Care Financing Administration (HCFA). Nevada's nursing facility surveyors also took part in that workshop. NHCA has plans to sponsor another Restraint Reduction Workshop in Las Vegas later this year.

Question. Why should seniors, most of whom have limited funds, buy non-qualified LTC insurance? Why are they taxed on $ they receive if they are put into a care home?

Answer. In 1996, Congress passed and the President signed into law the Health Insurance Portability and Accountability Act. Among many other things, this legislation gave preferential Federal tax treatment to "qualified" long term care insurance policies. That is, under the new law, purchasers of long term care insurance policies which meet new Federal standards are entitled to certain tax benefits (e.g. tax deductibility of some premiums and exclusion from income of policy benefits).

Although some seniors may be attracted to the lower premiums that non-qualified long term care insurance policies might offer, purchasers should also consider what they are giving up when they purchase a non-qualified policy. The Federal tax treatment of non-qualified policies is unclear. But qualified policies offer well defined Federal tax advantages. Qualified policies also meet new Federal standards for long term care insurance policies designed specifically to protect long term care insurance consumers. Seniors in the market for long term care insurance should, of course, consult with family, insurance professionals, and/or financial planning professionals.

With respect to the question about the taxation of long term care insurance policy payments to policy holders, with the implementation of the Health Insurance Portability and Accountability Act, seniors who collect benefits from a qualified long term care insurance policy will not be taxed on policy benefits.

Question. Why does Medicare pay more for medical equipment such as wheelchairs, walkers, canes, etc.? Why are nursing homes allowed to keep such equipment and resell items patients donated upon death or departure?

Answer. I respectfully suggest that this question would be more appropriate for the Health Care Financing Administration, the agency that administers Medicare and Medicaid.

Question. It's the people who are in nursing homes who need the help to be heard so quality care is the solution. Do you have any light on the staff/patient ratio for the level of skill care?

Answer. The Federal Government has developed a system linking appropriate staffing resources and reimbursement for skilled nursing facilities. This system, the Resource Utilization Groups III (RUGs III) will, I believe, in time become the standard for long term care staffing. It is my understanding that compliance with the RUGs III staffing standards would require a significant increase in Nevada's nursing facility staff and reimbursement.

Question. Currently, to get Medicaid (one) must spend down. So someone who may need nursing home care for 6 months must deplete life savings to qualify and then not have any financial resources to return to independent living. Difficult choice.

Answer. The Nevada Health Care Association (NHCA) and the American Health Care Association (AHCA) support changing the current State and Federal long term care programs to the requirement that Americans must "spend down" to poverty in order to get financial help with long term care services. AHCA has developed "SecureCare," and outline for long term care reform that would move long term care from "welfare" to health care—and help senior citizens avoid bankruptcy as the likely consequence of needing long term care.

○

MANCHESTER COLLEGE LIBRARY
3 9315 01036664 6

362.16 Un3m
United States. Congress.
Senate. Special Committee
The many faces of long-term
care

DATE DUE

ISBN 0-16-056532-4
90000
9 780160 565328